Praise for *The Thyroid S*

"This book has had a profound impact on the way [...] tients, and on my perception of the connection between the brain and hormones. If you're a woman, get this book. If you're a man with a woman in your life, get this book. If you're a man, get this book. The idea is—get this book." —MONA LISA SCHULZ, M.D., Ph.D., author of *Awakening Intuition*

"Practical advice . . . helpful right down to the appended reading list . . . The thyroid can affect both body and mind. [Dr.] Arem writes clearly about how the gland can disturb a person and personal relationships. He relays much useful information." —*Booklist*

"Dr. Arem provides solid explanations for symptoms of hypothyroidism in patients with normal blood levels of thyroid hormones and particularly addresses the needs of women who have thyroid and hormonal disorders." —GILLIAN FORD, author of *Listening to Your Hormones*

"This book will be of tremendous help to the many people with thyroid disease and residual depressive symptoms. Dr. Arem elegantly addresses the important interplay of thyroidology and psychiatry." —LAUREN MARANGELL, M.D., president, Brain Health Consults and TMS Center

"*The Thyroid Solution* presents a new and interesting perspective on the interaction between the thyroid gland and the brain. The text draws upon the deep clinical experience of the author that provides vivid personal examples." —E. CHESTER RIDGWAY, M.D., former head, Division of Endocrinology, Metabolism and Diabetes, the University of Colorado Health Sciences Center

"Clear, comprehensive, and incredibly useful . . . the best thyroid resource I have ever read." —KATHLEEN DESMAISONS, Ph.D., author of *Your Last Diet!*

"Dr. Arem is an incredible physician who has spent years researching and working with patients in clinical practice to identify the root causes of thyroid disease. In his book, Dr. Arem uncovers those root causes and lays out an innovative program to help you overcome thyroid dysfunction." —AMY MYERS, M.D., author of *The Thyroid Connection* and *The Autoimmune Solution*

BY RIDHA AREM, M.D.

The Thyroid Solution
The Protein Boost Diet

THE THYROID SOLUTION

THE

THYROID

SOLUTION

(THIRD EDITION)

A Revolutionary Mind-Body Program for
Regaining Your Emotional and Physical Health

RIDHA AREM, M.D.

BALLANTINE BOOKS

NEW YORK

As of the time of initial publication, the URLs displayed in this book link or refer to existing websites on the Internet. Penguin Random House LLC is not responsible for, and should not be deemed to endorse or recommend, any website other than its own or any content available on the Internet (including without limitation at any website, blog page, information page) that is not created by Penguin Random House.

2017 Ballantine Books Trade Paperback Edition

Published in the United States by Ballantine Books, an imprint of Random House, a division of Penguin Random House LLC, New York.

BALLANTINE and the HOUSE colophon are registered trademarks of Penguin Random House LLC.

Earlier editions of this work were originally published in hardcover in 1999 and trade paperback in 2007 by Ballantine Books, an imprint of Random House, a division of Penguin Random House LLC.

ISBN 978-0-425-28640-1
Ebook ISBN 978-0-425-28686-9

Printed in the United States of America on acid-free paper

randomhousebooks.com

4 6 8 9 7 5 3

*To the very special people who enriched my heart with love:
my very dear parents, my beloved wife, and my two wonderful sons.
It is my hope that this book will inspire my sons to
dedicate themselves to helping and loving others.*

PREFACE TO THE
2017 EDITION

When the first edition of this book was released, patients suffering from a thyroid hormone imbalance or an autoimmune thyroid disease, whether or not they had been diagnosed, had very limited resources to learn about their condition and understand and validate their symptoms and suffering. Millions of thyroid patients throughout the world were misunderstood, misdiagnosed, and made to feel like their symptoms were all in their heads. The link between thyroid disease and mood disorders, including depression, and the effects of thyroid hormone imbalance and autoimmunity on mood, behavior, appetite, and women's hormonal health were seldom discussed in books or by the media.

Some thyroid patients chatted on the Internet, sharing their experience to try to understand their symptoms, and refused to believe that they were crazy. Books about thyroid disorders basically chronicled the symptoms and signs of the conditions in a medical-textbook format, without describing the real-life issues and challenges faced by thyroid patients or providing ways to understand and cure the effects of thyroid disease.

When the first edition of *The Thyroid Solution* was published in 1999, I received thousands of emails from patients around the world, thanking me for writing the book. I continue to hear how it has changed the lives of so many people suffering from thyroid disorders. Because my vision of the impact of thyroid disease on a person's health and life and my comprehensive and futuristic approach to caring for thyroid patients go beyond what has been taught by conventional medicine, many conventional doctors, including endocrinologists and even leading thyroid experts, expressed disagreement with my vision and approach, which did not surprise me at all.

Over time, however, increasing numbers of these physicians have come to understand my vision and adopt my successful approach to caring for thyroid patients. Increasingly, thyroid patients are not treated based on laboratory testing only. More doctors now carefully listen to their patients' symptoms and are more aware that suffering may linger even after blood test results become normal with treatment. More doctors are showing compassion and providing more ways to alleviate the symptoms. Despite the progress we have witnessed, it is still not enough.

Since the previous edition of this book, I have gained more knowledge from both the patients I cared for and the expanding medical research published in the past few years. The first edition had triggered great interest among researchers in understanding further how the thyroid system affects our health and our physical and mental well-being. In addition, the growth of knowledge about how a disturbed immune system (which is the root of most cases of thyroid hormone imbalance) can affect physical and mental well-being has validated further the benefits of the comprehensive mind-body approach that I have taken to treat patients suffering from thyroid disease. Major advances have been made in recent years in recognizing the importance of good nutrition, the use of mind-body techniques, and supplementation of vitamins, antioxidants, and probiotics, as well as the fine-tuning of medications. We now know more about the contribution of immune system reactivity to the symptoms patients experience and the link between thyroid disorders and other autoimmune conditions such as lupus, rheumatoid arthritis, and Sjögren's syndrome. We also know more about the interaction between the immune system and brain functions, and have expanded our knowledge about how female hormonal issues and thyroid disease can be interrelated and how to overcome them. Knowing better how weight is regulated, the importance of thyroid hormone to appetite and metabolism regulation, and how thyroid hormone works to promote fat burn has allowed me to provide thyroid patients with the best means to win the weight battle. We have gained more knowledge in the field of anxiety, depression, and other mood disorders and the relationship between these disorders and the thyroid system, as well as the contribution of immune system reactivity to these mental conditions. We also know more about what triggers and perpetuates autoimmune reactions that affect the thyroid, and the roles of stress, environment, and vitamins and antioxidants in maintaining optimal health of the thyroid gland and the immune system. Given this current knowledge, physicians who care for thyroid patients should theoretically not only treat the thyroid hormone imbalance but also provide the best possible support for the immune system and the mind. Unfortunately, many healthcare professionals still continue to primarily focus on just prescribing thyroid medications and ignore the hidden roots of thyroid disease and the consequent suffering.

The book has been extensively revised and rewritten to include this knowledge, as well as the many new practical ways for thyroid patients to reach and maintain optimal wellness. Over the past few years, I have refined the T4/T3 combination treatment protocol for hypothyroid patients who have had lingering symptoms of fatigue and depression. I have learned more about the importance of the ratios of the two hormones for maximum benefits. For a T4/T3 combination treatment to be fully effective, it has to be tailored to the needs of the individual patient. In this new edition, you will learn how using compounded slow-release T3 instead of synthetic T3 will allow your doctor to titrate the dose of T3 in a more precise way to address your symptoms. You will also learn how to avoid falling into the trap of being treated with extreme approaches that will not allow you to achieve wellness. I will discuss in depth the ongoing controversy concerning normal ranges for thyroid tests, how you can easily be misdiagnosed, and how you can prevent this from happening.

Thyroid disease is in fact much more common than it was estimated to be in the past, and its incidence seems to be rising as a result of pollution and other environmental factors. Despite an increased awareness of how common thyroid disease is in our population, despite the many more books on thyroid disorders that are now available, despite the many articles published in health and women's magazines and on the Internet, and despite all the interest that has been generated since the publication of the first edition, there is still more to be done with respect to educating both the public and the medical community on this truly hidden epidemic. It is my hope that this new edition of *The Thyroid Solution* will enhance knowledge on these issues and be helpful to people throughout the world.

CONTENTS

INTRODUCTION

Several years ago, I saw two patients, Stacy and Maria, whose experiences ultimately inspired me to write this book.

Stacy came to me for a second opinion on her ailment, called Graves' disease, an autoimmune disorder that results in an overactive thyroid. She asked me to recommend a book for "civilians" dealing with the psychological and emotional aspects of thyroid disease. Stacy had already studied all the books suggested by the Thyroid Foundation of America, the principal patient resource organization for thyroid conditions. She had also browsed through the health and medicine sections of a number of large bookstores. Stacy had been suffering from her thyroid condition for four years, and the consequent mental and emotional symptoms had contributed to the collapse of her marriage and the loss of her job. She was determined to learn how her thyroid condition had affected her mind and how she was likely to feel in the future. Although I mentioned a number of scientific studies, I realized that I did not know of any books on this important topic directed at a general audience.

Shortly after Stacy's visit, I saw Maria, a young lawyer who had been suffering from weight gain, fatigue, and lack of motivation for approximately a year. "I am so tired and exhausted," she told me. "I have trouble focusing at work and often have trouble remembering what I just said. I have no motivation to do anything. My weight has been creeping up and I haven't been able to lose any weight even though I eat very little. All I do when I get home is lie on my couch and do nothing."

Maria recognized that she was suffering from depression, and her doctor had prescribed an antidepressant, but it did not help much. Because she was aware that depression and tiredness could also be symptoms of a thyroid imbalance, she began to wonder whether her symptoms were thyroid-related.

Maria had already seen two endocrinologists, but her standard thyroid blood tests came back in the normal range. I determined through my examination, precise testing, and an ultrasound of the thyroid that Maria was suffering from low-grade hypothyroidism caused by an autoimmune thyroid condition called Hashimoto's thyroiditis, and I prescribed levothyroxine (T4-only medication). But like many patients suffering from low thyroid, Maria's symptoms persisted despite the medication. When I switched Maria to a treatment combining T4 and T3 (the two hormones that the gland normally produces), she felt much better, as her fatigue and lack of motivation had improved, but was still not feeling her best. I had begun paying attention to the effects of foods, stress, antioxidants, and other factors that are likely to affect the health of the immune system and the way it affects a person's body and brain. When Maria started following a gluten- and dairy-free eating plan, taking the antioxidants I recommended, and practicing yoga, she regained her usual energy, enthusiasm, and vitality. She was also able to lose weight.

In the course of Maria's treatment, she asked me a number of good questions, among them where she could go to learn more about autoimmune thyroid disease, how thyroid disease and immune system reactivity affect the brain, and how these conditions can alter mood and behavior. Again, there was no book I could recommend that addressed, in layperson's terms, the intricate relationships among thyroid ailments, emotions, and thought patterns. My increasing awareness that patients like Stacy and Maria needed a way to learn more about their condition compelled me to write the first edition of this book in 1999.

The intent of *The Thyroid Solution* is threefold. First, it aims to introduce readers to the many ways that the thyroid can affect brain chemistry. In recent years, scientists have made remarkable headway in showing how brain chemicals, such as the well-known neurotransmitter serotonin, can influence everything from mood to appetite. Yet even many physicians do not understand how essential thyroid hormones are to normal brain chemistry. It is time for thyroid hormones to be recognized as key brain chemicals whose actions and effects are similar in many ways to those of serotonin and other neurotransmitters. These effects include regulating emotions and mood and aiding communications between mind and body, including regulating metabolism, sexuality, fertility, appetite, weight, and mental clarity.

Second, this book will show you the detailed intricacies that exist between the immune system, the thyroid gland, and the brain and will highlight the importance of reducing immune system reactivity if you are suffering from an autoimmune thyroid disease. Since the root of most thyroid hormone imbalances is an agitated immune system attacking your thyroid gland, many physical and mental symptoms and health effects of thyroid disease are directly or indirectly related to inflammation chemicals produced by the immune system. You will learn how to make the immune system less agitated and less reactive so that you can reach optimal physical and mental wellness. You will learn how nutrition, sleep, stress, antioxidants, the health of your gut, probiotics, and environmental factors (including overlooked environmental contaminants) can affect your immune system health and will influence your thyroid condition and its consequences.

Third, this book aims to provide thyroid patients, as well as their partners, families, and friends, with useful, practical information that may help them understand and cope with the difficulties and emotional suffering induced by thyroid diseases. *The Thyroid Solution* details a comprehensive mind-body program that will help you halt the escalation of symptoms and become well again. It also teaches you how to work with your doctor to obtain an accurate diagnosis, to achieve and maintain an optimal thyroid balance with treatment, and to overcome the lingering symptoms of thyroid disease.

At least one in ten Americans—more than thirty million people—suffers from a thyroid condition. Thyroid hormone imbalance, along with its fraternal twin, clinical depression, may be the common cold of emotional illness. Yet most victims don't realize that thyroid ailments have any mental or emotional components. They just know that they don't feel like themselves and haven't felt right for a long time. This book is directed to these individuals, and I am confident that it can help them regain their emotional health.

Addressing Conditions and Concerns

Like any organ in the body, the thyroid gland can be affected by a wide range of disorders—from the common and rampant condition called Hashimoto's thyroiditis, the leading cause of hypothyroidism (underactive thyroid), to rare and unusual conditions such as Riedel's thyroiditis (a condition in which fibrous tissue replaces healthy thyroid tissue). The main function of the thyroid gland is to produce thyroid hormones (T4 and T3), crucial chemicals that affect metabolism and other bodily functions. Thyroid hormones are also part of the brain chemistry mix that regulates mood, emotions, cognition, appetite, and behavior.

A complete home reference book of thyroid diseases would describe in detail all thyroid conditions, both unusual and common. But that would leave little room to detail the hidden and often misunderstood effects of the most common thyroid disorders, which affect millions of people. These disorders, which often lead to a thyroid hormone imbalance, are frequently induced by the immune system attacking the thyroid gland; they are considered the most common autoimmune disorders. For that reason, the main focus of this book will be these conditions.

The Thyroid Solution differs from many other thyroid books in that it depicts thyroid patients' real-life challenges, which I have come to know fully and understand while helping patients heal for more than twenty-five years. This is the first book to explain the hidden suffering that many patients have difficulty expressing and the first to provide new ways of addressing and heal this suffering. It is my hope that their stories will help you identify symptoms that you may have dismissed as unrelated to a thyroid condition. Further, their stories of regaining physical, mental, and emotional wellness may inspire you to find the answers and treatments you need.

How You Can Use This Book

Part I of *The Thyroid Solution* describes the emerging knowledge about the thyroid-mind connection and how thyroid imbalance is likely to affect your physical health, mood, emotions, and behavior. It highlights the types of thyroid conditions that could result in a thyroid imbalance and outlines their potential effects on your emotional and physical health. Here you'll find out how to recognize hypothyroidism and hyperthyroidism and work with your physician to obtain the proper diagnosis. Part I also shows you how neuroscientists have come to view the thyroid gland as an "annex to the brain," since the brain uses thyroid chemicals for a wide range of brain functions. You will learn a great deal about fatigue caused by thyroid problems and the mental effects induced by a reactive immune system. I will provide important information concerning the two most common autoimmune thyroid conditions, Hashimoto's thyroiditis and Graves' disease, and the links that may exist between them. You will also learn how dealing with stress, maintaining a healthy and stable mood, and coping with life depend to a great extent on whether the thyroid functions properly and on whether the right amount of thyroid hormone is properly delivered and dispersed in the brain. Stress and thyroid imbalance go hand in hand: thyroid imbalance affects your perception of stress, and stress can trigger an imbalance. This relationship between the thyroid, the immune system, and brain chemistry is intricate, and stress management is important in preventing flare-ups of thyroid imbalance. You will learn how the effects of thyroid imbalances are both physical and mental, although many physicians tend to only focus on the physical effects. You will also learn the many deplorable reasons why thyroid conditions often remain undiagnosed and misdiagnosed. One reason is that patients suffering from a thyroid imbalance and/or autoimmune thyroid disease often have symptoms of mood disorders and anxiety and therefore may be misdiagnosed as depressed or anxious. An imbalance of thyroid hormone in the brain can be caused by either a malfunctioning gland or a disruption in the way the hormone is dispersed in the brain. Either way, different types of depression and anxiety disorders can result. Thyroid hormone balance in the brain is crucial for maintaining stable mood and behavior. Many people suffering from depression who have not fully responded to conventional antidepressants experience miraculous mood-boosting effects when taking the right form and amount of thyroid hormones in conjunction with those antidepressants.

You will also learn about the most popular lab tests for measuring how much thyroid hormone you have in your system. Here we also examine a major controversy in the field: can you have a thyroid imbalance even though your blood tests seem normal? You will find an extensive summary of other medical conditions that may increase your risk of suffering from a thyroid condition in the future. These are the same conditions that you will need to watch for if you have already been diagnosed with Hashimoto's thyroiditis or Graves' disease.

Part II presents in-depth information about how thyroid imbalances may affect your weight, sex life, and relationships.

Thyroid hormone is one of the most potent chemicals that regulate fat burn and how much body fat you have. Weight issues are quite common whether you suffer from a low thyroid or an overactive thyroid. You may even continue to struggle with weight problems after correcting the thyroid imbalance. You will acquire the necessary knowledge that will help you understand how to halt the weight gain trend triggered by thyroid disease. This knowledge will also help you understand the fundamentals of my science-based diet, which will help you achieve your weight loss goals. Because thyroid imbalances can intrude in your personal life and affect both your sex life and relationships with devastating effects, it is important for you to learn how to discuss these intimate effects with your doctor. Such effects do not necessarily end after the imbalance has been treated, so you will also learn how to cope with these problems and how to ask your partner for the support you need.

Part III is devoted to women's health issues. Optimal thyroid health is necessary for increasing the likelihood of conception and carrying out a healthy pregnancy. During pregnancy, a thyroid hormone imbalance, even a minimal one, or an iodine deficiency may lead to serious pregnancy complications and can negatively affect the development of the fetus and the health of the newborn. You will learn practical tips that will help you maintain optimal thyroid balance prior to and during pregnancy. You will also learn about the connections between thyroid disease and issues such as infertility, miscarriage, postpartum depression, and premenstrual syndrome and menopause. A thyroid imbalance will cause or intensify premenstrual syndrome during the reproductive years and will affect the way a woman feels at menopause. Nearly 10 to 12 percent of postmenopausal women will experience hypothyroidism. Because the symptoms of menopause and those of thyroid imbalances share many similarities, it is important for women to know when to suspect a thyroid condition and when to consider estrogen therapy.

Part IV is the most practical section of *The Thyroid Solution*. You will learn how to work with your doctor to obtain the most appropriate treatment for your condition. You will also learn about some of the most common problems that can arise during the course of treating both hypothyroidism and hyperthyroidism, from side effects associated with the use of conventional thyroid drugs to the many problems associated with radioactive iodine treatment for Graves' disease. You will learn how to prevent or reduce the memory lapses and other cognitive problems, as well as depression, that may persist after thyroid imbalances have been treated. These lingering effects of thyroid disease often haunt millions of people even after their blood tests have returned to normal from treatment with thyroid medication, and you may need to be persistent in seeking a cure for them. Many of my patients have benefited from following the "Circle of Wellness" model I provide for recovering from the long-term effects of a thyroid imbalance.

If you suffer from hypothyroidism, thyroid-related depression, fibromyalgia, or lingering effects, and if you have been searching for a way to alleviate your symptoms and regain overall health, an innovative treatment protocol that I have developed which combines two thyroid hormones (T4 and T3) may well revolutionize the way you treat your thyroid condition. *The Thyroid Solution*, even in its first edition, is the first book for laypeople to discuss this treatment and show its benefits. In this new edition, I will show how your doctor can design a T4/T3 treatment specifically tailored to your needs.

In this new edition, I will also provide you with details on my healthy, science-based, immune-system-friendly diet (the ThyroLife Diet), which has helped thousands of thyroid patients struggling with their weight to lose weight efficiently. The eating plan in this diet will help you maintain an optimal metabolism whether you have a weight issue or not.

Finally, I detail my comprehensive mind-body program to help you achieve and maintain optimal physical and mental wellness while being treated for your thyroid condition. You will learn about important lifestyle choices you make every day that can prevent or alleviate thyroid-related effects. We look at the optimal diet for thyroid health—a diet that, not coincidentally, also supports the health of other glands and organs. You'll learn about the most thyroid-friendly nutrients, food sensitivities, the benefits of antioxidants and essential fatty acids for immune system and thyroid health, probiotics, and how to exercise when you have a thyroid disease. I also pay special attention to the thyroid-specific mineral iodine and medications that can affect your thyroid.

A Mind-Body Approach to the Thyroid

Ultimately, this book lets readers know what I try to emphasize to my patients: Thyroid disease isn't purely physiological—it is a biopsychiatric, mind-body ailment. A thyroid imbalance can be controlled just as a mental disorder can, by correcting brain chemistry (in this case, either too much or too little thyroid hormone) and restoring patients' wellness and peace of mind. My book also lets readers understand that immune system reactivity and the damaging inflammation chemicals that the immune system produces contribute to the many physical and mental symptoms of thyroid disease. In essence, the suffering of thyroid patients is in most instances due to both imbalanced thyroid hormone levels and negative effects from an agitated, sensitive, and reactive immune system that is disturbing brain and body functioning. Unless these two sources of suffering are addressed in a meticulous way, patients will be left with a wide range of annoying, impairing, and detrimental effects.

If I had my way, everyone who has not been feeling at his or her best for some time would routinely be tested for thyroid disease. Those patients diagnosed with a thyroid disease who, after a reasonable period of treatment with medications, didn't feel like their old selves again would benefit from the mind-body program that I detail in this book.

Thyroid dysfunction can inflict brutal blows to the brain and create changes that have long-term—and sometimes permanent—effects on your physical and mental health. When I treat the long-term emotional and mental effects of thyroid disease, I use both medication and personal therapy—the best of laboratory and listening-based patient care. My intention with *The Thyroid Solution* is to bring groundbreaking information and hope to all thyroid patients who are still suffering from mental anguish and who have not been understood by their physicians.

THE THYROID SOLUTION

PART I

THE EMERGING MIND-THYROID CONNECTION

How a Tiny Endocrine Gland Intimately Affects
Your Mood, Emotions, and Behavior

1

THYROID IMBALANCE

A Hidden Epidemic

Could you have an overactive or underactive thyroid and not even know it? Millions of Americans—and a high percentage of women in menopause and perimenopause (the decade or so before menopause during which hormonal, emotional, and physical changes begin)—do. A thyroid imbalance is not always easy to recognize. Physicians continue to argue whether a minimal thyroid imbalance affects mental and physical health. But the truth is that it does—and big time.

Do you have any of the following symptoms?

- Always fatigued or exhausted
- Irritable and impatient
- Feeling too hot or too cold
- Depressed, anxious, or panicky
- Bothered by changes in your skin or hair
- At the mercy of your moods
- Inexplicably gaining or losing weight
- Losing your enthusiasm for life
- Sleeping poorly or insomniac

Are you feeling burned out from having acted on an excess of energy for several months? Are you listless, forgetful, and feeling disconnected from your friends and family? Are people telling you that you've changed? Are you taking Prozac or a similar drug for mild depression but still feeling that your mind and mood are subpar? Or have you been treated for a major depression in the past?

If you suffer from more than one of these symptoms or answered yes to one or more of these questions, you could be one of the many people with an undiagnosed thyroid condition. Although some of these symptoms may seem contradictory, all of them can be indications of a thyroid imbalance.

You could also be one of the many people who has been treated for a thyroid imbalance but still suffers from its often-overlooked, lingering effects—effects that may continue to haunt you even after treatments have presumably restored your thyroid levels to normal. If you've ever been treated for a thyroid imbalance, answer these questions:

- Do you still suffer from fatigue?
- Do you feel better but still not quite your old self?
- Do you have unusual flare-ups of anger?
- Are you less socially outgoing than you used to be?
- Are you less tolerant of the foibles of family and friends?
- Do you suffer from occasional bouts of mild depression?
- Do you have frequent lapses in memory?
- Are you often unable to concentrate on what you're doing?
- Do you feel older than your real age?

If you've had a thyroid problem in the past but still answer yes to one or more of these questions, it is quite likely that your symptoms are thyroid-related. You don't have to suffer any longer. *The Thyroid Solution* will show you how you can work with your physician to heal these lingering symptoms.

The Hidden Suffering

At any given time in the United States, more than 30 million people suffer from a thyroid disorder, more than 10 million women have low-grade thyroid imbalance, and nearly 10 million people with thyroid imbalance remain undiagnosed. Some 500,000 new cases of thyroid imbalance occur each year.[1] All of these people are vulnerable to mental and emotional effects for a long time even after being diagnosed. Incorrect or inadequate treatment leads to unnecessary suffering for millions of these people. But these are numbers. Behind the numbers are the symptoms and ravaging mental effects experienced by real human beings.

For the past two decades, we have witnessed a major increase in the recognition and detection of thyroid diseases. This stems in part from improved medical technology, which has led to the development of sensitive methods of screening and diagnosing thyroid disorders. It also stems from the increased public awareness that thyroid disease may remain undiagnosed for a long time and that even mild thyroid dysfunction may affect your health.[2] It is also likely that thyroid imbalance has become more common as a result of deleterious effects related to our environment. Medical associations such as the American Association of Clinical Endocrinologists have conducted public screenings for thyroid disease, much as cholesterol testing has become available in shopping malls and other public places. At any given time, more than half of patients with low-grade hypothyroidism remain undiagnosed. In a thyroid-screening program involving nearly two thousand people that I directed in the Houston area,[3] 8 percent of those tested had an underactive thyroid. Many people screened had never heard of the thyroid gland but rushed to be tested when they recognized that they were suffering many of the symptoms listed in the announcement of the screening. In a statewide health fair in Colorado conducted in 1995, 9.5 percent of the 25,862 participants who were screened for thyroid imbalance were found to have an underactive thyroid and 2.2 percent had thyroid hormone excess.[4] The public's awareness of thyroid disease was boosted by press reports about former president George H. W. Bush and his wife, Barbara, Russian president Boris Yeltsin, and Olympic track champion Gail Devers when they were diagnosed with thyroid disease. Thanks to these factors, people with unexplained symptoms are becoming increasingly likely to ask their physicians whether these symptoms might be related to an undiagnosed thyroid disorder.

As an endocrinologist who has focused his research, teaching, and patient care on thyroid conditions, I realized early on in my practice that taking care of thyroid patients was not as easy as I had expected. Treating and correcting a thyroid condition with medication may not always make the patient feel entirely better. I discovered that to care fully for my patients, to help them heal completely, I had to treat their feelings as well as their bodies. If they didn't feel better even though their lab tests said they were cured, I learned to listen to them, believe them, and work with them to help them become wholly cured. In taking care of thyroid patients, the physician's role is not merely to address physical discomfort, test the thyroid, and make sure blood test results are normal (indicating normal amounts of the various thyroid hormones in the bloodstream). Addressing the effects of thyroid disorders on the mind, addressing the health of the immune system (often the root of the thyroid condition), helping patients cope with their condition, and counseling them sympathetically are equally important.

Many physicians treat dysfunctioning thyroids, but few of them listen to the person attached to the gland. They concentrate on the blood tests, and once your lab results become normal, for these physicians your case is closed. Yet you may go on to suffer for years from a variety of physical and mental symptoms related to the thyroid condition. Research has shown that patients with thyroid imbalance continue to have symptoms even after their thyroid hormone blood levels have become normal with treatment.[5] Physicians should be treating the still-suffering patients in a more comprehensive way for as long as it takes for the physical and mental effects to subside. The reality today, however, is that millions of patients suffer needlessly while their doctors continue to treat thyroid disease as a simple physical disorder rather than what it is: a complex blow to the body and brain.

In general, primary care physicians have not been adequately trained to detect and manage thyroid disease and may lack the expertise needed to diagnose and treat a wide range of thyroid disorders.[6] They also receive little teaching on the effects of thyroid disease on mental health or on understanding the interplay between the mind, the thyroid, and the immune system.

The majority of practitioners of internal medicine and family medicine complete their residency without having had some form of training in endocrinology (the field of hormones). When they leave their training programs, they have inadequate knowledge of thyroid disorders and inadequate experience in diagnosing and treating these disorders. As a consequence, they seldom look for subtle indications of thyroid disease.

Often a primary care physician ignores the thyroid gland in a routine examination and fails to examine the gland by touch. Yet the simple touch examination, or palpation, of the thyroid gland is quite important in finding clues to the presence of thyroid disease. Often physicians are not taught how to palpate the thyroid gland during their training. Many physicians would admit that they were never taught the right way to examine the thyroid gland and do not do the exam routinely in their practice.

Because both the physical and mental symptoms of thyroid disease masquerade as signs of many other illnesses, getting the proper diagnosis can sometimes take a long time. Often symptoms are misdiagnosed and viewed as trivial. Until patients find the right doctor, they are left alone to deal with devastating effects, which may include depression or even upsetting changes in personal behavior. Thyroid imbalance can quickly escalate into a destructive brain chemistry disorder—as powerful and pervasive as major depression, an anxiety disorder, or manic-depression.

Once the brain has been denied thyroid hormone or oversupplied with it because of thyroid disease, it takes a long time to recover. If the symptoms are ignored, they can intensify. A vicious cycle occurs wherein the patient gets depressed, the thyroid disease worsens, physical and emotional effects multiply, and mental health suffers further. This cycle is not widely understood or recognized, and many physicians do not know how important it is to halt the cycle—or, indeed, *how* to halt it.

As we will see, thyroid disease is more often than not related to your immune system attacking your thyroid gland and causing inflammation in the gland. Beyond the effects on the gland itself, the inflammation chemicals put out by the immune system are dispersed throughout your body and can produce a wide range of both physical and mental effects. You end up having multiple symptoms related not only to thyroid imbalance but also to a quite reactive, inflammation-generating immune system.

The Thyroid and the Mind

The Swiss artist Arnold Böcklin (1827–1901) painted a portrait of a woman who appeared quite depressed. Her unsmiling face was sad and lifeless, and her eyes had a detached look. The most striking thing about her appearance, however, was that the front of her neck was swollen. The swelling was so evident that Böcklin drew attention to it with his use of color and lighting. As a layman, he recognized that she had a physical illness and that she was depressed, but it is doubtful that he made a connection between her thyroid and her depressive state. In fact, we did not begin to understand this connection until the late nineteenth century.

Even before the thyroid gland was shown to play a role in regulating metabolism, it was recognized as "the gland of the emotions." In fact, the relationship between the thyroid gland and the mind was thought for years to have merely an anatomical basis: the thyroid is physically close to the brain. The thyroid was believed to protect the brain from overheating, which could result from increased blood flow to the brain when a person was upset. Dr. Robert Graves was the first to provide the classic description of what is now known as Graves' disease. In his description of this "newly observed affection of the thyroid gland in females,"[7] he highlighted symptoms of the nervous system and used the term *globus hystericus* because of the many psychiatric manifestations exhibited by his patients. Dr. Caleb Parry, who had recognized the condition before Graves but expired before his observations were published, wrote: "In more than one of these [patients], the affliction of the head has amounted almost to madness."[8]

For decades, in fact, Graves' disease was considered to be a mental illness rather than a true thyroid disorder. The early label "crystallized fright" illustrates that this condition was seen as some kind of mental illness that follows a psychological trauma. Among the first physicians to focus on the physical symptoms of the condition was Baron Carl Adolph von Basedow. In 1840, he described four patients with protruding eyes, goiter, and rapid heartbeat. He was also the first to describe pretibial myxedema, a brownish swelling over the legs that occurs in a small number of patients with Graves' disease. Whereas the term *Graves' disease* has prevailed in the English-speaking world, *von Basedow's disease* is the term used in Germany and some other European and African countries.

Nearly half a century after Graves' observations, the British physician Dr. William Gull[9] described for the first time the physical and mental consequences of an underactive thyroid. His writings suggested that some of the effects of hypothyroidism were significant mental changes leading to a severe slowing of the mind. Since then it has become clear that the main function of the thyroid gland is to produce thyroid hormone, which regulates the functioning of our body and at the same time is a bona fide brain chemical that regulates mood, emotions, and many other brain functions. Doctors now have come to understand that the basis of the thyroid-mind connection, which was, for a long time, a mystery, is at least in part related to too little or too much thyroid hormone circulating in the body. A patient with a thyroid imbalance may experience physical effects such as skin problems, irregular heartbeat, congestive heart failure, high blood pressure, muscle dysfunction, and gastrointestinal disturbances. Thyroid hormones regulate the metabolic rate, a concept so well popularized that most people associate thyroid imbalance with metabolism and weight problems. And yet, for many people, the emotional and mood-related consequences of a thyroid imbalance are more drastic than the physical ones.

Paradoxically, whereas nineteenth-century physicians first described and demonstrated the significance of such mental symptoms, many modern-day physicians who treat thyroid patients tend to view thyroid disease only as a glandular disorder with *physical* symptoms only.

Why Thyroid Imbalances Are Frequently Unsuspected

Let's take a look at the main reasons why doctors do not diagnose or misdiagnose thyroid imbalances.

Stress, depression, anxiety, tiredness, and other emotional or mental states can mask a thyroid imbalance. Your doctor may perceive symptoms caused by a thyroid imbalance as trivial, primarily because many of us complain of varying degrees of tiredness,[10] lack of interest in life, and weight problems. Quite often, thyroid imbalance makes you suffer from symptoms of depression. Depression is the most common condition seen in general medical practice and also the most common mental effect of thyroid imbalance. Researchers estimate that, at any given time, 10 percent of the population suffers from depression; over a lifetime, the prevalence may be as high as 17 percent.[11] Most patients with mental health problems seek help from primary care physicians rather than psychiatrists.[12] Quite often these physicians have received no training or inadequate training in assessing, detecting, and managing subtle mental disorders. Doctors accurately diagnose fewer than 50 percent of patients with unequivocal depression.[13] Even among those who are correctly diagnosed with depression, only a small portion receives adequate treatment for a sufficient time.[14] The financial pressures placed on doctors and the bureaucracies of the current healthcare system have made doctors unable to spend additional time talking to patients who may be depressed. They do not have the time or they do not get reimbursed for that time. Getting into the emotional aspects of somebody's life can be a drain on physicians' energy, so many will actually avoid trying to understand the root of a patient's anxiety or depression. Internists and family practitioners may feel uncomfortable dealing with mental anguish and may stick to the familiar territory of performing a physical examination, performing laboratory tests, and prescribing medications.

When obvious stress is present, such as a difficult divorce, a stressful job, or other personal problems, your doctor is unlikely to consider a thyroid dysfunction as a possible cause of or a contributing reason for your symptoms. He may tell you, "You're doing too much, it's all stress!" if you complain about tiredness, feeling down, anxiety, and weight gain. Your close relatives and your doctor become convinced that the overwhelming stress and life situations are responsible for the symptoms. Yet, as we'll see in Chapter 4, stress itself can trigger a thyroid imbalance and contribute to depression. Stress generated by the effects of thyroid hormone imbalance can lead to an escalating cycle of stress-illness-stress. Stressful life events may then be blamed for what are really thyroid-related symptoms, allowing these symptoms to linger and intensify. I recommend that everyone who has experienced a major stress, such as a difficult divorce or the death of a loved one, and has ongoing symptoms have his or her thyroid tested.

You might have read or heard about symptoms of thyroid imbalance and come to the conclusion that your symptoms are likely to be due to a thyroid condition. If you ask your doctor to test your thyroid, he or she may resist the idea. Molly, who had gained a lot of weight and was exhausted from her hypothyroidism, told me:

> Before I was originally diagnosed as being hypothyroid, I had read about it in a magazine. I kept telling my family physician that I had a lot of these symptoms. He never checked my thyroid. He told me, "You just want thyroid hormone because you think it will make you lose weight." That wasn't what I was looking for at all. I was just looking for an answer to why all these things were happening to my body. He finally agreed to do tests, and sure enough, I was hypothyroid.

You need to be persistent and have your doctor obtain the tests needed to uncover the root of your symptoms.

Doctors are even more likely to miss a thyroid problem and misdiagnose you if you have previously suffered from depression, panic attacks, or any other mood disorder. Symptoms of a thyroid imbalance are then likely to be attributed to the mood disorder, and the physician searches no further. One patient told me, "I learned quickly after I had been in the psychiatric hospital the first time what not to tell doctors, because once they hear that you had a mental condition, they disregard everything else you say."

Patients with thyroid imbalance may see a psychiatrist rather than a medical practitioner for depression and anxiety. Because depression and anxiety disorders can cause the same physical symptoms as thyroid imbalance, psychiatrists are likely to come up with a psychiatric diagnosis when they see a thyroid patient. One study showed that when psychiatrists use conventional psychiatric criteria to assess hyperthyroid patients, they diagnose nearly half of the patients as depressed or suffering from an anxiety disorder.[15] Unfortunately, some psychiatrists do not always look for a thyroid condition as a possible reason for their patients' fatigue, lack of interest in life, and inability to function as before.

The apparently close link between depression and thyroid imbalance has wide-ranging consequences. For a person like Rachel, a young wife and real estate agent I treated recently, uncovering that link was crucial for overall health and happiness. Before her true, thyroid-related condition was identified and treated, Rachel showed many of the signs of clinical depression. "I was always tired," she related.

> I couldn't exercise anymore, and that was very frustrating. I would come home and fall asleep. If I wasn't sleeping, I was doing nothing more than watching TV. I didn't cook. I didn't clean. I didn't even let the dog out. I also put on twenty pounds in one month and lost a lot of hair, which was terrible for my looks and my self-esteem. I just had no willpower. I had to take a broker's license test, which cost my firm $2,000, but I couldn't even get motivated to study for it. I just wanted to go home and put on my nightgown and sit there on the couch. I lost interest in having any social life with my husband. I didn't want to see anyone. We quit going out. Our sexual relationship went to zero, too.

Given Rachel's symptoms, it is not surprising that for a long time she was diagnosed as depressed. Yet many of these same symptoms are associated with an underactive thyroid, and when Rachel was treated for her thyroid imbalance, she began to improve. "I gradually woke up and began to feel good," she said. "I didn't feel groggy or rushed anymore. I started eating right. I was more active and doing moderate exercise, and I lost thirty pounds. My husband and I went dancing, and I reunited with my friends again. They all asked, 'Where were you?'" For Rachel to fully answer that question, she would need to understand more about the interplay of thyroid, mind, and mood. Clearly, an underactive thyroid frequently causes depression, and an overactive thyroid tends to result in an anxiety disorder. Nevertheless, anxiety is also common in hypothyroid patients, and some patients with an overactive thyroid suffer from depression.[16]

Patients aren't totally aware of the full range of their symptoms or don't communicate them to their doctors. You may unintentionally hinder a proper diagnosis by failing to volunteer all of your complaints to your doctor. The statement "I'm tired and exhausted" usually reflects only surface symptoms. The symptom of fatigue may hide a multitude of feelings and emotional problems that patients may be reluctant to reveal. Most people have difficulty analyzing and clearly expressing how they feel or how their mind has been affected. Often we are not taught to recognize how our hearts feel, and many of us are taught to ignore or discount our emotions. We frequently lump all discomfort and mental suffering into "I'm tired, I'm exhausted, and I can't function the way I used to." Also, we tend to dismiss any mental or physical dysfunction as temporary.

Many people experiencing fatigue, lack of interest in life, and an inability to function as they once did suffer for years. They adjust to these feelings and are able to work and take care of responsibilities at home. But inside they are hurting. They have to struggle to appear normal to those around them. They live in a state of denial or self-dismissal and may not seek help or treatment for their symptoms.

Some of this self-dismissal stems from the stigma our culture puts on any and all mental conditions. The prevailing view that mental suffering is less serious than physical suffering may cause some people with a thyroid imbalance to hide their anxiety, depression, or pain and not seek medical help. Others may fear ridicule from friends and relatives if they do seek treatment.

One patient who was suffering from lingering depression due to hypothyroidism told me, "I knew I was depressed and something was inadequate within me. I didn't want my family to know. I didn't want my company to know. I didn't have health insurance coverage for depression treatment, so I couldn't afford proper help." Many patients are afraid to seek psychiatric care because they may later encounter significant difficulties in obtaining certain types of insurance.

A second-year law student whom I evaluated for a possible thyroid disorder had suffered from a severe anxiety disorder for two years. He had correctly diagnosed his anxiety disorder a year earlier but had not reached out for help. "I could not go see a psychiatrist because later on, when I sit for my bar exams, just having a record saying I saw a psychiatrist will affect my entire career." This patient turned out to have an overactive thyroid due to Graves' disease.

I cannot emphasize enough how important it is for you to seek help as soon as possible after the onset of your symptoms rather than accepting them and doing nothing about them.

The wide range of physical symptoms can mask a thyroid imbalance. If your symptoms are predominantly physical, your doctor may focus on the organ or organs involved instead of searching for a general body imbalance and an underlying condition. He or she may end up treating you for specific symptoms and fail to diagnose the thyroid condition that is causing the symptoms. For instance, rapid heartbeat is a common symptom of an overactive thyroid that often leads physicians to consider heart disease. But if the heart evaluation is normal, doctors often dismiss the patient as anxious.

Judy, a forty-one-year-old divorced woman whose mother had died three years previously, was experiencing many symptoms of anxiety and depression. Even more disturbing to her were frequent palpitations and weakness in her arms and legs. Overactive thyroid can cause muscle weakness, which should not be confused with the intermittent general weakness accompanying acute anxiety. In Judy's words:

> I had been experiencing rapid heartbeats for about three years. I was nervous and impatient. I had shaky hands. My doctor told me it might be nerves. He put me on the anxiety-reducing drug Xanax. One time I got up at night to go to the bathroom, and when I started walking, I felt like I was going to fall over. I felt like I was losing control. I was nauseous and my heart was beating fast. I called a friend and asked him to come and get me. When I went in the first time, the doctor in the emergency room said I was under tension.
>
> I kept having the same symptoms. I went to the hospital several times, and the doctors gave me a beta-blocker to slow my heart down, but it wasn't enough. I kept waking up at night with palpitations.

The doctors ended up scheduling a twenty-four-hour heartbeat-monitoring test.

It took a long time for Judy to be diagnosed with Graves' disease. The physicians who saw her on numerous occasions were focusing on her heart. After her overactive thyroid was treated, all her symptoms, including the rapid heartbeat, resolved.

Thyroid hormone imbalance affects the functioning of most bodily organs. How severely it affects organs, however, differs from one person to the next. Imagine two people having the same level of hypothyroidism. They may have some symptoms in common, such as dry skin, constipation, and weight gain. One of them, however, may have severe headaches, which then become the main concern for both the patient and the physician. Joint and muscle pain is another symptom that often triggers unnecessary testing and leads to the wrong diagnosis. Doctors frequently consider neurological or rheumatological conditions in such patients rather than a thyroid disorder.

Patients who undergo repetitive testing for rheumatological or neurological conditions and are referred to different specialists often become frustrated because the testing fails to produce a firm diagnosis. In the meantime, the patients' symptoms of depression and their feelings of being out of control may increase. Undiagnosed thyroid patients typically go from physician to physician, searching for the reason for their symptoms.

Gynecological and hormonal symptoms can mask a thyroid imbalance. Women with a thyroid imbalance frequently seek help from their gynecologists because their symptoms, both physical and mental, have evolved concurrently with the onset of heavy or irregular menstrual periods or loss of menstrual periods. Their symptoms, including the menstrual problems, are often attributed to gynecological or hormonal changes. They are often told that they are becoming menopausal or are perimenopausal.

Janet had been suffering from hypothyroidism for more than two years, but her gynecologist focused on Janet's heavy bleeding. Janet ended up having a hysterectomy after having unsuccessfully tried various hormonal treatments. According to Janet:

The gynecologist gave me hormone samples to try for three months. I was still having heavy periods, and nothing felt better, so I went back. I got another type for three months. Four times I went and tried different hormones. Then I had a hysterectomy. I kept gaining weight. My hair was falling out. I felt out of control. I said, something is not right here. Finally, after the hysterectomy, a doctor diagnosed me with hypothyroidism.

Angela, a thirty-five-year-old sales manager in a department store, told of how she suffered from numerous symptoms for which she could find no explanation for a long time:

After I had my second child, I stayed home for the first year of his life, and then I went back to work. There were times that I had a feeling of ill-being, sinking. If I didn't lie down and go to sleep, I felt like I was going to fall down and sleep where I was. I developed more symptoms, such as the migraines. My internist put me on Valium, which I stopped because it made me feel drowsy, but I then began to take Xanax twice a day and another drug for anxiety.

Angela was also suffering from impaired short-term memory, moodiness, anger, and frustration, partly due to thyroid hormone imbalance and partly as a result of anxiety from not knowing what was happening to her. When her menstrual periods became heavier and started lasting seven to eight days, she became concerned that all her symptoms were gynecological.

She says, "My mother told me, 'Your symptoms sound like you have early menopause. Go and see your gynecologist!' I complained to my gynecologist about my periods getting longer. She suggested using hormones to correct the problems, but my symptoms grew worse."

Angela's experience shows how the mental suffering due to hypothyroidism may be incorrectly attributed to reproductive hormonal problems. When estrogen or progesterone treatments do not help alleviate your symptoms, it is very important to get tested for a thyroid imbalance.

Thyroid symptoms are often dismissed as unimportant "female complaints." In recent years, the question has arisen as to whether internists and family practitioners are adequately trained to provide care for women and to understand their health needs fully. Women's health considerations differ from men's because of differences both in reproduction and in hormonal, psychosocial, and socioeconomic factors.

A study published in the *Journal of Women's Health* in 1993 suggests that the detection of thyroid abnormalities among fifteen- to sixty-four-year-old women often depends on the competence of family and general practitioners and gynecologists. The study showed that women in general receive the majority of their healthcare from family and general practitioners (54.9 percent), while internists accounted for only 21.5 percent and gynecologists for 23.6 percent of visits.[17] However, women's general physical examinations were largely performed by gynecologists (57.3 percent).

An American College of Physicians task force has defined the minimum competencies for physicians who take care of women and has recommended enhancing the competencies pertaining to women in the field of internal medicine. Competency in the field of thyroid disease is not emphasized enough, despite the fact that thyroid disorders predominantly affect women. Women are more likely than men to be misdiagnosed, perhaps because many doctors often attribute women's complaints to anxiety. Because of time constraints, some doctors may dismiss women who express "too many symptoms" when they detail their history. They may misperceive the emotional effects of a thyroid imbalance as "typical female complaints." Or they believe the symptoms are hypochondriacal. Such prejudices can result in failure to diagnose a thyroid imbalance.

Leslie Laurence and Beth Weinhouse, in *Outrageous Practices: The Alarming Truth About How Medicine Mistreats Women*, recount the story of a woman with an overactive thyroid caused by Graves' disease. It was twenty years before a physician finally made the correct diagnosis.[18] According to the patient, "They didn't look thoroughly enough because I'm a woman."

The consequences of dismissing the symptoms of thyroid imbalance in women are probably more severe than is the case with any other common condition that doctors deal with. The complex interplay between premenstrual hormonal changes, menopause, the postpartum period, reproduction, and thyroid imbalance has not been significantly addressed in women's healthcare. We need to raise our awareness of the deficiencies in providing optimal care for women afflicted with thyroid disease.

Your Doctor May Not Get the Right Test or May Overlook Abnormal or Borderline Results

The search for a correct diagnosis is lengthy in many patients. To determine whether you have a thyroid imbalance, you must be tested for the level of

TSH (thyroid-stimulating hormone), the pituitary hormone that regulates the functioning of the thyroid gland. The TSH test is much more reliable for detecting an underactive thyroid than the measurement of thyroid hormone levels in the blood. If your doctor relies only on the T4 and T3 measurements and fails to order the appropriate test (TSH), you may not be properly diagnosed for hypothyroidism. Jane, a twenty-eight-year-old nurse, told her primary care physician about her classic symptoms of a thyroid imbalance: fatigue, weight gain, decreased sexual desire, hair falling out, dry skin, and lack of concentration. On her insistence, he ordered a T4 test (which measures the level of T4, one of the two thyroid hormones produced by the thyroid gland). Her results came back within the normal laboratory range, whereupon he declared that Jane could not have thyroid disease. However, he had not checked her TSH.

She says, "Being told that nothing was wrong with me made me think I might be crazy. I have a history of people trying to deny me my feelings, trying to tell me that what is going on in my body is not real." When her TSH level was later measured by an endocrinologist, she was diagnosed as hypothyroid.

Even if your TSH level has been checked, your doctor may interpret slightly abnormal or borderline results as trivial and not significant. You may be denied treatment even though low-grade thyroid imbalance could be promoting many of your symptoms. I will address in Chapter 7 the significance of borderline and marginally abnormal thyroid tests, as well as the controversy on what should be considered a true normal range for TSH. If you have symptoms of thyroid imbalance and your test result is in the gray zone of normalcy, you need to be persistent in pursuing the possibility that your symptoms could be thyroid-related—more so if other family members have been diagnosed with a thyroid condition or other immune-related disorders.

As you can imagine, having your doctor dismiss your symptoms as unimportant, transient, or irrelevant could generate a great deal of anxiety. Not only would you question your own experience and judgment, but you would still be suffering from the very real problems that caused you to go to your doctor in the first place! You may feel that you are perceived as a hypochondriac or even come to think you are imagining things. Yet at some level, you do know that your body is not acting the way it should. When thyroid patients ultimately obtain a proper diagnosis that confirms that there is something medically wrong with them, they are almost universally relieved that their symptoms were not just "in their mind" and that they were not "going crazy."

The challenges faced by thyroid patients are not limited to having their concerns dismissed and failing to receive a correct diagnosis. Often thyroid patients do not receive comprehensive care that addresses all the intricacies and effects of immune system reactivity as well as the physical and mental effects of thyroid disease. Thyroid disease can affect every single aspect of your mental health, yet this is not recognized or addressed by many health-care professionals. Conventional doctors often limit their treatment to just prescribing one thyroid hormone medication without seeking to perfect the treatment, which is typically required for patients to feel their best. As a re-sult, many thyroid patients wind up on high doses of thyroid medications that are not necessarily conducive to long-term wellness.

Frustrated and even desperate, people may turn to the Internet for help, but the information they find there is in many instances not quite accurate and at times potentially harmful. Thyroid patients may become trapped in a cycle of misinformation provided by individuals who lack meaningful knowl-edge about how they should be treated. Unfortunately, many thyroid pa-tients, patient advocates, and even physicians who have no real expertise in the field of thyroid disease and autoimmunity have written books providing inaccurate, distorted, and occasionally even dangerous recommendations. In essence, because of their dissatisfaction with the care they receive from con-ventional healthcare professionals, thyroid patients have become targets of manipulation for unqualified people who have no expertise in the field and who are looking merely to make money off people's illnesses. Throughout this book I will provide you with the information you need to ascertain that you are getting properly diagnosed and receiving optimal treatment. I will also provide you with my detailed and comprehensive mind-body program that has helped thousands of patients struggling with thyroid disease.

Important Points to Remember

- Thyroid imbalances have such a wide range of effects on body and mind that thyroid conditions can hide or masquerade as many physical and emotional disorders.
- At any given time, more than half the people suffering from a thyroid imbalance are either undiagnosed or misdiagnosed.
- Do not necessarily rely on your primary care physician to detect and treat your thyroid disorder. Many primary care physicians have been in-adequately trained in this field or lack the expertise to deal with com-plex cases. Be persistent in asking for the right testing and follow-ups.
- If you are experiencing emotional problems, talk about them openly with your doctor. Discuss *all* of your symptoms. Much of the suffering caused by a thyroid imbalance can be easily corrected.
- Remember, although thyroid disease can cause depression, anxiety, and mood swings, you may *not* need a psychiatrist.

2

I'M TIRED OF BEING TIRED

Could It Be My Thyroid?

Most people associate thyroid disease with slow metabolism and weight gain issues. The reason is that the chemicals that the thyroid gland produces (thyroid hormones) have a tremendous say in how much fat you burn, even at rest, and how much body heat you generate. But these hormones also have a huge influence on your energy levels simply because they regulate most of the biochemical reactions that make your body and brain function optimally. A disturbance in these hormones makes your entire body less energetic, and lack of energy is also linked to metabolism and weight.

Since the beginning of my career in thyroid disorders and metabolism, fatigue has been one of the main reasons patients come to see me. They desperately want to find out if their fatigue and the resulting impaired quality of life have anything to do with their thyroid. Fatigue is in fact the most common symptom of any thyroid imbalance. More than ever before, people are seeking help from their primary care physicians and from hormone specialists, called endocrinologists, to determine whether their fatigue is thyroid-related or not. All this is because of the increased public awareness of thyroid disease and its symptoms. Unfortunately, many people's concerns are dismissed because their thyroid levels appear normal, and so they remain tired even though they have a bona fide thyroid condition.

For many thyroid patients, the root of the thyroid imbalance is the immune system's attack on the thyroid gland. Their immune system becomes overly activated and produces inflammation chemicals that, beyond damaging their thyroid gland, affect physical and mental well-being in numerous other ways.[1] Immune system reactivity explains why patients treated with thyroid medication may continue to struggle with lingering fatigue and other annoying mental and physical symptoms. For mental and physical thyroid symptoms to fully resolve, thyroid patients often need more than just thyroid medication. They need more in-depth care of their immune system in order to make it less agitated and reactive. Because the mind, thyroid, and immune system are so interconnected, thyroid patients need to embrace the mind-body program I will detail throughout this book. Not only will this help reduce inflammation throughout the body, but it will make thyroid hormone work more efficiently for overall wellness.

Jessica's Thyroid Journey

Jessica, a forty-two-year-old corporate executive, came to see me for a second opinion concerning her thyroid condition and persistent fatigue. At the age of thirty, two months after she delivered her second child, she began suffering from fatigue, lack of interest and motivation, trouble focusing, hair loss, and difficulty losing the weight she'd gained during her pregnancy. Since then her fatigue and exhaustion, often worse in the afternoon, had persisted: "I usually wake up tired and try to get as much done as I can, then I hit a slump and I can't do anything. There are days I don't even feel like getting dressed."

Searching for the cause of her fatigue, Jessica visited numerous doctors. They all reiterated that she was not suffering from a thyroid disease and that the results of her thyroid tests were in the acceptable range. It took Jessica five years to finally be recognized as suffering from low thyroid when her thyroid test results suddenly showed up slightly abnormal for the first time. Although she felt somewhat better after being prescribed thyroid medication, her fatigue, difficulty focusing, concentrating, and irritability had not fully resolved. She also continued experiencing weight gain, lack of interest, anxiety, waves of mental fogginess, and tiredness, all affecting her quality of life.

Finally she flew from Denver to see me, and I determined that her low thyroid was caused by an autoimmune condition called Hashimoto's thyroiditis. Although her persistent fatigue was partially caused by suboptimal thyroid medication treatment, her reactive and agitated immune system was producing inflammation chemicals that were affecting her energy level and mental well-being in other ways. Therefore, in addition to perfecting her thyroid medication treatment, I focused on improving the health of her immune system in order to reduce the inflammation that haunts most thyroid patients today. Miraculously, after two months of treatment, Jessica's vitality returned, her exhaustion and fatigue dissipated, and her mental clarity significantly improved. With a smile on her face, she told me: "I feel like I am a new person now."

The Desperate Search for Why You Are Tired

Feeling tired is an extremely common symptom in the general population. Roughly one in five people complain about feeling tired. In fact, fatigue has become the second-leading cause of physician visits, after pain.[2]

Too many people say they are fed up with healthcare professionals dismissing their fatigue as an insignificant complaint. Fatigue is often attributed to stress, lack of sleep, or lifestyle factors, rather than to an underlying medical condition. The search for the cause of fatigue can be tedious for the physician because a wide range of conditions must be considered and there may be multiple factors responsible for the fatigue, requiring an extensive medical evaluation.[3]

Conditions frequently considered by health professionals in patients suffering from long-standing fatigue include anemia, liver disease, diabetes, depression, cancer, heart disease, or chronic infection. The reality is that almost every lingering medical condition can lead to fatigue. Often, unfortunately, no medical condition is uncovered, leaving you frustrated and wondering why you are tired. For many, the source of their fatigue is related to a thyroid condition that remains unidentified for years before effective help is obtained. What is important to keep in mind is that even if you have been diagnosed with and treated for a medical condition that causes fatigue, you could still easily be suffering from a coexisting thyroid condition that is contributing to your persistent fatigue. Conversely, if you are a thyroid sufferer and continue to struggle with fatigue, it is possible that a coexisting condition is involved.

The following are potential causes of fatigue:

Hormonal imbalances
• Thyroid imbalance and autoimmune thyroid disease (i.e., Hashimoto's thyroiditis)
• Adrenal insufficiency
• Pituitary deficiencies (such as shortage of growth hormone)
Sleep disorders
• Sleep apnea
• Sleep deprivation
• Narcolepsy
Anemia (iron deficiency, pernicious anemia, etc.)
Autoimmune disorders
• Lupus
• Polymyositis (a rare muscle disease), dermatomyositis (a rare disease causing weak muscles and a skin rash)
• Sjögren's syndrome

- Polymyalgia rheumatica
- Rheumatoid arthritis
- Other autoimmune conditions

Infections (Lyme disease, Epstein-Barr virus, HIV, and many others)

Mood disorders

- Depression
- Chronic stress
- PTSD

Chronic fatigue syndrome

Fibromyalgia

Medications (beta-blockers, antidepressants, and many others)

Chronic medical conditions

- Liver disease
- Kidney disease
- Heart disease
- Diabetes

Toxicity (from drugs, heavy metals, alcoholism, or other sources)

Food sensitivities

Cancer

Thyroid Disease on the Rise

More than ever before, people are suffering from thyroid problems. Thyroid disease is currently viewed as the most common disorder related to the endocrine system. Experts often disagree on how many Americans actually suffer from some form of thyroid imbalance, with many standing behind the number 13 million, which I consider an underestimate.

The major differences in estimates occur because the medical community has not reached a consensus on the real normal reference range for the blood tests that allow doctors to diagnose a thyroid imbalance. Although the range for what is normal has been narrowed over the years, some doctors still view many patients who have bona fide thyroid disease and suffer from symptoms as "normal," even though they are not. If the conventional range for blood testing is ever narrowed further, millions who are currently viewed as not having a thyroid condition will suddenly be considered to have one. In my opinion, it is very likely that roughly 50 million Americans suffer from some form of thyroid disease. After so many years of diagnosing and treating thyroid patients, I have come to the conclusion that conventional thyroid tests are only useful in diagnosing clear-cut thyroid imbalances. Indeed, normal thyroid test results by no means exclude the possibility of a thyroid imbalance. Currently, about 80 percent of people suffering from a thyroid imbalance are women, and the most common thyroid imbalance is hypothyroidism.[4]

The number of autoimmune thyroid disease cases seems to be rising in the United States. It is likely that increased stress partly accounts for this. In addition to stress, our environment plays a role: infections, a lack of antioxidants, and environmental contaminants are among the most significant environmental factors linked to thyroid disease. On top of that, what we eat (and don't eat) contributes to immune system reactivity.

Not all thyroid conditions result in thyroid imbalance or are associated with an immune system attack on the thyroid gland. Moreover, enlargement of the gland or lumps within the gland are quite common. For instance, thyroid nodules (lumps), defined as isolated growths within the gland, are quite common and affect more women than men.[5] In many cases, the nodule has been present for a long time before it is discovered, although it can be detected by your doctor through a neck examination. If you have a thyroid nodule, you may not necessarily have any symptoms, but you may suffer from difficulty swallowing, hoarseness, a feeling of pressure in the neck, or even neck pain.

Thyroid nodules that can be detected through manual examination affect roughly 3 to 7 percent of the population. Nowadays, with routine thyroid ultrasounds, it is estimated that small nodules—less than 1 cm in size—are found in as much as 20 percent of the population.[6] Nodules are also quite often detected incidentally when magnetic resonance imaging (MRI) or a computerized tomography (CT) scan of the neck is performed for other medical reasons. A greater number of people seem to be affected by thyroid nodules than ever before, although this may have to do with more routine use of ultrasound imaging and a greater awareness of thyroid disease than with any increase in their actual frequency.

Roughly 15 percent of lumps bigger than 1 cm are cancerous, although small nodules can be cancerous as well. Most nodules do not produce excess thyroid hormone (resulting in hyperthyroidism), but some do; these are known as toxic nodules. If you have thyroid gland inflammation or a thyroid hormone imbalance, you may also have a nodule. The main concern about having a thyroid nodule, whether small or big, is the possibility of thyroid cancer. There is some indication that thyroid cancer is becoming more prevalent than it was years ago. Recent reports have indicated that thyroid cancer has become the second most common cancer in women after breast cancer, while one or two decades ago it was considered the sixth or seventh most common cancer in the general population. It is likely that environmental chemicals and nutritional factors have contributed to the increase in thyroid cancer.

What Is the Thyroid Gland and What Does It Do?

The thyroid is a butterfly-shaped gland situated in the lower part of the front of the neck. It is one of several endocrine glands, which release into the bloodstream substances that have a wide range of functions and effects throughout the body.[7] The hormones produced by the thyroid gland reach every cell in your body, regulating their activity and biochemical functions.

Your thyroid produces two different hormones, T3 and T4. Both thyroid hormones are made up of two molecules of the amino acid tyrosine. The difference between T3 and T4 is that T4 contains four iodine atoms, while T3 contains three. T3 is more potent than T4 with respect to its biochemical effects. The thyroid gland produces much more T4 than T3, but cells have the ability to convert T4 into the more active thyroid hormone, T3. In fact, 80 percent of all the T3 you produce in your body comes from T4; only 20 percent is produced by the gland itself. Both thyroid hormones are stored in large quantities inside the thyroid gland. When released into the bloodstream, they become attached to proteins, with a small fraction of thyroid hormone remaining in a free form, ready to be used by cells for regulatory functions. Normally, the levels of thyroid hormone available in the free form remain constant and perfectly balanced at all times. Consequently, the optimal functioning of your body cells depends both on an optimally functioning gland and also on whether the body's cells are healthy enough to produce enough T3 from T4.

A Needy and Vulnerable Gland

While optimal thyroid function is crucial for your overall well-being and health, the gland is still vulnerable to inflammation because quite a few environmental and nutrition-related factors can impair its performance.[8] The table below shows the many general factors that can affect the health and function of the thyroid.

FACTORS THAT IMPAIR THYROID HORMONE PRODUCTION

Nutrient deficiencies
Environmental damage to the thyroid gland from viruses, bacteria, or toxins
Certain foods
Immune system attacks on the thyroid
Neck radiation
Surgical damage
Genetic conditions that impair the ability of thyroid cells
to produce the right amounts of thyroid hormone

Micronutrients for Optimal Thyroid Function

The health of the thyroid gland requires balanced amounts of a long list of minerals, vitamins, and antioxidants that have the ability to support thyroid function and prevent damage to thyroid cells (the normal process of producing thyroid hormones results in significant quantities of toxic chemicals, called free radicals, and antioxidants prevent these from damaging thyroid cells). A deficiency of any of these micronutrients can also make the gland struggle in fulfilling its critical function of producing thyroid hormone.[9] While the thyroid gland needs many micronutrients, there are several that play specific and crucial roles in the process of thyroid hormone manufacture; those are the ones I will discuss in this section.

- Tyrosine
- Iodine
- Selenium
- Iron
- Zinc
- Copper
- Vitamin A
- Vitamin E
- Vitamin C

Tyrosine. Tyrosine is the backbone amino acid of the thyroid hormones T4 and T3. Tyrosine is obtained directly from many protein sources. Your body also has the ability to convert phenylalanine, an essential amino acid (one of the amino acids that the body cannot produce on its own), to tyrosine. Foods rich in tyrosine and/or phenylalanine include soy, eggs, dairy, meats, seafood, and nuts. I don't recommend tyrosine supplementation, as an excess in your body can lead to adverse effects including headaches, fatigue, skin rashes, rapid heartbeat, and irritability. Choose a thyroid supplement that does not contain any tyrosine.

Iodine. Your thyroid gland requires adequate amounts of iodine to properly produce the right amount of thyroid hormone. When the gland doesn't receive enough iodine, thyroid cells enlarge and begin to proliferate, resulting in an increased thyroid gland size (a condition called goiter) and the gland becomes unable to produce the needed amount of thyroid hormones, possibly leading to hypothyroidism.

Despite increased public awareness and government iodization programs worldwide, iodine deficiency remains a significant problem. Roughly 200 million people in the world suffer from iodine deficiency and its resulting health consequences. Although iodine deficiency is not as common in the United States as in other parts of the world, there is some evidence suggesting we may be experiencing a resurgence of this public health issue. For many people in the United States, iodine intake is low. Part of the reason for this may be the amount of fast food consumed in this country, as fast food is typically very low in iodine. And people following strict weight loss diets seem to be at a greater risk of suffering from iodine deficiency. The U.S. Food and Drug Administration does not require food packaging to list iodine content, making it difficult for consumers to monitor and regulate their own iodine intake. Given these factors, it is unsurprising that iodine consumption may remain overlooked in many people.

The slowing of thyroid function related to iodine deficiency is even worse if you already have thyroid inflammation or if you've suffered previous thyroid damage of any kind. Even if your thyroid gland is healthy, iodine deficiency may cause a state of low-grade hypothyroidism, with fatigue, weight gain, constipation, depression, and impaired memory. Iodine also helps flush toxins such as fluoride, mercury, and lead from your body. These toxins tend to naturally accumulate in the thyroid gland and impair the thyroid hormone manufacturing process.

In the diet, iodine is primarily obtained from clams, shrimp, haddock, halibut, oysters, salmon, canned sardines, beef liver, pineapple, canned tuna, peanuts, eggs, whole-wheat bread, seaweed, grains, iodized salt, and other iodine-enriched food products. To avoid iodine deficiency, use iodized salt instead of traditional table salt. However, the most reliable way of getting adequate iodine is by taking a multivitamin/antioxidant mix with appropriate amounts of iodine. Adults need to consume 150 to 500 mcg of iodine a day for the gland to produce the right amount of thyroid hormone. For children, 90 mcg a day is needed. Avoid too much iodine, as this can have detrimental effects on thyroid function.

Many pregnant women are not getting enough iodine on a regular basis. Over a third of pregnant women still have urinary iodine levels consistent with mild iodine deficiency. Yet iodine deficiency during pregnancy can contribute to impaired brain development in the fetus, miscarriages, and other health conditions in the newborn. Make sure that your prenatal vitamin includes iodine. If you are pregnant, you will need at least 220 mcg a day, and if you are lactating, at least 290 mcg per day.

Selenium. Found in nature, selenium is a trace mineral that has important functions in the body. Selenium is essential for the gland to produce the right amount of thyroid hormone. In fact, the thyroid gland has the highest concentration of selenium in the body. An antioxidant, it protects cells from the damaging effects of free radicals. Selenium has tremendous benefits for the functioning of the immune system, helping it be less reactive in people who are already suffering from thyroid disease. This micronutrient is also essential for clearing toxic chemicals from thyroid cells, preventing thyroid cell damage, and maintaining overall thyroid health. It is viewed as one of the micronutrients most necessary for both the production of thyroid hormone and the conversion of T4 to T3 in the thyroid gland and in other parts of the body.[10] This explains why your blood and cellular T3 levels become low when you are deficient in selenium. Selenium deficiency can also induce a state of general inflammation in your body, affect your mood, cause insulin resistance, and contribute to infertility, miscarriage, and other hormonal issues. If you suffer from both iodine and selenium deficiency (a more common situation in certain parts of the world), your thyroid gland can become severely damaged, leading to hypothyroidism and a condition called cretinism in children. Foods rich in selenium include shellfish, crab, kidney, poultry, dairy, and liver. That being said, selenium can easily be lost in food processing, putting you at risk of getting less than you need. In addition, too much thyroid hormone in your body, as a result of an overactive thyroid or medication overdose, can easily make you become deficient in selenium, especially if your nutritional selenium intake is marginal. With well-balanced nutrition, you should be getting between 30 and 85 mcg of selenium daily, though this may not be enough to reduce immune system reactivity. I recommend that you get at least 100 mcg of selenium to prevent thyroid cell damage and keep your immune system less reactive. Make sure you do not take supplemental selenium exceeding 300 mcg a day, as selenium excess can cause diarrhea, fatigue, hair loss, and a color change in the fingernails. Too much selenium can also cause functional damage to your thyroid. If you are not getting the right amount of selenium in your diet, you should consider taking a thyroid supplement that includes the right amount of selenium.

Zinc. Zinc is an essential trace mineral and is crucial for optimal thyroid hormone production, both ensuring proper functioning of the thyroid gland and preventing damage to thyroid cells. Research has shown that zinc deficiency can induce low thyroid hormone levels in animals. Patients with Down syndrome are more prone to suffer from hypothyroidism as well as zinc deficiency, and it is likely that zinc deficiency is a major contributing factor to hypothyroidism in these patients.[11] If you suffer from a combined deficiency of selenium and zinc, significant thyroid gland damage can occur, leading to low thyroid function. Excessive zinc intake can also affect the absorption of other important trace minerals, such as copper and manganese, affecting thyroid function. Foods rich in zinc include dairy, poultry, beef, crab, oysters, spinach, nuts, beans, pumpkin, and squash.

Iron. Iron is another trace element necessary for thyroid hormone production. Iron deficiency is quite common, perhaps more in women than men, particularly those who experience heavy menstrual periods. You are also more likely to suffer from iron deficiency if you have a malabsorption issue or gastrointestinal inflammatory disease. Iron deficiency can cause anemia and sleep disturbances, and can contribute to low thyroid function, especially in people who also suffer from iodine, selenium, or zinc deficiency or in people with already damaged thyroid glands. Foods rich in iron include liver, spinach, lentils, beans, dark chocolate, oysters, and olives. If you have a thyroid condition such as an autoimmune thyroid disease, you need to make sure that your iron levels are in a very good range in order to avoid worsening thyroid function. If you are taking thyroid hormone medication and you need iron supplementation, make sure that the iron supplement is taken late in the day, several hours after taking the thyroid medication.

Copper. Little attention has been paid to this trace mineral, yet it plays an important role within the thyroid gland, where it is involved in processing iodine for the manufacture of thyroid hormone. Copper deficiency is uncommon, as copper is found in many food sources. However, people with gastrointestinal disorders may suffer from copper malabsorption and copper deficiency. Foods rich in copper include whole-grain cereals, legumes, oysters, organ meats, fruits, leafy green vegetables, and many other foods. Taking too much copper can impair thyroid function, however; if you are taking a thyroid supplement, make sure that the amount of copper it includes does not exceed 2 to 3 mg a day.

Vitamin A. Vitamin A is crucial for optimal thyroid hormone production. It is essential not only for the manufacture of thyroid hormone but also for thyroid hormone to work efficiently in the cells. Foods rich in vitamin A include liver, fish oils, leafy green vegetables, milk, eggs, fruits, and cereal. If you have an autoimmune thyroid disease, I recommend that you take a natural supplement that includes the right amount of vitamin A in the form of beta-carotene.

Vitamin E. Vitamin E is a powerful antioxidant that helps in the process of converting T4 to T3 in the thyroid gland. Vitamin E is also important for maintaining brain health and cognitive functions.[12] Foods rich in vitamin E include green leafy vegetables, almonds, sunflower seeds, egg yolk, avocado, and spinach. Supplementation should not exceed 400 IU per day, as vitamin E excess can cause significant negative health effects, including heart problems and an increased risk of bleeding.

Vitamin C. Vitamin C helps with the conversion of T4 to T3. It also has powerful antioxidant properties that help thyroid cells remain healthy. Food sources of vitamin C include peppers, guavas, green leafy vegetables, broccoli, berries, citrus fruits, tomatoes, and peas.

Cruciferous Vegetables: How Much Is Too Much?

There's a lot of information (and misinformation) out there about foods that may lower thyroid function. There are certain foods, known as goitrogens, that can impair the manufacture of thyroid hormone and can lead to a goiter (enlarged thyroid gland). The most common goitrogens are:

- CRUCIFEROUS VEGETABLES
  Broccoli
  Brussels sprouts

Cabbage
Cauliflower
Collard greens
Horseradish
Kale
Mustard greens
Turnips

OTHER FOODS
Soybeans
Soy products
Pine nuts
Flaxseed
Canola oil
Millet
Spinach
Radishes
Peaches
Strawberries

The effect of these foods on thyroid function in humans is probably not great unless you consume them on a daily basis and in large amounts.

The majority of the vegetables in the list above fall into the group known as cruciferous vegetables. These naturally contain considerable amounts of different types of organic compounds called glucosinolates, which are ultimately converted to isothiocyanate molecules.[13] These have the ability to impair the uptake and processing of iodine in thyroid cells and decrease thyroid hormone production. Research on pigs showed that it takes roughly the equivalent of sixty pounds of cruciferous vegetables for these compounds to affect the animal's thyroid function.[14] Clearly, then, eating normal amounts of these vegetables is not likely to affect thyroid function in people not suffering from thyroid disease. Furthermore, cooking these vegetables, as opposed to eating them raw, significantly reduces their impairing effect on the thyroid. Another good reason not to avoid cruciferous vegetables altogether is that many of these foods contain isoflavones, substances that have tremendous anti-inflammatory and antioxidant properties. Isoflavones such as quercetin and kaempferol also have detoxifying properties and support the immune system, which is of great importance to people suffering from autoimmune thyroid disease. The upshot is that the effects of cruciferous vegetables on the thyroid are minimal when you cook them and eat them in moderation. They can play a role in a well-balanced diet, and there's no need to deprive yourself of them.

If you have a thyroid condition, however, you have to be cautious about not overconsuming raw cruciferous vegetables every day. One way people might do that without realizing it is in juice, as juicing raw vegetables has become quite popular these days. Although I believe that raw vegetable juice is okay for thyroid patients, I recommend limiting it to four or five days a week and paying careful attention to the amounts consumed, as excessive quantities might further affect the gland's ability to produce thyroid hormone if it is already damaged by Hashimoto's thyroiditis and related inflammation.

A lot of attention has been paid to soy as well. Soy foods have become increasingly popular in the Western world because they contain isoflavones, in particular genistein and daidzein, which are phytoestrogens (that is, they are plant-based substances that act like estrogens in the body). Soy protects against heart disease, osteoporosis, breast cancer, and prostate cancer, can help with hot flashes, lowers insulin resistance, and reduces inflammation. However, in large quantities, soy can impair the manufacturing of thyroid hormone and in particular the production of T3, the most active form. Research has shown that the phytoestrogen intake typical of soy consumption in Western cultures does not cause deterioration of thyroid function even in patients with low-grade hypothyroidism. However, consistent consumption of soy in high amounts can produce low thyroid function in animals, and feeding infants soy-based formula can lead to the formation of a goiter.[15] People who consume one to two servings of soy on a daily basis for extended periods of time can increase their risk of low thyroid function, especially if they have thyroid disease. If you already have low-grade hypothyroidism and regularly eat significant amounts of soy, equivalent to 16 mg a day of phytoestrogens, this can worsen the function of the thyroid.[16] Indeed, genistein and daidzein both impair the manufacture of thyroid hormone.[17] Unlike isothiocyanates in cruciferous vegetables, the goitrogenicity of the isoflavones in soy is not reduced when the soy is cooked. Eat soy in moderation, not more than three or four times a week, even if your thyroid gland is healthy.

Toxic Chemicals That Affect Thyroid Gland Function and/or Thyroid Hormone Efficiency

The thyroid is a very sensitive gland. It can be affected by immune attacks, various infections, and exposure to radiation. The gland and its function can also be negatively affected by many environmental factors, such as toxic chemicals, that disrupt the endocrine system. Unfortunately, we come into contact with many endocrine disruptors every day through the air that we breathe and the products that we consume. Substances such as insecticides, herbicides, and fungicides can affect the functioning of the thyroid gland in different ways and trigger thyroid imbalance. One way is to impair the uptake of iodine by the cells in the thyroid gland. They can also be toxic to the thyroid itself; animal research has shown that exposure to DDT and amitrol can cause goiter and hypothyroidism. The longer you work in or are exposed to a toxic environment, the more likely it is that you will have a thyroid imbalance. You can even be affected if you have regular contact with people who work in such environments: one study has shown that more than 10 percent of spouses of people whose work involves pesticide application have a thyroid imbalance.

Even if your thyroid gland produces adequate amounts of thyroid hormone, many environmental toxins make thyroid hormone less effective at doing its job in your body. These endocrine disruptors can mimic actual hormones in the body, blocking cell receptors and preventing the actual hormones from binding to them. This can cause serious thyroid hormone inefficiency and slowing of metabolism. It is important for thyroid patients to be aware of which chemicals to look out for, as they could be contributing to the thyroid disorder as well as to persistent and annoying symptoms that have gone unresolved despite taking thyroid medication.

Here is a list of some of the most widespread environmental toxic chemicals that can affect thyroid health, thyroid hormone efficiency, and thyroid autoimmunity:

- **Perchlorate and lithium.** Found in drinking water, they can impair thyroid hormone production. Contamination of tap water with perchlorate is becoming a serious health hazard. Widespread industrial waste is the root of this contamination. As we've seen, cells in the thyroid gland need iodine to manufacture thyroid hormone. In essence, when you have perchlorate in your system, the thyroid ends up picking up perchlorate instead of iodine. This makes the gland unable to produce the needed amount of thyroid hormone. Lithium can also lower thyroid hormone levels by interfering with the release of thyroid hormone by the gland. Lithium may trigger and/or worsen thyroid autoimmunity.
- **Pesticides.** Several classes of pesticides, including organochlorines (for example, DDT, heptachlor, lindane, and chlordane), fungicides (including Benomyl and Mancozeb), and herbicides (such as paraquat), interfere with thyroid hormone production.[18] They can also exacerbate immune attack on the thyroid.
- **Perfluorooctanoic acid (PFOA) and perfluorooctanesulfonic acid (PFOS).** These substances are found in consumer products such as carpet cleaners, nonstick cookware, and some fabrics. Chronic exposure correlates with the occurrence of thyroid disease. It is also a cause of slow metabolism and obesity.[19]
- **Tributyltin chloride (TBTCl).** This chemical is used as a bactericide, fungicide, and pesticide, and it is also found in many anti-fouling paints, plastics, and tap water. It has been shown to have a negative effect on

thyroid function and impair thyroid hormone action in the cells. Even in trace amounts, it promotes slow metabolism and weight gain.

- **Triclosan.** Triclosan is an antifungal and antibacterial agent found in many consumer products such as soap, hand sanitizers, toothpaste, and detergents. Triclosan is structurally similar to thyroid hormone. Some studies have demonstrated a decrease in thyroid hormone levels following ingestion of triclosan. Note that the FDA has banned triclosan in antibacterial soaps and body washes sold to consumers.

- **Polychlorinated biphenyls (PCBs).** The production of PCBs was banned in the United States back in 1979, but these organic pollutants are still found today in rivers, lakes, and even water in urban areas. They can impair thyroid hormone production and thyroid hormone action in the cells.

- **Bisphenol A (BPA).** An organic synthetic compound found in many plastics and sometimes also dumped into rivers and lakes, BPA blocks T3 receptors and impairs thyroid hormone action in the cells. It also slows down metabolism and causes insulin resistance.

The Pituitary: Master of the Thyroid Gland

Your thyroid gland cannot produce adequate amounts of thyroid hormone without getting a signal from the master gland, the pituitary gland, which is a tiny structure located at the base of the brain. The pituitary gland regulates the functioning of many endocrine glands including the thyroid gland, the adrenal glands, and the ovaries. It produces a chemical hormone called thyroid stimulating hormone (TSH) which makes thyroid cells manufacture and release T4 and T3. If your pituitary gland becomes inflamed or destroyed, it may lose the ability to send the command to the thyroid, making the thyroid gland become sluggish. The end result is called pituitary hypothyroidism, or central hypothyroidism. If your pituitary gland is healthy, it will increase the production of TSH when it senses that your thyroid gland is not working well. When your thyroid is damaged or unable to perform optimally, TSH levels tend to increase. In contrast, if your thyroid gland overproduces thyroid hormone, TSH levels decline. The pituitary gland has the ability to sense any minor changes in your thyroid hormone levels and this is the reason TSH blood testing is the most sensitive way to determine whether you have a normal thyroid function or not.

Thyroid Hormone Imbalance: Fatigue and Beyond

To understand how thyroid hormone imbalance can affect both your physical and mental health and how it can have devastating effects on your quality of life, you need to know what thyroid hormone regulates in your body. It turns out that thyroid hormones actually play a role in every single aspect of the body's biological functions. They regulate your energy level and dictate how much fat you burn and how much heat your body generates in order to maintain a stable and optimal temperature.[20] They also meticulously regulate the following:

- The levels and functioning of neurotransmitters in the brain that control mood, emotions, appetite, memory, and anxiety states
- Sexual function
- Cholesterol and blood sugar
- The proper functioning of the cardiovascular system
- The proper functioning and motility of the GI tract
- The health of the hair, skin, nails, and bone
- The functioning, endurance, and performance of muscle cells
- The proper functioning and synchronization of reproductive organs (ovary, testicles, uterus)
- Brain development and growth of a developing fetus, and growth after birth
- Proper functioning and health of the immune system
- The functioning of other endocrine glands such as the pituitary gland, the adrenal glands (which produce the vital energy hormone cortisol), and the pancreas (which produces insulin)

Clearly, for your body, brain, and immune system to function in an optimal way, you need to have well-balanced levels of the two active thyroid hormones, T4 and T3. A thyroid imbalance in the form of low thyroid levels (hypothyroidism) occurs whenever the thyroid gland fails to produce 100 percent of the needed amounts of thyroid hormones. An imbalance in the form of too much thyroid hormone in your system (hyperthyroidism) is usually the result of either overproduction by the thyroid gland or taking too much thyroid hormone to treat hypothyroidism.

Considering the significant role thyroid hormone plays in the body, it's obvious that thyroid hormone imbalance can affect not only your energy and weight but also your mood, emotions, appetite, weight, skin health, nails, hair, and GI tract. It may increase your risk of cardiovascular disease, muscle dysfunction, osteoporosis, and infertility. It can also put pregnant women at a higher risk of miscarriage and pregnancy complications, and preterm delivery, and potentially lead to developmental problems in children.

The Epidemic of Low-Grade Thyroid Hormone Imbalance

Most of those in the medical community view a very minute impairment of thyroid gland function leading to a very small insufficiency or excess of thyroid hormone in your body as a trivial abnormality. In fact, most doctors consider minor thyroid hormone abnormalities as subclinical conditions (conditions that do not cause any clinical effects). I disagree with this view. I strongly believe that these low-grade abnormalities are bona fide medical conditions that can lead to serious clinical consequences that can affect people's quality of life.[21] Low-grade thyroid imbalances affect at least 8 to 10 percent of the population, with low-grade hypothyroidism being more common than low-grade hyperthyroidism. Low-grade thyroid hormone imbalance is actually the root of the fatigue and suffering experienced by millions of people. The consequences for energy level, mood, and mental clarity are obvious. Low-grade thyroid hormone imbalance can also make you vulnerable to depression, anxiety symptoms, panic attacks, forgetfulness, and difficulties with focusing and concentration. The effects on your metabolism can be striking as well and might lead to weight gain and even metabolic syndrome.

The Many Faces of Thyroid Fatigue

Carefully listening to my patients over the years has taught me that the fatigue caused by thyroid imbalance can be devastating, going far beyond merely being tired. There are some clues that your fatigue may be linked to thyroid disease. Thyroid-related fatigue is often a mix of physical and mental fatigue associated with waves of mental grogginess, which my patients frequently call "brain fog." The fatigue may not be constant; it can fluctuate throughout the day, often becoming more pronounced in the afternoon. You may actually go through cycles of worsening and improvement of energy levels. A person suffering from physical fatigue will say, "I cannot do it. I feel tired. I want to do it, but I can't." A person suffering from mental fatigue will say, "I do not feel like doing it." Mental fatigue is typically associated with lack of motivation, lack of interest, sleep issues, pains and aches, emotional instability, and cognitive impairment.

Most people and even doctors believe that thyroid-related fatigue is simply the effect of thyroid hormone imbalance. In fact, thyroid fatigue has many faces and is experienced in different ways by different patients. The reason is that thyroid fatigue is not always caused by just an imbalance of thyroid hormone. It is often the result of a mix of effects related to imbalanced thyroid hormone levels and effects related to autoimmunity, sleep problems, and thyroid hormone inefficiency. Because of all these factors, a thyroid condition can make you feel tired, depressed, moody, unpredictable, anxious, and exhausted. It can significantly impair your quality of life.

- Thyroid hormone imbalance (excess or deficiency) makes you feel physically tired because thyroid hormone regulates physical bodily functions.

- Thyroid hormone imbalance causes mental fatigue, lack of motivation, and lack of interest because thyroid hormone regulates brain neurotransmitters.
- In autoimmunity, the immune system, which is attacking your thyroid, also produces different types of inflammation chemicals that affect your brain and other parts of your body. When these chemicals reach brain cells, they affect their function, promoting fatigue, mental fog, and waves of depression.
- Thyroid disease affects your sleep, causing insomnia, disturbed sleep, sleep deprivation, and sleep apnea. In turn, these sleep issues have a significant negative effect on your energy and will make immune system reactivity worse, engendering a major vicious cycle of fatigue, immune system attack, and thyroid hormone instability.

Throughout my many years of caring for thyroid patients with different levels of thyroid imbalance, I have noticed those suffering from thyroid symptoms are rarely concerned about the direct or indirect health consequences of thyroid imbalance. They are actually almost always seeking help because their quality of life has become affected. Thyroid imbalance can interfere with work performance, life enjoyment, and relationships. As I see it, an impaired quality of life is a very common consequence of having a thyroid imbalance, even if the imbalance is minimal. Yet scientific research showing how thyroid imbalance impairs quality of life has been limited because the effects cannot be measured or quantified precisely. As a result, most healthcare professionals caring for thyroid patients do not believe that thyroid disease can negatively affect quality of life. Unfortunately, what they overlook is that it's not just the thyroid hormone imbalance that plays a role here, but also the inflammation chemicals released by the immune system. These can have devastating effects on energy level, mood, emotion, behavior, and metabolism. Moreover, these immune system effects are not usually addressed by healthcare professionals.

Immune-System-Related Fatigue

When your immune system attacks your own thyroid, your body is showered with many inflammatory chemicals called cytokines. In addition to affecting the thyroid gland, these substances also have negative effects elsewhere in the body, including the brain. The inflammation generated by the immune system has a tremendous effect on both physical and mental energy. Even more significant, immune system reactivity can actually intensify as thyroid hormone levels become imbalanced; it's as if the thyroid imbalance makes the immune system even angrier and more reactive, and symptoms worsen.

When this cascade occurs, thyroid patients can experience major, debilitating fatigue, including fibromyalgia and adrenal fatigue.

Fatigue and Thyroid-Related Depression

The thyroid hormones T4 and T3 influence mood, emotions, appetite, and cognition because they regulate levels of important brain chemicals such as serotonin, noradrenaline, and dopamine.[22] This explains why any minute insufficiency or excess of T3 in the brain can cause depression, anxiety, problems with concentration, memory issues, and poor attention span. This also explains why even a low-grade thyroid imbalance can make you prone to depression and irritability.[23]

All it takes for depression symptoms to resolve or improve is the right thyroid medication treatment (see Chapter 20 on my T4/T3 protocol). Depression can present itself in many different forms, but the most common types are chronic mild depression, major depression (an extreme form of depression that can lead to suicidal thoughts, a severe feeling of disconnection, insomnia, and loss of appetite), and manic-depression (bipolar disorder). Many people think that depression just involves intense feelings of sadness, but in reality the central feature is a blunting of feelings that is not always associated with sadness.

Thyroid imbalance–related depression is more often than not a mild or low-grade depression. It may be associated with a slowing down of energy and a decline in motivation, interest, and drive. It can make you eat (or overeat) as a way of seeking comfort, you may sleep more than usual, and you may suffer from anxiety. You are also more likely to experience anger, irritability, and low stress tolerance, making you perceive minor stressors or daily tasks as unbearable and overwhelming.

The fatigue of low-grade depression related to thyroid disease is a frustrating chronic condition that, in extreme situations, can impair your ability to function as you used to. As the day goes on, your fatigue and low mood are exacerbated, making you want to just lie on the couch. In many thyroid patients, energy and enthusiasm will pick up from time to time, but this is often only temporary.

The Thyroid-Fatigue-Sleep Connection

Poor sleep quality, sleep deprivation, and interrupted sleep are often contributing factors to fatigue in thyroid patients. These sleep issues not only directly compromise your energy level but make your immune system more reactive and damaged as well.

There are many ways thyroid disease can affect sleep patterns. Depression and anxiety can make you experience difficulties falling asleep and can even cause insomnia. When you do fall asleep, it may be difficult for you to remain asleep for more than a few hours at a time.

Thyroid imbalance can be associated with sleep apnea, an intermittent cessation of breathing during sleep. There are two kinds of sleep apnea. In obstructive sleep apnea, the soft tissue at the back of the throat collapses temporarily during sleep; this is more common in overweight people, and, as we have seen, thyroid imbalance can cause weight gain. In central sleep apnea, there is a disconnect between the breathing center in the brain and the diaphragm. With either type, you can wake up several times each night, seemingly for no reason. Sleep problems may be worse if you are going through the transition to menopause.

When thyroid imbalance affects your sleep, you will have even lower energy levels during the day. Insufficient or interrupted sleep can present serious health risks and cause excessive daytime sleepiness, making it harder to carry out your daily activities. Correcting the thyroid imbalance by taking the right medications, losing weight, and beginning appropriate treatment for sleep apnea will help. You also need to follow a strict sleep schedule and use a relaxation technique such as meditation in order to help improve your overall sleep quality.

The Icing on the Cake: Cellular Hypothyroidism

Having perfectly normal thyroid hormone levels in the blood is important but not sufficient for the cells to function properly. As I explained earlier, the most abundant thyroid hormone in the blood and throughout the body is T4. Thyroid hormones are incorporated into the cell, where T4 changes into either T3 (the active form of thyroid hormone) or reverse T3 (a biologically inactive hormone). If cells are inefficient at producing the right amount of T3 and instead produce reverse T3, there will not be enough T3 in the cell to perform its regulatory functions properly. I view this situation as a state of tissue or cellular hypothyroidism, somewhat akin to having low blood levels of thyroid hormones.

The process of producing T3 depends on many factors. One is the amount of selenium in your cells. If you are deficient in selenium, your cells become unable to produce normal amounts of T3 and instead produce more of the inactive reverse T3. In addition, a buildup of free radicals in the cells, to the point where the physiological intracellular antioxidant system is overwhelmed, will lower your T3 levels.[24] It turns out that thyroid patients almost universally have a tremendous buildup of free radicals in their cells, impairing the conversion of T4 to T3. Environmental factors that can add to the free radical buildup include heavy metal toxicity (mercury, cadmium, and lead), allergies, cigarette smoke, exposure to industrial chemicals, or overly intense exercise. Environmental pollutants that have also been implicated in tissue or cellular hypothyroidism include herbicides, BPA, PCBs, triclosan, perchlorate, pesticides, fungicides, and water contaminants such as trihalomethane, benzene, arsenic, bromide, fluoride, and dioxin, along with the artificial sweetener sucralose (Splenda) and other food additives. Sleep deprivation and stress increase the body's production of the stress hormone cortisol, and too much cortisol impairs the conversion of T4 to T3. Depression, weight gain, and even eating too much sugar, saturated fat, and trans fat can increase the number of damaging free radicals. A final factor that increases free radical damage is the inflammation chemicals released by the immune system. This explains why patients suffering from an autoimmune thyroid disease such as Hashimoto's thyroiditis are likely to have a more severe form of cellular thyroid hormone imbalance. In Chapter 3 I will detail how the thyroid gland can be affected by the immune system and how immune system reactivity can affect your physical and mental health.

Important Points to Remember

- If you have become tired for no apparent reason, you may be suffering from a thyroid imbalance and/or an autoimmune thyroid disease such as Hashimoto's thyroiditis.
- There is a wide range of factors that can make your thyroid gland unable to produce a normal amount of thyroid hormone. You need to pay attention to essential micronutrients, what you eat and don't eat, and environmental factors that can affect your thyroid gland.
- Thyroid hormones regulate the functioning of almost every single system in your body. This explains why thyroid imbalance can cause a long list of both mental and physical symptoms.
- The fatigue caused by thyroid disease has to do not only with thyroid hormone imbalance but also with inflammation chemicals generated by the immune system.
- Thyroid fatigue is more often than not a mix of physical fatigue and mental fatigue. Sleep problems associated with thyroid disease often add to your fatigue.

3

WHEN THE IMMUNE SYSTEM
STRIKES THE THYROID

Aunique and amazing interplay exists between the thyroid gland and the immune system. An attack on the thyroid gland by the immune system will trigger more immune system agitation, impairing thyroid function even more, creating a seemingly endless vicious circle. The problem is that the thyroid gland is one of the body parts most vulnerable to immune system attacks, which can result in thyroid hormone imbalance, but the health of the immune system *depends* to a great extent on perfect thyroid hormone balance. So imbalanced thyroid hormone levels make the immune system more reactive and damaging to the thyroid gland and other body parts.

The Immune System and What Happens When It Goes Wrong

The root cause of most types of thyroid hormone imbalances and of many symptoms of thyroid disease is an immune system reacting to the thyroid gland and producing inflammation chemicals that affect not only your thyroid but the rest of your body. In this chapter, I will detail the different types of autoimmune thyroid conditions and their effects. But first let me explain how the immune system works in normal circumstances and what makes it become reactive to your own body parts.

The immune system is made up of a number of body parts working together to protect the body against disease. I like to compare it to a watchdog that is always on high alert. The spleen, thymus gland, lymph nodes, and bone marrow all have immune functions, as they serve as sites for the production or storage of specialized cells that target and kill harmful bacteria, viruses, parasites, and anything else foreign to the body. The immune system must be able to identify a broad range of infectious organisms and foreign particles in order to attack and destroy them.

To accomplish this, it uses a complicated process of chemical signaling and is equipped with a memory system that recognizes anything that belongs to the body. It swiftly and continuously reacts to and fights anything it recognizes as foreign until eradication. The immune system uses a variety of strategies to accomplish this, including the production of targeted proteins known as antibodies or immunoglobulins. These are proteins that are specifically designed to bind to certain molecules associated with infectious organisms, foreign bodies, and even foods.

Your immune system is constantly working to differentiate between "self" and "not self." Ideally, the immune system is designed to prevent you from getting sick; it destroys only foreign cells, things that are "not self," and does not attack your own organs and tissues. However, in some instances the immune system fails to recognize what belongs to you and views certain molecules in your own organs as foreign. This results in the immune system attacking and fighting cells that contain these molecules, a process known as *autoimmunity*. Resulting from an overactive immune system mistakenly attacking normal cells, autoimmune diseases can cause dramatic dysfunction in an organ or body system. It turns out that the most vulnerable body part to immune system attacks is the thyroid gland, explaining the high rate of thyroid disease in the general population. The two main autoimmune thyroid diseases, which are also the most common causes of thyroid imbalance, are Hashimoto's thyroiditis, the most prevalent disorder that can result in thyroid hormone deficiency, and Graves' disease, the most common root of excessive thyroid hormone production and hyperthyroidism.

What Is Hashimoto's Thyroiditis?

Hashimoto's thyroiditis is a chronic, ongoing autoimmune attack on the thyroid gland that causes inflammation and destruction of thyroid gland cells. Eventually the damaged thyroid cannot produce sufficient amounts of thyroid hormone. In other words, this condition can cause a constant state of hypothyroidism, or low thyroid. Hashimoto's thyroiditis actually affects the thyroid gland in different ways. Sometimes the autoimmune attack infiltrates cells and causes only mild cell damage. In extreme cases, the attack will destroy thyroid gland cells altogether, causing more severe hypothyroidism.

The incidence of Hashimoto's thyroiditis in females has multiplied tenfold over a thirty-two-year time frame. However, it is impossible to know for sure if this increase is due to more cases of autoimmunity or simply to a better understanding and awareness of the condition, leading to more diagnoses. Official reports from the American Thyroid Association based on epidemiological studies indicate a 1–2 percent incidence of Hashimoto's thyroiditis in the general population. In my view, this estimate severely underestimates the true frequency of the autoimmune condition. In part this is because the estimate is based on blood testing for thyroid antibodies, when there are millions of patients who suffer from Hashimoto's thyroiditis but test negative for thyroid antibodies. An ultrasound imaging of the thyroid is a much more sensitive and precise diagnostic tool, as it typically indicates evidence of inflammation even when the antibody screen is negative.[1] Just from screening and epidemiological studies, we know that roughly 8 to 10 percent of people have clear-cut, low-grade hypothyroidism with abnormal results on a thyroid blood test (TSH)[2]; the majority of these people have underlying Hashimoto's thyroiditis. Counting people with low-grade hypothyroidism who have normal blood test results, the prevalence of this condition would certainly exceed 15 percent of the entire population.

Autoimmune thyroiditis is the most common thyroid condition diagnosed in children as well. Children are the most at risk for acquiring the disease if they have a genetic predisposition; in these children, environmental factors can trigger the disease. As in adults, Hashimoto's thyroiditis often leads to hypothyroidism, which can cause delayed growth, a goiter, and a wide range of other symptoms, including fatigue, mental grogginess, trouble concentrating, exacerbation of ADD, depressive symptoms, overeating, and significant weight gain.

Approximately 25 to 60 percent of children with Down syndrome have low-grade hypothyroidism, and research has shown that about a third of children with Down syndrome have positive anti-TPO antibodies, an immune marker for Hashimoto's thyroiditis.[3] The appearance of antithyroid antibodies occurs much sooner in patients with Down syndrome than in others, so children with Down syndrome should have thyroid testing, including anti-TPO testing, on a regular basis from an early age.

What Is Graves' Disease?

Graves' disease, also an autoimmune thyroid condition, typically results in an overactive thyroid and affects 1 to 2 percent of the population. The antibodies that attack the thyroid stimulate the thyroid gland and make it produce excessive amounts of thyroid hormone. It is the most common cause of hyperthyroidism in both adults and children. Graves' disease affects women five to seven times more frequently than men. The damaging antibodies of Graves' disease can also attack the eyes. Graves' eye disease, also called thyroid orbitopathy, is the result of inflammation of the structures around the eyes, including the eye muscles.

What Makes You Vulnerable to Autoimmune Thyroid Disease?

Triggers for autoimmune thyroid disease include your genetic predisposition to autoimmunity, how much iodine you consume, stress, medications, and several types of infections. A complex interaction between environmental conditions and genetic predisposition can lead to Hashimoto's thyroiditis, Graves' disease, or both.

Your Genes Have a Say . . .

Extensive studies of large populations as well as family and twin research have proven that our genes play a role in the occurrence of autoimmune thyroid conditions. Although Hashimoto's thyroiditis and Graves' disease cause opposite reactions in the gland, people affected by one or the other have some common genetic vulnerability. One out of three families in which two or more members suffer from autoimmune thyroid conditions have cases of Graves' disease as well as Hashimoto's thyroiditis.[4] There is no single gene responsible for autoimmune thyroid disease; rather, a number of genetic factors are involved. Some of the susceptible genes are unique to Graves' disease, some are unique to Hashimoto's thyroiditis, and some are present in both conditions.[5] This explains why members of the same family may have either Graves' disease or Hashimoto's thyroiditis. This also explains why some people can have both Graves' disease *and* Hashimoto's thyroiditis, causing the gland's function to fluctuate over time. The genetic predisposition to autoimmune thyroid disease is an important factor—but not the only one—in determining who is vulnerable to a thyroid imbalance. In fact, the genetic factor is of very small importance compared to other factors. The California Twin Study has shown that if one of two identical twins has Graves' disease, the other twin only has a 17 percent chance of having it as well.[6] Although that other twin is also predisposed to having Hashimoto's thyroiditis or other autoimmune conditions, the risk is less than 20 percent.

Two tests that are used when Hashimoto's thyroiditis and other autoimmune thyroid conditions are suspected are the thyroglobulin antibody and the anti-TPO antibody tests. Thyroglobulin is a big molecule that stores thyroid hormone inside the thyroid gland. Thyroperoxidase (TPO) is one of the enzymes that facilitates the manufacture of thyroid hormone. In autoimmune thyroid disease, the immune system also produces antibodies called IGG4. If you have high levels of IGG4, thyroglobulin, and anti-TPO antibodies, you have a good chance of passing on your genetic predisposition to your offspring.

Having Any Autoimmune Condition Will Put You at a Higher Risk for Autoimmune Thyroid Disease

Genetic predisposition to autoimmune thyroid disease overlaps with the genetic predisposition to virtually all autoimmune conditions.[7] This means that having one of the conditions in the list below will make you more likely to have Hashimoto's thyroiditis or Graves' disease. It also means that if you have an autoimmune thyroid condition, you need to watch for the occurrence of any of these autoimmune conditions at any time of your life. (See details in Chapter 7.)

- Adrenal insufficiency (Addison's disease)
- Vitiligo
- Alopecia areata
- Celiac disease and gluten sensitivity
- Type 1 diabetes
- Multiple sclerosis
- Pernicious anemia
- Myositis/dermatomyositis
- Lupus
- Rheumatoid arthritis
- Sjögren's syndrome
- Scleroderma
- Ankylosing spondylitis
- Psoriasis/psoriatic arthritis
- Myasthenia gravis
- Crohn's disease
- Ulcerative colitis
- Autoimmune hypophysitis (attack on the pituitary gland)

Being a Woman Makes You More Vulnerable to Thyroid Disease

Women are seven to ten times more likely to have autoimmune thyroid conditions than men are, and the reason lies in genetic factors coupled with the effects of sex hormones. The fluctuation of hormones such as estrogen and progesterone plays a role in triggering these disorders. This is illustrated by the fact that before puberty, both sexes are equally likely to develop an autoimmune disease, whereas during and after puberty, women become more vulnerable to such conditions. Having been pregnant makes you more vulnerable to Graves' disease than if you had never been pregnant. Researchers believe that this is related to the effect of high sex hormone levels during pregnancy. Some evidence indicates that estrogen aggravates autoimmune thyroiditis,[8] while testosterone might suppress the immune attack.

The Older You Get, the More Susceptible You Are to Immune Attacks on the Thyroid

With aging, the vital balance that keeps the immune system harmless to your organs becomes precarious, and this may also make you susceptible to auto-immune thyroid disease as you grow older. As you age, you are at greater risk of having Hashimoto's thyroiditis. Thyroid antibodies increase with age, and an increase in thyroid antibodies puts you at a greater risk of having an auto-immune thyroid disease. Women's risk increases even more when they reach the transition to menopause.

Stress Could Trigger Immune Attacks on Your Thyroid

In recent years, there has been a noticeable increase in the frequency of auto-immune thyroid disorders. People are more stressed-out these days, and it is likely that stress accounts for some of this increase.[9] In Chapter 4 I will ex-plain how stress can act on the immune system to trigger and perpetuate thyroid imbalance.

Your Race and Ethnicity May Have a Say

There is a correlation between race and the probability of an autoimmune thyroid disease, with Caucasians being the most at risk, followed by Mexican Americans and African Americans.

Smoking Puts You at Greater Risk for Graves' Disease

Smoking has disturbing effects on the health of your immune system. If you are genetically predisposed to autoimmune thyroid disease, nicotine can cause a buildup of free radicals in the cells of your immune system, making it more likely to be reactive.[10] The risk of Graves' disease decreases over time after you quit smoking.

Consumption of Iodine Can Affect Your Risk

Countries where most of the population gets sufficient iodine, as opposed to countries where most of the population is iodine deficient, show higher rates of hypothyroidism and probably thyroiditis as well. Moving from a country that is iodine-deficient to a country that is iodine-sufficient increases the number of thyroid antibodies in your system and the probability of hypothyroidism. Consuming too much iodine puts you at risk for having autoimmune thyroid disease as well.[11]

Infections Can Trigger Autoimmune Thyroid Disease

Infections are among the most significant environmental factors that have been linked to autoimmune thyroid disease. Among the infectious agents that have been implicated are Coxsackie B virus, *Yersinia enterocolitica*, and *Escherichia coli*. Also, infections with *Helicobacter pylori* (the bacterium that results in gastritis and ulcers) have been found in a high percentage of people with autoimmune thyroid disease.[12]

Your Nutrition Could Be a Trigger or a Contributor

The kind of food you eat can affect your immune system and make you more susceptible to autoimmune reactions involving the thyroid. A deficiency in important nutrients—essential amino acids, vitamin A, folic acid, vitamin B_6, vitamin C, vitamin E, vitamin D, zinc, copper, selenium, and omega-3 fatty acids, just to name a few—can make the immune system more prone to attacking your thyroid gland.[13] A wide range of toxic environmental contaminants can directly affect the health of your thyroid, as we saw in Chapter 2; these chemicals can also alter the health of your immune system, making it more agitated and reactive.[14] Quite likely they are responsible for the steady increase in the prevalence of autoimmune thyroid disease. Moderate alcohol intake seems to decrease the risk of Graves' disease and Hashimoto's thyroiditis, but heavy drinking increases the likelihood that your immune system will become disturbed and attack your thyroid. Lack of exercise is another factor associated with a greater risk of autoimmune thyroid disease. Research has also shown that radiation exposure can trigger autoimmune thyroid disease.[15]

Could You Have Both Hashimoto's and Graves'?

As I explained earlier, the immune system can attack the thyroid gland in two ways: inflammation and destruction (Hashimoto's thyroiditis) or inflammation and stimulation (Graves' disease). Although the end result of the two types of attacks is different, the root of the thyroid problem is the same. The genes that make you predisposed to one are the same as the genes that make you predisposed to the other. This is why some people are affected by Hashimoto's thyroiditis while others from the same family can be affected by Graves' disease. This also explains why a patient suffering from thyroid autoimmunity can be simultaneously affected by both conditions; such a patient can have low, high, or normal thyroid levels depending on which one is predominant at any given point, and the relative balance can change with time. The immune system attack on the thyroid gland is a dynamic process that can change from day to day, week to week, or month to month. Numerous patients with Hashimoto's thyroiditis who have concomitant Graves' disease can have bouts of hyperthyroidism followed by bouts of hypothyroidism and swings in thyroid levels over time, the thyroid gland's function truly being at the mercy of the immune system. This explains why patients with Hashimoto's thyroiditis and low thyroid can abruptly shift to Graves' disease and thyroid overactivity, while in patients suffering from Graves' disease, it is not uncommon to see Hashimoto's thyroiditis take over, making the gland shift from overactivity to underactivity.[16] Therefore, if you have Hashimoto's thyroiditis and are treated with thyroid medication, it is crucial that you be carefully monitored with thyroid testing on a regular basis.

3 CASES OF HAVING BOTH HASHIMOTO'S THYROIDITIS AND GRAVES' DISEASE

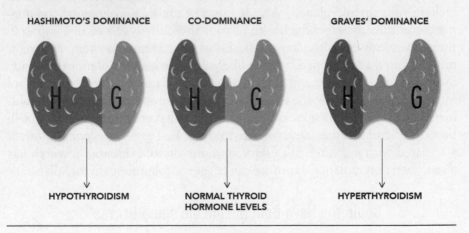

HASHIMOTO'S DOMINANCE   CO-DOMINANCE   GRAVES' DOMINANCE

HYPOTHYROIDISM   NORMAL THYROID   HYPERTHYROIDISM
                          HORMONE LEVELS

Do I Have Hashimoto's Thyroiditis?

The inflammation associated with Hashimoto's thyroiditis often, but not always, results in a swollen thyroid gland (a goiter). The size of the swelling varies from one person to another. In extreme cases, the goiter can be seen with the naked eye.

During a careful gland touch examination, an experienced doctor will be able to tell whether your gland is enlarged and/or inflamed by immune attacks. The surface of the thyroid gland is typically irregular and lobulated. The inflammation of Hashimoto's thyroiditis can make your gland become tender and even painful. You may experience bouts of pain, discomfort, and even a choking sensation. This reflects flare-ups of immune system reactivity triggered by stress, sensitivity to certain foods, nutrient deficiencies, or poor sleep.

Quite often, Hashimoto's thyroiditis does not affect the function of the thyroid gland and thyroid tests will be normal. The conventional belief in the medical community is that having Hashimoto's thyroiditis with normal thyroid gland function does not cause symptoms and does not require treatment. However, through taking care of so many patients afflicted by Hashimoto's thyroiditis I discovered that the disease does in fact cause a wide range of symptoms, some annoying but others potentially severe, even when thyroid levels have not been affected. These symptoms, not recognized by doctors for years, are actually caused by immune-system-generated inflammation chemicals affecting mind and body.[17] These can include fatigue, a feeling of weakness, weight gain, body aches, hair loss, mental sluggishness, forgetfulness, emotional instability, anxiety, and even depression.

Sonya, a high school teacher, suffered from fatigue, lack of enthusiasm, anger, irritability, and difficulty focusing for four years. She had seen an endocrinologist who detected a goiter and diagnosed her with Hashimoto's thyroiditis, as she had tested positive for antithyroid antibody, but her thyroid blood tests were perfectly normal, so the doctor told her that there was nothing he could do for her condition. Eventually she came to see me, and I recommended a thyroid- and immune-system-friendly eating plan as well as supplementation with several antioxidants, probiotics, omega-3 fatty acids, and vitamin D. I did not prescribe any thyroid medication, as her thyroid function testing was perfectly normal. Three months later, when she returned to my office, she had lost approximately fifteen pounds and was feeling much better. Her lack of enthusiasm, irritability, anger, and fatigue had markedly improved. Sonya insisted that I repeat her thyroid antibody testing; amazingly, the antibody level—the marker of immune reactivity to her thyroid— had come down dramatically.

The Drastic Inflammation Effects of an Angry Immune System

Whether you have Hashimoto's thyroiditis or Graves' disease, your immune system perceives certain molecules in your thyroid gland as foreign, and as a result, it attacks your thyroid as if it does not belong to your body. In Hashimoto's thyroiditis, the immune system produces anti-TPO antibodies; a blood test for these antibodies is used to diagnose this condition. In Graves' disease, the immune system produces both thyroid antibodies and a unique antibody called thyroid-stimulating immunoglobulin (TSI), which has the ability to stimulate thyroid cells, causing thyroid hormone overproduction.

The thyroid hormone imbalance caused by the immune system's attack on your thyroid gland is not the only reason you experience thyroid symptoms such as fatigue, mood changes, or mental fog. While attacking your thyroid through these antibodies, the immune system also releases multiple inflammation chemicals that have drastic effects on your brain and body. Antibodies and inflammation chemicals can induce multiple physical and mental symptoms and seriously affect the quality of your life whether your thyroid hormone levels are normal or not. Generally speaking, women with thyroid disease who have high anti-TPO antibody levels have the most thyroid symptoms; the anti-TPO antibody level is a marker for immune system reactivity.

The symptoms of autoimmunity are the result of the abundant release of antibodies and nonspecific inflammation chemicals, called cytokines, such as tumor necrosis factor alpha (TNF-alpha) and interleukin-1, 6, 12, and 17. Cytokines are small proteins important in cell signaling. Produced by immune system cells, they are released whenever the immune system reacts to an infection or to the introduction in your body of what is perceived as a foreign molecule, particle, or organ of any kind.[18] Inflammation chemicals cross the blood-brain barrier and interact with brain cells, causing toxicity and affecting the activity of neurotransmitters such as dopamine, serotonin, and norepinephrine, which are involved in mood, mental energy, and behavior.[19] When you produce high levels of these potent inflammation chemicals, you end up having low mental energy; you feel unable to make the effort to do or obtain something. These substances also promote a wide range of chemical changes in the brain that end up making you feel depressed and affected by mental fog and cognition issues.

Hashimoto's thyroiditis and Graves' disease, like most autoimmune disorders, are real causes of depression and anxiety.[20] Recent research comparing the incidence of depression and anxiety among Hashimoto's thyroiditis sufferers and healthy people without thyroid disease clearly demonstrated a significantly higher incidence of depressive disorders, anxiety, and panic attacks among patients with Hashimoto's thyroiditis. It is now becoming clear that suffering from depression and having a hard time recovering from depression, even with antidepressants, is related to high levels of inflammation chemicals produced by the immune system. A study published in the *Journal of Neurology, Neurosurgery, and Psychiatry* has shown that inflammatory markers can be used to diagnose depression and predict a response to treatment in people suffering from inflammatory conditions.[21]

In addition to affecting brain functions, nonspecific inflammation chemicals promote general body inflammation and a buildup of free radicals in many body parts, affecting normal cell functioning and lowering your physical energy level. They induce a rise in your cortisol level, causing yet more cellular dysfunction, which can affect your appetite, metabolism, and cause you to experience fluid retention and bloating. The more reactive your immune system is, the more you become afflicted by systemic general body inflammation causing a wide range of both physical and mental symptoms. In extreme cases, immune system reactivity can lead to thyroid-related fibromyalgia, a debilitating condition that can produce exhaustion, depression, severe sleep disturbances, and diffuse joint and muscle pain. Research has shown a correlation between anti-TPO antibody levels and the occurrence of fibromyalgia in thyroid patients.[22] How severely you will be affected by inflammation chemicals produced by the immune system has to do with your genes, which determine whether you are more or less susceptible to the mental and physical effects of these substances.

Hashimoto's encephalopathy is an extreme but fortunately rare form of immune system reactivity that can occur in patients suffering from Hashimoto's thyroiditis. While most experts consider this to be a rare condition, it is likely that many people suffer from this disorder but remain undiagnosed. Hashimoto's encephalopathy is a neuromental condition likely to be caused by very high levels of inflammation chemicals and antibodies that have a direct and toxic effect on the brain. Over a few days, you begin to have personality changes, sleep problems, difficulty talking, disorientation, and severe concentration and memory issues. You may experience psychotic behavior and seizures. Even your muscle functions can be affected by the deleterious effects of inflammation chemicals in your brain. The symptoms range from mild to extremely severe and can be intermittent, meaning that they get better and then recur. Patients with Hashimoto's encephalopathy often have very high levels of antithyroid antibodies. If you are diagnosed with this condition, you will be prescribed corticosteroids to control or resolve your symptoms.

How to Support Your Immune System Naturally

As we have seen, the immune system affects how you feel both physically and mentally when you are suffering from an autoimmune thyroid disease. Obviously, the thyroid imbalance that the immune system has caused can produce a wide range of symptoms, but the immune system will amplify and add more inflammation-related effects. The two are connected, as I explained at the beginning of this chapter, because the thyroid imbalance caused by the immune system attack has, in turn, a major effect on immune system reactivity, simply because the health of the immune system depends, to a great extent, on perfect thyroid hormone balance. To restore your wellness and quality of life, both physical and mental, your treatment program must focus on continued thyroid hormone balance, with thyroid medication tailored to your needs. Equally important, though, is stabilizing your immune system, and making it less reactive.

Elisa, a thirty-two-year-old nurse, had been diagnosed with an underactive thyroid eight years earlier and was being treated with levothyroxine, a T4-only medication. Her dosage had been adjusted multiple times and her thyroid levels were now perfectly normal, but she continued to suffer from multiple lingering problems, including fatigue, low-grade depressive symptoms, and an inability to lose weight. Having heard that the combination of T4 and T3 treatment might be the solution for her lingering symptoms, Elisa came to see me in hopes that a new and more tailored medication treatment for her underactive thyroid would help her feel better. My examination and testing showed that she had been suffering from Hashimoto's thyroiditis.

I changed her T4-only medication to a combination of T4 and T3, which I adjusted over the following four months. I also recommended a comprehensive program that included natural supplements and nutritional suggestions as well as practicing tai chi. At a follow-up visit four months later, her thyroid tests (including free T4 and free T3) were perfectly normal, but Elisa said that the new treatment had done nothing for her persistent irritability, lack of energy, and brain fog. When I asked Elisa if she was taking her supplements and paying attention to her eating plan, she responded, "I am too busy to remember to take my supplements. I thought taking the right medications would be enough." I reemphasized the importance of embracing the entire mind-body program. Two months later, she returned to my office and the first thing she told me was, "Dr. Arem, you saved my life! I have been good with my nutrition, I have been taking my omega-3 fatty acids and the supplements that you recommended, and I actually lost five pounds since I last saw you." What is remarkable is that her thyroid hormone levels were identical to what they had been during her previous visit. The only thing that differed was a lower antithyroid antibody level (the immune marker for Hashimoto's thyroiditis).

Over the years, I have dealt with hundreds of patients with Hashimoto's thyroiditis who have perfectly normal thyroid test results but continue to suffer from disturbing symptoms including fatigue, depression, irritability, anger, and cognitive changes. What makes their physical and mental symptoms totally disappear is actually what makes the immune system less reactive and produce smaller amounts of inflammation chemicals.

Clearly, the symptoms described by Hashimoto's sufferers cannot always be blamed on the thyroid hormone imbalance. Many of them are related to the immune system and can persist even when the thyroid imbalance has been corrected. Here are the eight measures I often recommend to my patients suffering from thyroid autoimmunity:

1. Switch to a thyroid- and immune-system-friendly low-glycemic, high-fiber eating plan that is low in saturated and trans fats, is high in polyunsaturated fats and omega-3 fatty acids, and includes multiple sources of protein. Trans fats and saturated fats make the immune system more agitated; omega-3 fatty acids, in contrast, calm the immune system down.

2. Take into account food sensitivities by eliminating the foods that your immune system reacts to. I often recommend food sensitivity testing to make proper food elimination decisions (see Chapters 21 and 22). From my extensive experience with food sensitivity testing, I have found that most patients affected by autoimmune thyroid disease are sensitive to gluten and dairy (particularly dairy products derived from cow's milk).

3. Address sleep issues, such as insomnia, sleep deprivation, and sleep interruptions, as these can negatively affect immune system function.

4. Take a comprehensive mix of crucial vitamins, minerals, and antioxidants to support thyroid and immune system health. In Chapter 2 I explained the importance of certain minerals, vitamins, and antioxidants to keep thyroid cells as healthy as possible. Minimizing damage from high levels of oxidative stress is quite important in thyroid autoimmunity, as damage triggers more autoimmunity, meaning more inflammation chemicals.[23] In addition to providing the right ingredients to thyroid cells for optimal health, the antioxidant mix should include several micronutrients with anti-inflammatory properties that have the ability to improve the health of the immune system. These micronutrients substantially reduce the free radical load in the cells of an already agitated immune system. You need to pay particular attention to selenium supplementation, as it is known to reduce immune system attacks on the thyroid in both Hashimoto's thyroiditis and Graves' disease. Selenium, as I explained in Chapter 2, is a potent antioxidant necessary for optimal thyroid function, thyroid health, and conversion of T4 to T3 in the body.

5. Correct any vitamin D deficiency and optimize vitamin D levels. Extensive research has clearly shown a link between low vitamin D levels and thyroid autoimmunity.[24] Roughly 80 to 90 percent of people with Hashimoto's thyroiditis suffer from vitamin D deficiency, which has been found to be a potential contributing factor to the occurrence of autoimmune thyroid disease. It is likely that a genetic association exists between the ability of the skin to produce vitamin D and the susceptibility to having an autoimmune thyroid disorder. It is very important to have your vitamin D levels tested periodically. If you are suffering from vitamin D deficiency, take the amount of vitamin D_3 (the active form of vitamin D) needed to achieve and maintain optimal 25-hydroxy vita-

min D levels (I recommend a level between 45 and 60 ng/dL). The requirement for vitamin D supplementation varies from one person to another, as the ability to absorb vitamin D is different from one person to another. Furthermore, be aware that interrupting vitamin D supplementation will result in a drop in your vitamin D levels, which will cause your immune system to start misbehaving, making your symptoms worse.

6. Take a probiotic supplement. More and more research is demonstrating that immune system health is strongly linked to gastrointestinal health, which in itself is greatly influenced by the microflora living in the GI tract. A perfect balance between good and bad bacteria is rarely maintained in humans. Bacterial imbalance causes clinical or subclinical inflammation, which can exacerbate immune system reactivity and lead to other health consequences, including irritable bowel syndrome, brain symptoms, and hormonal symptoms. For thyroid patients with an already agitated immune system, taking probiotics is essential to reducing your immune system's production of inflammation chemicals. Probiotics offer other benefits as well, including lowering cholesterol and triglyceride levels, reducing stress and anxiety, improving insulin resistance, and helping you with your weight loss efforts.[25] Research has shown that probiotics reduce the intensity of many gastrointestinal disorders, such as inflammatory bowel disease. Amazingly, bacterial imbalance in the GI tract can make you become allergic or sensitive to certain foods; the result is a vicious circle of intestinal inflammation leading to food sensitivities, which in turn further exacerbate inflammation. This can ultimately lead to what is known as leaky gut syndrome, which has a major impact on the level of inflammation in the rest of your body and your mood, anxiety level, weight, and energy level. It has been my experience that patients with Hashimoto's thyroiditis and Graves' disease are much more vulnerable to bacterial imbalance and subclinical GI inflammation. I cannot emphasize enough the importance of taking the right types and amounts of probiotics to help counteract the negative effects of food sensitivities and GI inflammation on your immune system. I also typically recommend that you eat less fat, as high-fat meals will promote the growth of bad bacteria, worsening your bacterial imbalance.

7. Omega-3 fatty acids. The benefits of omega-3 fatty acids are many: improving thyroid hormone efficiency, lowering bad cholesterol levels, and improving neuromuscular functions and cardiovascular health. Omega-3 fatty acids really help reduce inflammation in your body and lessen immune system reactivity. The typical Western diet is too high in omega-6 fatty acids, and the immune system becomes more agitated

when you have too much omega-6 in your system compared to omega-3. For this reason, you need to take a daily supplement that includes the right amounts of EPA (600 mg/day) and DHA (400 mg/day).

8. Stress. As we've seen, the immune system and thyroid balance affect brain function, mood, and behavior; the flip side of this is that the mind can have major effects on immune system health and reactivity. Stress and perception of stress can make the immune system agitated and reactive, which in turn can affect thyroid function and thereby impact both physical and mental health. In Chapter 4 I will describe in detail how stress, the immune system, and the thyroid interact.

Many patients ask me whether there are medications that can counteract thyroid autoimmunity and help with their symptoms. Several medications that have the ability to counteract inflammation chemicals in the bodies of people suffering from autoimmune disorders have been developed and have been shown to improve their quality of life and improve energy levels. A number of these target TNF-alpha, which regulates immune cells and exacerbates inflammation and autoimmunity. Several antibody medications are currently available to counteract TNF-alpha (Enbrel, Humira, Cimzia, and Remicade) and are effective in treating rheumatoid arthritis and inflammatory bowel disease. However, they are not useful or recommended for patients who only suffer from autoimmune thyroid disease, considering their potential side effects.

AHCC (active hexose correlated compound), a group of compounds derived from fungus, has been used by some health professionals to reduce inflammation and boost the immune responses in immune compromised individuals and cancer patients. However, I believe that AHCC could be harmful to people suffering from autoimmune disorders by making the immune system more reactive.

I recommend that you take curcumin in the form of a supplement in order to reduce the production and accumulation of inflammation chemicals in your body as well as for its other health benefits. (See Chapter 22 for antioxidants and other ingredients to support thyroid and immune system health.)

Low-dose naltrexone is an opioid blocker currently recommended to help prevent the relapse of alcohol and drug addictions and to help inflammatory conditions such as Crohn's disease, fibromyalgia, and multiple sclerosis. While the use of low-dose naltrexone might be expanded to other ailments in the future, there is currently no scientific basis for its use in autoimmune thyroid disease, and no data on long-term use. In my opinion, practicing a mind-body technique to slow down the reactivity of the immune system is safer and more effective.

Important Points to Remember

- Hashimoto's thyroiditis and Graves' disease are the leading causes of thyroid imbalance. Both conditions represent reactions of the immune system on the thyroid gland.
- Your genes account for some of the predisposition to having an autoimmune thyroid disease. The effect of stress and the environment, vitamin D deficiency, deficiencies of other vitamins and antioxidants, and infections is far from negligible.
- In autoimmune thyroid disease, like any other autoimmune condition, your immune system produces high amounts of inflammation chemicals that affect your body and mind and can result in multiple physical and mental symptoms even when your thyroid levels are perfectly normal.
- If you have Hashimoto's thyroiditis, you may also have coexisting Graves' disease. This can cause your thyroid to become unstable, and the result is that you shift from one type of thyroid imbalance to another.
- There are several natural measures that you should take to help your immune system become less reactive, including taking the right amounts of many antioxidants that have the ability to improve immune system function.

4

STRESS AND THYROID DISEASE

Which Comes First?

At the end of a lecture I gave to a third-year medical class, a student named John came up to me and said that his twenty-three-year-old wife, Christy, had been experiencing "odd symptoms" for the previous year and that her primary care physician could find nothing wrong with her. "I'm wondering whether she has a thyroid condition, because she has many of the symptoms you described," he said. In my first encounter with Christy, she told me what was happening to her. Her scenario was typical of what many thyroid patients go through.

Christy traced her symptoms to a period the year before when she and John had married and she had started law school. About that time, she began to gain weight and be extremely fatigued. At times, she felt her heart was beating fast; she was moody and would cry for no reason. Christy was having a hard time functioning and frequently felt "strange" in her body, which is often typical of panic attacks. She attributed her symptoms to the stress of being newly married and feeling torn between her husband and her studies. Her mother frequently blamed her for having brought her symptoms on herself, saying that Christy shouldn't have started law school and gotten married at the same time.

Her primary care physician was initially concerned that Christy's palpitations might indicate a heart problem, but her heart exams turned out normal. Once he learned more about Christy's schedule, the doctor, like her mother, suggested that her symptoms were due to stress. When Christy finally consulted me, I determined through blood tests that she had an underactive thyroid caused by Hashimoto's thyroiditis.

Christy told me:

Before this time, I was a relaxed person. But suddenly anything would set me off. Even little annoyances or problems seemed like the end of the world and had to be resolved right then. Even though I'm not a devoted cook, if John didn't finish the meal I served, I would fly off the handle. I overreacted to everything, and John wouldn't know from minute to minute what might set me off. This went on for an entire year.

Clearly the stress Christy was feeling was actually creating more stress. Her thyroid condition made her unable to deal with the minor stresses that had never affected her previously.

Christy had suffered unnecessarily for a year. She embraced my mind-body program and once her thyroid levels became well balanced with treatment, Christy became more able to deal equitably with the stress she faced.

"I don't get upset over silly things anymore. I'm feeling great, doing well in school now and at home without feeling stressed-out. John is happy, too. Recently he said, 'You're back; you're nice again.'"

Christy's story illustrates how dramatically thyroid hormone imbalance can affect a person's ability to deal with stressful events, even the small ones that would normally just be minor parts of daily life. Indeed, the relationship between stress and illness is more apparent in thyroid disorders than in any other medical condition. Thyroid disease is an ideal example of the interrelations between mind and body because it reveals how difficult it is to separate out whether the mind or the body is the origin of illness.

How your mind handles stress dictates whether you will recover quickly or fall into an emotionally and physically depleting stress-illness-stress cycle. Laid-back persons who handle difficult situations relatively easily are not likely to be swept up in such cycles. Those who find stressful situations difficult to bear might easily end up with a thyroid hormone imbalance once stress, and reactions to it, occur. *But these people should not be blamed for their illness.* They did not, as Christy's mother had told her, bring this illness on themselves. Different people handle stress differently, and you cannot avoid stress. It is an inevitable part of life.

Think of stress as a long bar with many notches in it. At one end of the bar are small notches that represent minor stresses, such as an argument with a colleague, a child spilling soda on the sofa, or too much paperwork. In the middle of this bar are bigger notches representing life events such as the loss of a job, feelings of financial insecurity, or marital troubles. At the opposite end of the bar are large gashes—traumatic events, such as being a victim of violence or abuse or serving in combat. How your mind and body respond to a stressful event, however, may have more to do with how you *perceived* the event than with the precise nature of the event.

You feel, integrate, and react to stressful events through responses in your brain chemistry. The body responds to happy or upsetting events in an area of the brain called the limbic system, the same area that controls mood and emotions. This is also the part of the brain where thyroid hormone is delivered in great amounts. Within the limbic system, thyroid hormone is a major chemical player.

Thyroid imbalance, whether from a deficiency or an excess of thyroid hormone, generates a myriad of emotional, mood, and cognitive effects and weakens the ability to cope with stress. Disturbed emotions inevitably generate new stress related to anger, irritability, depression, and maladjusted behavior. Upsetting situations that grow out of this regenerated stress are perceived in an amplified way, leading to a feeling of being constantly stressed out.

Even a laid-back person can easily fall into the stress trap if his or her thyroid gland becomes dysfunctional, simply because thyroid hormone is one of the chemicals that regulates how we perceive and emotionally respond to stress. Symptoms of thyroid imbalance are often confused with symptoms due to stress. The similarity between stress reactions and symptoms of thyroid hormone imbalance causes a problem that is common among thyroid patients: their imbalance may go unrecognized for a long time before it is considered as a possible reason for their suffering. Both patients and physicians blame the symptoms of thyroid imbalance on stress rather than on a chemical imbalance that is affecting the patient's body and mind.

How Stress Can Trigger Thyroid Disease

It is crucial to understand that a mental state or stress can trigger and worsen thyroid disease and that you can learn ways to help yourself get well. My thyroid patients often ask, "What caused or triggered this condition?" Even though stress is not the only possible catalyst, it is in many patients an obvious one.

Physicians Deepak Chopra, Andrew Weil, and Bernie Siegel have emphasized the importance of attitude and mind-related techniques (such as meditation and guided relaxation) to help avoid or overcome illness and have increased our understanding of the relationship between stress and illness. *Anatomy of an Illness,* Norman Cousins's account of his mind and spirit's triumph over illness, was among the first memoirs to bring to public awareness the incontrovertible connection between good spirits and good health.[1] Since its publication in the late 1970s, much research has supported this connection and further enhanced our understanding of how stress affects the mind and body. Under stress, the brain emits chemical messages that trigger major responses of the endocrine system. One such response, perhaps the most significant one, is the increase in production of the hormone corticotropin-releasing factor (CRF) by the hypothalamus. Normally, CRF enhances arousal and attention and makes your body and mind adjust better to stress and respond appropriately to it. CRF, by acting through the pituitary gland, will also make the adrenals produce excessive amounts of the stress hormone cortisol. In addition, too much CRF will affect neurotransmitters in the brain that regulate mood.[2] By this mechanism, too much CRF in the brain will make you prone to becoming depressed and panicky when you experience too much stress. If you handle stress well, the response of the endocrine system is minimal and short-lived. But if you are stressed for a long time; experience major upheavals, setbacks, or traumas; or have difficulties coping with stress, your endocrine system becomes chronically challenged and causes health problems.[3] How you react to stress depends somewhat on your personality makeup, on your genes, and also on whether you suffered from stressful events in early life. Infancy and childhood stress makes you more fragile when it comes to dealing with stress later in life and more vulnerable to depression, anxiety, panic attacks, and post-traumatic stress syndrome as a result of ongoing stress.[4] One of the most significant consequences of the endocrine system's response to too much stress or difficulty coping with stress is a disturbance of the immune system.[5] There are differences in the physiologic responses to stress between women and men. These differences make women more vulnerable to autoimmune disorders.

In studies conducted on the effect of arguing and hostility, psychologist Janice Kiecolt-Glaser showed that the more hostile people are during marital arguments, the more suppressed are their immune systems.[6] High levels of stress—and, more important, an impaired ability to cope with stress—will disturb your immune system and make it react to your thyroid gland as if it were a foreign structure, particularly if you have a genetic vulnerability for such reactions. In essence, stress will make your immune system lose the ability to differentiate between "self" and "not self." Stress will also weaken your immune system, which will make your body more vulnerable to infection, allergic reaction, and even food sensitivity.[7] When you're stressed, viral and bacterial infections stay with you longer. The immune system will attack the invading virus, but if the virus has a molecular structure that mimics the makeup of the thyroid gland, when the immune system produces antibodies to attack the virus, it will mistake the thyroid gland for the virus. The key player in the scenario is the immune system.

With that in mind, it is easy to understand that the difference between a person who successfully interprets and deals with stress and the rest of us is that the more relaxed among us are less likely to experience disturbances of the immune system and other ailments resulting from too much cortisol. The biochemical cascade that links the brain to the immune system is at the root of how mental stress triggers and perpetuates thyroid disease.

The Stress/Thyroid Escalation Cycle

A wide variety of stressful situations may serve as the trigger for an autoimmune attack on your thyroid. For example, when I saw my patient Ron for the first time, he had already been treated for hyperthyroidism due to Graves' disease. His symptoms lingered, however, and his hormone levels were still not in balance, so I asked him to describe the circumstances that led to his disorder. In his words:

> I was in the military and living near the base with my wife. I was working two jobs trying to put her through school. One job was teaching, which kept me busy from six in the morning until three in the afternoon. I slept from four until seven, then I'd get up and go to the commissary, where I would stock shelves until about one A.M. We had borrowed money from my wife's family to put a down payment on a house and were being pressed to pay back the loan. The pressure was unbearable. My boss in the teaching job was verbally abusive and openly belittled me. It was a totally stressful situation.

Ron traced his early symptoms to this time in his life. "I couldn't tolerate the heat. I was sweaty all the time, and my heart pounded constantly. I had muscle contractions and chest pains. At night, I would be sleeping and then jump out of bed. I went to the doctor at the base. He kept saying it was stress-related and I might want to see a psychologist."

As is often the case, Ron became short-tempered and found it hard to control himself around his children. He quit his second job, which made it more difficult to repay the loan. That situation, in turn, put even more pressure on him. His symptoms lingered. Each time he went back to the doctor, he was told his condition was stress-related. Unable to cope any longer, he left the army.

The Escalation Cycle

In many patients like Ron, detailed histories obtained when they are finally diagnosed reveal that major stress events, sometimes quite remote, probably triggered their conditions. Doctors may blame this event for the patient's symptoms. This misdiagnosis or lack of diagnosis may lead to lingering symptoms and finally escalation and perpetuation of the stress. Often physicians are faced with a Gordian knot: they can only guess whether symptoms are primarily due to a thyroid imbalance. If the treatment does not get to the root of the problem or find a way to break the cycle, however, the symptoms will go on endlessly.

Much of the cycle of symptoms takes root in the period before the patient is diagnosed. A mild dysfunction triggered by a stressful event becomes a more severe dysfunction with more stress. The additional stress results in illness, leading to more stress. The onset of one disease giving rise to another that subsequently affects the first is the pattern doctors face in diagnosing and treating autoimmune thyroid disease. Yet this escalating cycle could easily be halted in its early stages if both physicians and patients became more aware of it. Interrupting this cycle by diagnosing the thyroid imbalance early and addressing the stress issues related to it prevents unnecessary physical and mental suffering, personal problems, and undue stress, enabling the patient to feel better faster.

Kimberly's struggle with a thyroid condition illustrates the perils for the patient entangled in the cycle. An attractive thirty-four-year-old woman, Kimberly was referred to me for Graves' disease by her gynecologist. Kimberly was certain that her symptoms had begun some two years earlier, approximately four months after she started a new job. Prior to that, she was happy and relaxed. She said:

> I thought the job would take me further in my career in management, but the pressure was too much. After trying to keep up, I began to realize it wasn't the right job for me. My self-esteem began to suffer.
>
> I was stressed out and became anxious and depressed. I seemed to be sick all the time and exhausted, which I related to being ill for most of the winter. I became belligerent, uncooperative at work, and angry and overactive at home. My husband thought I was having a breakdown. He insisted I see a psychiatrist.

Kimberly slowly became entangled in a chain of events that affects many thyroid patients, sometimes for years, both before and after diagnosis. The psychiatrist treated her with antidepressants, which can cause patients with an overactive thyroid to feel worse. Kimberly noticed a puffiness around her eyes, and she lost weight. But because these symptoms were insignificant in relation to the problems that seemed to be pulling her world apart, she ignored them. The antidepressants did not help, so the psychiatrist put Kimberly on an antianxiety medicine. Meanwhile, her self-confidence was eroding daily at work, and the humiliation leaked into all areas of her life. Eventually she was fired.

At this point, Kimberly "went a little crazy," to use her expression. She interviewed for many jobs but came across as insecure and unfocused. No one would hire her. To fill the void, she tackled hundreds of extra tasks at home and performed them badly. Her husband had to take over the management of the children's activities. Arguing with her husband became part of Kimberly's daily life. The loss of her job and the reduced income became a source of marital tension. At some point, she began to suffer rapid heartbeats and consulted a cardiologist. He diagnosed her symptoms as stress-related. Her psychiatrist noticed that Kimberly had developed tremors and suggested she see a neurologist. Tests came back negative. Even so, Kimberly says, "I cried. I didn't care that there was nothing wrong. I just wanted someone to help me."

Kimberly's disease was spiraling. From the time the stress of the new job triggered her Graves' disease to the mood disorder that followed and the physicians' confusion about the root of her problem, Kimberly had run around the circle of thyroid disorder many times, with each symptom leading inevitably to the next. Depression followed stress, a disturbed immune system caused a worsening of the overactive thyroid, stress and the effects of hyperthyroidism led to exhaustion, and uncontrollable behaviors caused low self-esteem, which produced further stress. The cycle became self-reinforcing.

An astute gynecologist was the first physician to consider testing Kimberly's thyroid. By treating Kimberly's thyroid condition and addressing the stress issues, we were eventually able to interrupt this stress cycle. It wasn't quick and easy, however. The mental anguish had altered Kimberly emotionally, affecting her brain chemistry. Organically, she had gone through a change. It took weeks to normalize her thyroid hormone levels. Kimberly gradually regained her equilibrium through much support from home, good therapy, and an antidepressant medication. Sadly, her troubles could have been stopped at many points if both she and her doctors had not been confounded by the confusing mind-body symptoms of thyroid disease.

Until quite recently, researchers were unable to determine conclusively that stress is a major trigger of Graves' disease. This is ironic because, in the first cases of Graves' disease ever diagnosed, it was noticed that major stress had precipitated the cycle. The Irish physician Caleb Parry, the first to recognize the condition, described "Elizabeth S., aged 21," who "was thrown out of a wheelchair in coming fast down a hill . . . and was very much frightened. From this time she has been subject to palpitations of the heart and various nervous affections. About a fortnight after, she began to observe a swelling of the thyroid gland."[8]

It is often difficult for researchers and physicians to determine whether stress has been precipitated by thyroid imbalance or vice versa. There is just no way to pinpoint when the thyroid condition began in an individual unless blood levels of thyroid hormones were measured before the onset of stress.

Despite these difficulties, researchers have been able to establish a clearcut link between stressful events and the onset of Graves' disease. One study, for instance, concluded that factors such as change in work conditions, change in time spent on work, and hospitalization of a family member for a serious illness (factors that could not have been caused by the thyroid condition) were all associated with the occurrence of Graves' disease.[9] Another study conducted at the University of Tokyo on 228 patients with newly diag-nosed Graves' disease concluded that stress increased the occurrence of Graves' disease 7.7-fold in women.[10] The study also showed that smoking (perhaps an indication of stress) increased the risk for Graves' disease, too. Divorce, marital difficulties, death of loved ones, and financial troubles are also possible triggers of Graves' disease.

The difficulties facing researchers are even greater with Hashimoto's thy-roiditis. Many patients with Hashimoto's thyroiditis have a minimally under-active gland, causing tiredness, depressive symptoms, weight gain, dry skin, and a feeling of being colder than usual. Because the symptoms of Hashimo-to's thyroiditis are more insidious than those of Graves' disease, few research-ers have seriously attempted to establish that stress could trigger this condition or the resulting imbalance. However, in my many years of experi-ence, I have been able to correlate stress with the onset of symptoms of Hashimoto's thyroiditis in numerous patients.

Nevertheless, endocrinologists routinely see patients with hypothyroid-ism whose symptoms began "coincidentally" with either stress (or what the patients described as stress) or depression. As with Graves' disease, physi-cians must wonder whether the stress or depression triggered Hashimoto's thyroiditis and the resulting underactive thyroid, or vice versa. Does the sharp increase in Hashimoto's thyroiditis at menopause occur only because of hormonal changes, or does it also occur because stress and depression are more common around this phase of the reproductive cycle? Does the high frequency of thyroid imbalances after delivery of a baby result only from an immune system temporarily vulnerable because of hormonal swings, or do the stress of having to care for a new baby and the concomitant depression contribute to triggering the imbalance?

The effects of depression on the immune system are similar to those caused by stress. Therefore, the sequence of chemical interactions that leads to the triggering of an autoimmune thyroid disorder is also likely to occur during depression. Physicians are only beginning to pay attention to this sce-nario. A recent study showed that women suffering from postpartum depres-sion are more likely to have Hashimoto's thyroiditis than women who do not experience postpartum depression—even when the hormone levels of the depressed women are normal.[11] Also, women with Hashimoto's thyroiditis, whether they are perimenopausal or postmenopausal, are afflicted three times more frequently with depression, even if they do not have a thyroid imbalance.[12] Clearly, depression and autoimmune reactions to the thyroid have the same root in the immunoendocrine system. Depression and the stress that often precedes depression could be the trigger of the immune at-tack on the thyroid, resulting in Hashimoto's thyroiditis and underactive thy-roid.

Another extremely important component of the relationship between Hashimoto's thyroiditis and mental stress is illustrated by a study that revealed that people hospitalized for depression have a higher frequency of Hashimoto's thyroiditis than the general population, even when their thyroid hormone levels are normal.[13] Another study confirmed this association in an Italian community, showing that autoimmune thyroid disease was three to four times more common among patients with mood and anxiety disorders.[14] Until recently, physicians have blamed hypothyroidism for causing depression and assumed that treating the underactive thyroid would reverse the depression. But sometimes the opposite is true: in many people, when physicians treat the thyroid imbalance, the depression—which might have been the source rather than the consequence of the thyroid imbalance—persists unless treated and addressed in its own right and unless immune system reactivity has been tempered by natural measures detailed in Chapter 3. Physicians should begin to suspect that depression, a form of major stress, might be the triggering event in many patients with Hashimoto's thyroiditis. Those patients exhibit the same escalation phenomenon described in patients with Graves' disease. For people suffering from either condition, steps to halt the cycle are the same: correct the thyroid hormone imbalance and address issues of stress and depression.

The accompanying diagram on page 64 illustrates the complex set of interactions between brain chemistry and the thyroid that can contribute to the stress-illness escalation cycle. Cascades of biochemical interactions can lead to escalation of symptoms and adverse effects. Stress can make the brain send chemicals to the immune system, which in turn can attack the thyroid gland, resulting in thyroid imbalance.

- A thyroid imbalance can disturb brain chemistry, affect mood, and alter the ability to cope with stress, making the effect of stress on the immune system worse.
- A thyroid imbalance makes the immune system more reactive, and this causes more inflammation chemicals to be produced.
- As the immune system is attacking your thyroid (or any other part of the body), it produces nonspecific inflammation chemicals (see Chapter 3) that affect brain chemistry and function, making it harder to deal with stress. This in turn exacerbates immune system reactivity.

As you can see, each one of these effects feeds into another effect, making the escalation of autoimmunity, stress, and imbalance endless and self-perpetuating.

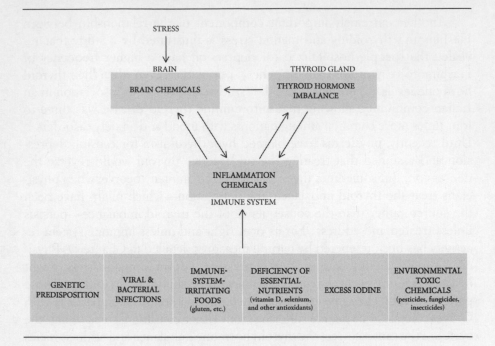

The Brain and Thyroid Function

The amount of thyroid hormone produced by the thyroid gland compensates for the amount used by cells. The amount of thyroid hormone manufactured by the thyroid gland is primarily governed by the pituitary gland, which is situated at the base of the brain and produces thyroid-stimulating hormone, or TSH. The amount of TSH delivered to the thyroid gland tells the thyroid how much thyroid hormone to manufacture.

The pituitary gland senses any increase or decrease in thyroid hormone levels in the blood and reacts to the change by adjusting the production of TSH. Therefore the pituitary sees that the levels of thyroid hormones in the circulating blood remain normal and constant—and sees that the right amount of thyroid hormone is delivered to organs and to the brain. For instance, if the thyroid gland becomes damaged and produces less thyroid hormone than normal, the pituitary senses the decrease in thyroid hormone levels and releases more TSH. This stimulates the thyroid gland to produce more hormone and correct the deficiency.

But the brain, when necessary, can have a say in how much thyroid hormone should be produced. Some areas of the brain, including those involved in regulating mood and behavior, can control the function of the pituitary. The intermediary between these regions of the brain and the pituitary is the hypothalamus, which communicates with the pituitary by emitting a chemical called thyrotropin-releasing hormone, or TRH. These areas of the brain send messages to the thyroid gland by making the pituitary increase or decrease the production of TSH. For example, the body's perception of cold is transmitted to the brain through brain chemicals that communicate with the pituitary, telling it to increase the TSH level as a reaction to low temperature so that the thyroid produces more thyroid hormone and the body will generate more heat. If you starve yourself or fast for a prolonged time, or face extreme physical stress such as surgery or a major illness, your brain instructs the pituitary to produce less TSH so that your thyroid manufactures less thyroid hormone. This defense mechanism slows your metabolism and the rate of organ destruction. The brain is, in effect, protecting the body against starvation by lowering its metabolic rate. This also explains how the thyroid slows its function if you are suffering from an eating disorder, such as anorexia nervosa. The brain perceives an eating disorder as a potential threat to the body's energy reserves and will make the thyroid lower metabolism and preserve as much energy as possible for survival. After a major stressful event, such as a war situation, the brain may send signals to the thyroid gland to increase its production of thyroid hormone for a long time, which, in theory, will allow the person to be hypervigilant. (See the diagram below showing how the brain regulates the thyroid system.)

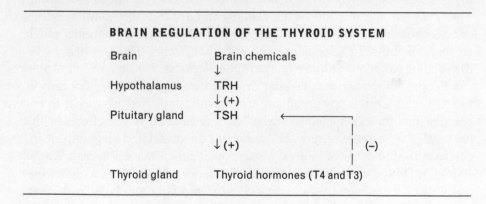

BRAIN REGULATION OF THE THYROID SYSTEM

Brain	Brain chemicals
	↓
Hypothalamus	TRH
	↓ (+)
Pituitary gland	TSH
	↓ (+)
Thyroid gland	Thyroid hormones (T4 and T3)

The Thyroid and Postwar Syndromes

Many people who have been engaged in combat subsequently experience a multitude of mental and physical symptoms, such as shortness of breath, fatigue, headaches, chest pain, rapid heartbeat, diarrhea, troubled emotions, and sleep disturbances. These symptoms have been noted among veterans since the American Civil War and have been seen after most major wars, including the Vietnam War and the Persian Gulf War.[15]

Postwar psychoneurosis or, more familiarly, post-traumatic stress syndrome, is a complex condition that mixes depression, anxiety, and a host of other symptoms. Although many studies have been devoted to finding the cause for this syndrome, few researchers have carefully studied the possible link between thyroid function, wartime stress, and subsequent thyroid disease. Evidence supports the notion, however, that this syndrome reflects, to a great extent, the levels of both thyroid hormones and cortisol that were produced in response to the stress of combat.

When you experience a major stress that you interpret as a significant threat, the brain relays a chain of signals to the endocrine system that may go on indefinitely, provoking significant emotional response, impaired cognition, and mood changes. One of the typical reactions is the stimulation of the thyroid gland to produce higher amounts of thyroid hormone. This prolonged stimulation explains why you remain superalert, frightened, and anxious for a long time after a major event such as combat or physical or sexual abuse. The effects of the increase in thyroid hormone levels in relationship to the levels of cortisol explain to a great extent the symptoms experienced by people suffering from post-traumatic stress syndrome, such as those who fought in combat or lived through a war.[16] Similar reactions occur after a natural disaster, an epidemic, a rape assault, a catastrophic illness, or an accident.

Combat veterans who experienced major stress have persistently high thyroid hormone levels at times and can feel extremely anxious as a result. They are unusually watchful or wary, angry, and irritable; they may have sleep or concentration problems. In essence, high levels of thyroid hormone, which are part of the self-preservation response that occurs during a major life-threatening situation, produce this extreme alertness.

People who experience combat or live in war-torn areas are not only at risk for experiencing post-traumatic stress syndrome. They also seem to become at risk for experiencing Graves' disease because of the effects of the stress on the immune system. For instance, doctors noted a significant increase in the incidence of Graves' disease during the Franco-Prussian War of 1870–71. During and following World War I, doctors observed a higher frequency of Graves' disease. For instance, at Camp Upton in New York, doctors noted that many people who were labeled as having a war neurosis had clear-cut symptoms of Graves' disease. The same doctors found that an overactive thyroid was responsible for some of the cases of "war neuroses" that they were treating.[17] During World War II, an increase in the frequency of overactive thyroid was also noted among refugees from Nazi prison camps and among the people of occupied Denmark.[18]

Former president George H. W. Bush may be an example of someone involved in a wartime situation who ended up suffering from a stress–thyroid imbalance–stress cycle. Did, in fact, the stress of the Gulf War trigger or unmask the president's Graves' disease?

The speculation about stress triggering President Bush's overactive thyroid was prompted by the fact that his symptoms became evident approximately two months after the Gulf War cease-fire (February 24, 1991). While jogging at Camp David on Saturday, May 4, Bush experienced shortness of breath and an irregular heartbeat. This led doctors at Bethesda Naval Hospital to test his thyroid, which was found to be mildly overactive. Prior to the diagnosis, President Bush had experienced a few symptoms, which began two to three weeks before his admission to the hospital. Toward the end of March, he had decided to lose weight and exercise more. However, Bush's loss of seven or eight pounds over a two-week period was disproportionate to his dieting and exercise. His secretary had also noted a trembling of Bush's right hand, which caused some difficulty writing. Bush's entourage at the time—including his wife, his trusted aide Patty Presock, General Brent Scowcroft, and others on the White House and residence staff—had not noticed any emotional distress prior to diagnosis of the president's Graves' disease.

There has also been speculation that President Bush's overactive thyroid had preceded the war. Some news reporters described the president as animated by an incredible level of energy immediately after Iraq's August 2, 1990, invasion of Kuwait.[19] His heightened interest in sports activities at the time, his fast pace, and his overactivity led some to speculate that Bush might have been suffering from an overactive thyroid as far back as August 1990—almost six months prior to the war. This would put the onset of Graves' disease during the months of preparation leading up to the war, one of the most intense periods in Bush's presidency.

It must be noted that a number of alternative mechanisms have been identified that may well have played a more important role in triggering Bush's ailment. Two years before President Bush was diagnosed with Graves' disease, First Lady Barbara Bush had been diagnosed with the same condition. Cases in which partners are diagnosed with Graves' disease are known as "conjugal Graves' disease."[20] Conjugal Graves' disease may be due to environmental factors, such as toxins in the home or workplace, or even too much iodine and other chemicals in the water. The search for such factors in the White House was fruitless. Viral infections are also considered environmental in nature and can be implicated if there is a genetic predisposition, which both George and Barbara Bush could have.

(Coincidentally, the Bushes' dog, Millie, was suffering from lupus. When the news broke that the Bushes and their pet all had autoimmune disorders, the president's personal physician, Dr. Burton Lee, received numerous letters reporting cases of pets suffering from lupus whose owners have Graves' disease.)

There is increasing evidence that links infection, specifically infection by retroviruses, with Graves' disease. The possible link between a retrovirus and

Graves' disease can be measured through the level of antibodies in the patient's system.[21] It turned out that both the Bushes had significant levels of antibodies to the virus in their systems. These findings were never made public, however, perhaps because these results did not provide clear-cut proof that the virus was the direct cause of their condition. The medical evidence does strongly suggest, though, that in the cases of the president and Mrs. Bush, infection by a virus contributed to the Graves' disease.

Former president George H. W. Bush's case illustrates how difficult it is to prove that stress was a factor in triggering the condition. Did infection by a retrovirus cause Bush's Graves' disease, or did it result from stress generated by the Gulf crisis? Perhaps the most likely scenario is that it was a combination of the two.

Stress Management

Stress management should become a central part of any strategy for treating thyroid patients. Persons who have suffered thyroid imbalances are always on the brink of falling into an escalation cycle. Some need counseling and psychotherapy; others need antidepressants and antianxiety medications. But everyone benefits from perfect thyroid balance and relaxation techniques, which will help avoid the overwhelming stress that kicks off the cycle. Your brain has to show your thyroid and your immune system that it is in control.

The effect of stress on thyroid disease is not limited to triggering the disease and contributing to the prediagnosis escalation cycle described earlier. Stress can hurt you at all phases of treatment, including when thyroid hormone levels have returned to normal. For instance, patients with Graves' disease who have been successfully treated with a several-month course of an antithyroid medication (methimazole or propylthiouracil) may experience a remission of their disease and no longer require medications to maintain normal thyroid levels. Although the autoimmune disease can become dormant as a result of the treatment—and the physician and patient hope that it will remain dormant indefinitely—the condition will never go away. In such patients, stress and difficulties coping with stress can easily result in flare-ups of overactive thyroid, even after many years of remission. A report presented in 1995 at the Eleventh International Thyroid Congress in Toronto showed that in patients with Graves' disease, stress could promote a relapse of overactive thyroid.[22] And I have seen countless patients suffering from Hashimoto's thyroiditis and hypothyroidism who were doing well on a stable dose of thyroid medication but then experienced a sudden shift to Graves' disease and hyperthyroidism as a result of a stressful event such as a divorce or losing a job.

Stress undoubtedly increases the severity of the autoimmune attack upon the thyroid gland, even when the patient has been stabilized through adequate treatment. In one study of a large number of women whose glands contained dormant Graves' disease, researchers noted that many of the subjects became hyperthyroid during periods of stress. Once the stress went away, the functioning of the gland returned to normal.[23]

Recent research has also shown that if you are treated with medications for Graves' disease, you are less likely to respond to the treatment if you are experiencing a lot of stress, if you have a personality background of depression or paranoia, or if you have mental fatigue.[24]

Obviously no one can avoid negative events in life, but while you are having your thyroid condition treated, make sure you address your depression, engage in positive thinking, escape from stressful situations as much as you can, and practice relaxation techniques consistently. (For more details on relaxation techniques, see Chapter 18.)

People who have experienced a thyroid imbalance may continue to suffer adverse effects even after their thyroid levels have returned to normal. Patients who do not feel the same as they used to, despite normal blood levels, are often those who have experienced lengthy cycles of stress-imbalance-stress. These longtime sufferers often describe symptoms similar to those who were affected by an enormous trauma, such as being the victim of a crime or a combatant in war. For this reason, physicians consider the aftermath of thyroid imbalance a form of post-traumatic stress syndrome.

This sounds serious—and it is. Beyond the suffering the patient experiences before diagnosis and into the midst of the cycle, the healing must continue even after the disorder has been corrected. It is essential for friends and loved ones to understand that the thyroid patient may remain vulnerable to the effects of stress for some time. For these longtime sufferers, stress management is one of the most crucial steps toward recovery. Their brain chemistry has been altered, and their ability to cope with stresses, even small ones, has become precarious. They need to assume control again.

After the patient has fallen into a destructive cycle, it is possible to interrupt the spiral by boosting the effects of medication and easing the lingering mental symptoms that have not diminished over time. The combination of support—proper treatment and stress management—will halt the patient's anguish at the source.

"I'm stressed-out," "I can't cope with the pressure." Although statements like these are tossed around lightly, it is important to pay attention to these feelings, in addition to avoiding and managing stress. It is even more important for those who have an autoimmune thyroid condition or a genetic predisposition to this type of disorder. Like species that must live in water to breathe, these sufferers must consciously avoid and manage stress or they will get caught up in the vicious cycle of stress affecting the immune system, which in turn affects the thyroid imbalance generated by the immune system; in turn, the immune system becomes even more reactive, attacking the thyroid further.

Doctors diagnose thyroid disease more frequently than ever before. Many attribute this to wider availability of testing or improvements in technology, both of which have enabled us to conduct more sensitive diagnostic tests. It may also be because contemporary life brings greater stress and makes more demands on us. In 1930, Dr. Eli Moschowitz, in a review concerning psychiatric manifestations of Graves' disease, warned the medical community that "those influences that tend toward conflict and sensitization of the individual will breed Graves' disease" and suggested that Graves' disease was a "social disease and a product of higher civilizations."[25] I believe his prediction applies to Hashimoto's thyroiditis as well.

If increasing stress is at the root of the rise in thyroid disease, then people with thyroid problems must learn ways to cope better with stress. Relaxation techniques such as meditation, yoga, or tai chi can help prevent thyroid imbalance, especially if you have a family history of thyroid disease or other autoimmune conditions. Practicing stress management is essential for women who have reached menopause or have just delivered a baby, for people holding demanding jobs, and for people caring for demanding households.

There is no single best technique for stress management. The choice of a technique depends on whether you have other health conditions and on whether you can perform physical exercise. It could be deep-breathing exercises with meditation, sitting still while listening to soothing music, or mindful exercise such as yoga or tai chi. The ancient practice of tai chi has been shown to improve mood and emotions,[26] and could be one of the most efficient ways to preserve a healthy mind, immune system, and thyroid. For people with no physical impairment, I recommend tai chi most often. Relaxing your mind while exercising will boost your brain chemistry and make you feel in control again.

Most of us suffer from stress at work. Continuing stress at work will put you at risk for becoming a thyroid patient. It will also make you more likely to suffer from lingering symptoms, even if your thyroid condition has been properly treated. Stress management programs in the workplace will help you deal with stress and the symptoms of depression and anxiety. Use a cognitive behavioral technique at work to prevent depressive symptoms and panic disorder.

With thyroid conditions, the mind-body connection is not just part of the disorder; it is part of the treatment as well. The thyroid is the annex to the brain—the gland with which and through which the brain communicates. For this reason, it is very responsive to techniques that work on the body through the mind. As soon as you're diagnosed, you should begin working on your own to break your cycle of symptoms. You should expect your physician to control the thyroid hormone imbalance properly, but you as a patient must address your own stress issues. You must take responsibility for your healing regimen and become actively involved in getting yourself well.

Important Points to Remember

- Stress and an inability to handle stress can precipitate the onset of a thyroid disease.
- Thyroid imbalance, in turn, impairs your ability to deal with stress and makes you perceive trivial or annoying matters as more significant.
- The stress-illness-stress escalation cycle is a pattern commonly experienced by thyroid patients. The key is to recognize the cycle and halt it by obtaining diagnosis and rapid treatment.
- If you have been diagnosed with a thyroid imbalance, stress management techniques should be part of your treatment program to maintain optimal physical and emotional wellness. If you are genetically predisposed to thyroid disease, stress management techniques may prevent the onset of an imbalance.

5

HYPOTHYROIDISM

When the Thyroid Is Underactive

An enemy from within may ultimately have defeated Napoleon, one of history's greatest military leaders. Historians have noted that between 1804, when he was crowned emperor of the French, and his abdication in 1814, Napoleon experienced a steady mental deterioration that transformed him from an incisive, rapid decision-maker to a lethargic, hesitant man. He became unable to control his temper and lost such attributes as self-discipline, common sense, and the ability to work for long hours. His minister of marine, Denis Decrès, declared, "The Emperor is mad and will destroy us all."

What led some historians to conclude that the root of this dramatic deterioration was a severely underactive thyroid were the many changes to Napoleon's physical appearance that coincided with the alterations in his personality.[1] Napoleon gained a significant amount of weight. His face became round and his neck thicker. His long, straggly hair became sparse and fine. His hands became covered with fatty tissue and were described as "pudgy." Napoleon also suffered constantly from constipation and itchy skin, symptoms of an underactive thyroid. He changed from an impressively fit and vital leader to a prematurely aged man at forty-six, appearing completely worn out.

Obviously, doctors of Napoleon's time did not recognize hypothyroidism as a medical condition. Until fairly recently, similar scenarios of gradual deterioration to extreme levels of illness, ultimately leading to an inability to function, were common among severely hypothyroid patients, simply because doctors did not have accurate means by which to diagnose hypothyroidism. In fact, prior to the 1970s, when sophisticated testing to diagnose thyroid imbalance became available, underactive thyroid was believed to be a rare condition. Physicians often recognized it only after pronounced changes in a person's physical appearance and mental behavior had become evident. The diagnosis was frequently overlooked until patients needed to be hospitalized because of the effects of very severe hypothyroidism, including coma and insanity.[2] In some cases, the mental state of hypothyroid patients deteriorated to the extent that they became psychotic.[3] In 1949, Dr. R. Asher described his patients as having "myxedematous madness."[4] It turned out, however, that an underactive thyroid is one of the most common medical conditions that affect humankind.

In Chapter 4, I explained that the two most common causes of thyroid imbalance, Hashimoto's thyroiditis and Graves' disease, are disorders of the immune system. Hashimoto's thyroiditis is much more prevalent than Graves' disease. It affects more than 10 percent of the population and is the most common cause of an underactive thyroid. Numerous other conditions may also cause your thyroid to underperform:

- Treatment of an overactive thyroid with radioactive iodine or medications
- Surgical removal of part or all of the gland to treat nodules, goiter, Graves' disease, or cancer
- Transient hypothyroidism due to subacute thyroiditis, a viral illness that causes temporary partial damage to the thyroid gland (see Chapter 6)
- Transient hypothyroidism due to silent thyroiditis, an immune attack on the thyroid gland that also results in temporary damage to the gland (see Chapter 6)
- Previous radiation to the head or neck area
- Impaired blood supply to the thyroid after neck surgery for a nonthyroid-related problem
- Deficiency of iodine and/or essential micronutrients required for optimal manufacture of thyroid hormone (such as selenium, zinc, or vitamin A); see Chapter 2
- Eating excessive amounts of raw cruciferous vegetables and soy daily for extended periods of time
- Drug interactions (such as those from amiodarone, lithium, interferon, and interleukin-2)
- Absence or poor development of the gland (congenital hypothyroidism, childhood hypothyroidism)
- Genetic defects of enzymes that are essential for the manufacture of thyroid hormone
- Disorders of the hypothalamus or pituitary gland

Symptoms of Hypothyroidism

As thyroid hormone levels decrease, the functioning of most organs is affected. The person may begin to experience a multitude of physical symptoms, including:

- General tiredness
- Weight gain
- Aches and pains in joints and muscles
- Muscle cramps
- Constipation
- Dry skin
- Brittle hair
- Hair loss, including loss of eyebrow hair
- Feeling cold even in warm temperatures
- Milky discharge from the breast (galactorrhea)

The more severe the deficiency of thyroid hormone, the worse these symptoms become—and you may begin to experience other symptoms. If you have a significant deficiency of thyroid hormone, your voice may become hoarse, deep, husky, and slow; your speech may become thick; your face may become puffy; and even your hearing abilities may lessen. Your skin, especially on the palms of the hands, may become yellowish due to a buildup of the nutrient carotene in the blood. (The process that normally converts carotene into vitamin A in the body is slowed by hypothyroidism. In fact, if you are taking vitamin supplements containing beta-carotene, yellow palms could be an early clue that you have an underactive thyroid.) Also, your feet may swell and you may become short of breath even with minimal exercise. Your heart rate decreases, and your blood pressure may become high as a result of a loss of plasticity of blood vessels. It is estimated that high blood pressure occurs in as many as 21 percent of people with an underactive thyroid.[5]

Other important effects of an underactive thyroid on your health are those caused by high cholesterol. An underactive thyroid causes or worsens hyper-cholesterolemia. Research has shown that 20 percent of women older than forty with high cholesterol levels have underactive thyroids.[6] In addition to high cholesterol, low thyroid causes high homocysteine levels. The Third National Health and Nutrition Examination Survey has shown that high cholesterol and homocysteine are major reasons for the increased cardiovascular risk in patients with underactive thyroid.[7] For these reasons, patients with hypothyroidism should take folic acid (preferably as L-methylfolate such as Quatrefolic®) to lower homocysteine in addition to proper thyroid hormone treatment. Low thyroid also causes changes in clotting factors and produces inflammation in blood vessels that contribute to worsening of peripheral vascular disease.[8] Hypothyroidism can also cause anemia due to deficiency in iron, folic acid, or vitamin B_{12}. An undcractive thyroid lowers your defense against infections. Often, as you become hypothyroid, you become more vulnerable to fungal and viral infections and your reproductive function is affected. Heavy menstrual bleeding or even cessation of menstruation is not uncommon in severely hypothyroid women.

Many persons with severe hypothyroidism complain of numbness and a sensation of pins and needles in their hands or feet. These symptoms may indicate a hypothyroid-induced neuropathy, a degenerative nerve condition. Some studies have shown that more than 50 percent of severely hypothyroid patients have damage to their peripheral nerves and some suffer from the pins-and-needles sensation.[9] Another nerve-related condition that can occur in severe hypothyroidism is carpal tunnel syndrome, which is due to compression of the median nerve in the wrist. It causes tingling in your fingers and often resolves with thyroid hormone treatment.[10] Other neurological and muscle problems that can occur as a result of severe hypothyroidism include:

- Myopathy, a disorder of muscle tissue that can cause muscle weakness and result in high levels of creatine phosphokinase (CPK), a blood marker for muscle disease
- A delay in relaxation of the muscle following contraction
- An excessive increase in the bulk of muscles (in children)
- Seizures

With scvcrc hypothyroidism, you can also experience muscle coordination problems, which can prevent you from carrying out your usual daily activities. As a result of being unable to coordinate voluntary muscular movements (ataxia), you may experience loss of equilibrium, unsteadiness on the feet, lack of coordination of hands and feet, and trembling. You may also experience Dupuytren contracture (trigger finger) and decreased mobility of your joints.

Hypothyroidism can cause sleep apnea, which refers to a condition in which there is a temporary cessation of breathing during sleep. It is caused by the collapse of the upper airways during sleep. Sleep apnea causes the oxygen level in blood to decrease, and this will lead to disruption of the sleep pattern. Sleep apnea perpetuates weight gain and causes fatigue, daytime sleepiness, and cognitive impairment. You are more likely to suffer from sleep apnea if you are older, if you are menopausal, and if you smoke tobacco and consume alcohol. Being overweight puts you at ten times higher risk for having sleep apnea. Sleep apnea promotes insulin resistance and high blood pressure and increases your cardiovascular risk.[11]

Other physical symptoms that may indicate severe hypothyroidism—and that can lead to misdiagnosis—include gastrointestinal and respiratory symptoms such as:

- Decreased movement of the gastrointestinal tract, causing severe constipation
- Intestinal obstruction and, rarely, perforation (only in very severe hypothyroidism)
- Pleural effusion, an accumulation of fluid between the layers of the membrane that lines the lungs and chest cavity

The physical effects of hypothyroidism vary from person to person. In fact, you may experience symptoms related to only one organ. One patient may experience heart problems, whereas another may experience joint and muscle pain. A person with severe hypothyroidism who is not taking medication can slip into a state of myxedema coma, often triggered by exposure to cold, by medications that cause sedation of the brain, or by illnesses such as severe infection or stroke. A person in a myxedema coma has a very low temperature (hypothermia), may develop low blood sugar (hypoglycemia), and often needs a respirator. This condition is dangerous and can lead to death.

Mental Effects of an Underactive Thyroid

Likewise, the mental effects of hypothyroidism vary from person to person, even among those with the same severity of hypothyroidism. Alex may develop severe depression as a result of hypothyroidism, whereas Julia may have only mild, barely perceptible depression, and Bill may exhibit a significant number of anxiety symptoms. The reason for these differences stems from the fact that each person may be predisposed to a different type of response, depending on personality makeup and the existence of a mental issue that is either borderline or hidden. An underactive thyroid can cause any of the following mental symptoms:

- Depression
- Mental sluggishness
- Increased sleepiness
- Forgetfulness
- Emotional instability
- Loss of ambition
- Decreased ability to pay attention and focus
- Decreased interest
- Slowing of thought and speech

- Irritability
- Fear of open or public spaces (agoraphobia)
- Audiovisual hallucinations and paranoid delusions (rare, only in very severe hypothyroidism)
- Dementia (usually in long-standing severe hypothyroidism)
- Manic behavior

Contrary to common belief, hypothyroidism does not necessarily mean that the thyroid gland has completely stopped functioning. The deficiency could actually range from a minimal amount to a more significant loss, depending on the damage to the gland. Although the physical symptoms become more pronounced in severe cases of underactive thyroid, disturbances of mood and emotions are likely to occur even when the thyroid hormone deficit is minimal.

Today we have the tools to catch and treat even the mildest cases of hypothyroidism. Technological advances have enabled us to realize that hypothyroidism is a common condition. While severe hypothyroidism, representing the extreme end of the spectrum, affects 1.5 to 2 percent of the general population, low-grade hypothyroidism affects 8 percent of the population.[12] There are also people with seemingly normal blood test results whose thyroid is actually deficient (see Chapter 7). If one includes patients with borderline blood tests or tests that show up in the normal conventional range, the frequency of low-grade hypothyroidism may reach 10 to 15 percent of the population.

Although many people may have mild cases of hypothyroidism that remain stable throughout their lifetimes, some patients may experience a worsening of thyroid hormone deficit over time. Nearly 2 to 3 percent of people suffering from low-grade hypothyroidism progress to more severe hypothyroidism each year.[13]

Despite physicians' increased awareness of how common hypothyroidism is in the general population and the existence of precise testing of thyroid levels, many people still slip into the dark hole of hypothyroidism. If you suffer from any of the physical or mental symptoms described earlier in this chapter, have your doctor request a TSH (thyroid-stimulating hormone) test, which is the most sensitive test for detecting a thyroid imbalance due to a dysfunctioning gland.

Let's take a closer look at how the principal mental and emotional symptoms of an underactive thyroid play out in real life.

"EXHAUSTED AND OVERWHELMED"
Regardless of whether a person's hypothyroidism is mild, moderate, or severe, the most common—and most noticeable—symptom of an underactive

thyroid is fatigue. This tiredness typically has a physical component (from the slower metabolism) and a mental component (linked to depression). Depression and loss of brain power are the most common mental effects of an underactive thyroid. In Chapter 8, I will detail how hypothyroidism can either cause depression or be a major contributing factor to it, including low-grade depression, chronic minor depression, or in extreme cases major depression. Undoubtedly, fatigue is a universal symptom of depression. Hypothyroidism will also make you sleep more than you used to.

Hypothyroid individuals who sleep more than they formerly did often attribute the increased sleepiness to just being tired when, in fact, it could be related to depression. In many hypothyroid patients, tiredness and sleeping more than usual are expressions of lack of enthusiasm and loss of interest in doing things, even customarily pleasurable activities. When the deficiency of thyroid hormone worsens, the mental slowing and the depression become compounded by the slowing of your body. This may make you feel as if you are drowning in a hole. Patients suffering from an underactive thyroid may also experience significant anxiety symptoms and a wide range of cognitive impairments.

CRIPPLING ANXIETY

In my clinical experience, anxiety is a much more common symptom of hypothyroidism than physicians generally acknowledge. Because anxiety and panic attacks are typical symptoms of hyperthyroidism, some patients with an underactive thyroid may become confused when they experience these symptoms yet are told they are hypothyroid. Anxiety can have a crippling effect on a person with an underactive thyroid accompanied by tiredness and depression.

Although in many people the anxiety is related to the depression itself, in other people anxiety symptoms are prominent with little or no depression. Even then, however, thyroid hormone deficit and its effect on brain chemical transmitters result in anxiety. The fact that an underactive thyroid alters a person's mechanisms for coping with stress and lowers self-esteem may account for the prominence of anxiety as a symptom. Also, fears and self-doubt are often compounded by the awareness of defects in memory and concentration.

Hypothyroid people, especially women, often begin to feel they don't "look nice" and may be worried about being seen in public. Their anxiety may grow worse with the advent of other physical symptoms such as headaches, muscle cramps, pains, aches, and hair loss. Not knowing the cause of these symptoms increases their worries.

Marie, a twenty-nine-year-old nurse, had struggled through college with many of the effects of undiagnosed hypothyroidism. Because she suffered from so many symptoms of anxiety, a psychiatrist most likely would have diagnosed her condition as a generalized anxiety syndrome. She was extremely tired and depressed for almost two years before her thyroid problem was diagnosed. She suffered anxiety from having attempted to overcome her physical symptoms, as well as difficulties with memory and concentration, which hurt her performance in a very competitive school environment.

She explained:

I started getting really tired my first year in college. The exhaustion and the need to sleep for extended hours, after what other people would consider a normal day, would really affect my life. I didn't have the desire to do a lot of partying because I was too tired. I had to drive several hours to the hospital to do my clinical training, so I related the fatigue to all the hours of travel and the stress of work and studies. My hair was falling out. My skin and eyes were dry all the time. I had a lot of generalized aches and pains that I couldn't explain.

I was so afraid that I would not pass my exams, that I would be a failure. I had myself so worked up and anxious that one of my college professors called me and said, "What is going on? You're not yourself." I told her I was fine, but I was just a ball of nerves. She said, "No, you're not yourself. You are normally very calm. Now, you seem to be running on adrenaline." I told her it must just be the anxiety of having to take tests.

An impaired memory and a decreased ability to focus and concentrate aggravated Marie's struggle. Her concerns about being unable to accomplish certain tasks generated more anxiety and unrealistic fears, eventually leading to crippling panic attacks. Four to six weeks after she started thyroid hormone treatment for her underactive thyroid, she began to feel much better. Four months later, when her thyroid test results were normal and stable, her depression and anxiety symptoms had greatly improved. Her memory and concentration returned to normal. All her physical symptoms resolved except for the hair loss, which persisted for more than six months after correction of the underactive thyroid.

Clearing the Mental Fog

Although you may be able to describe physical symptoms such as joint pain or muscle cramps in a relatively straightforward manner, when you try expressing in detail a subtle deficit in your cognitive abilities, you immediately realize the extreme difficulty of the task. A few years ago, one patient described the mental effects of hypothyroidism to me as "a brain fog." An underactive thyroid can leave you unable to remember details, names, or even events. As a result of low thyroid levels, your brain loses some of the power it normally has to grasp and process a thought. You may comprehend a con-

cept while reading a book or listening to someone talk; then immediately afterward, you may be unable to fully describe it. The concept becomes blurred
in your mind. Often when you try to express a thought, you cannot think of
the right word, whereas before, you used to quickly review several words and
easily pick the most appropriate one. Concentration difficulties are unequivocally the most significant and disturbing mental consequence of low thyroid.

Lisa, an undergraduate student who was considering law school, became
depressed and experienced many of the symptoms of hypothyroidism. "After
my baby was born," she said, "I went into a funk. I was exhausted and blue.
Sometimes I would get angry at my two older sons for no reason, which was
not typical of me."

When Lisa first came to me, her mental dysfunctions had grown more
debilitating, and she was no longer considering law school because of the
cognitive impairments she was experiencing. She said:

> I have lost the ability to concentrate. I ask a question and forget the answer im-
> mediately, and I have to ask again. It is humiliating. I think of one thing and
> then another, and I can't stay focused long enough to think either thing through.
> I have tried to hide my memory loss so no one would know how bad it is, but
> it's gotten to the point where I can't hide it any longer. I become easily con-
> fused. Now I am even afraid to drive, because I suddenly get disoriented.

Difficulties with memory and concentration are often symptoms of depression and anxiety disorders as well. But when the patient has an underactive thyroid, impaired cognition is worse and aggravates the anxiety.

Anne, a twenty-four-year-old secretary who had moderate hypothyroidism, had suffered from both depression and symptoms of anxiety for three
years. But what made her seek medical help was her worsening memory loss.
Her husband had become disabled four years earlier as a result of a car accident, which contributed to her general depression. In her words:

> Before diagnosis, I definitely experienced a higher level of anxiety than I ever
> had before. I would begin ruminating on things and wouldn't be able to let
> them go for days. I would be worried about trivial things. I know when I am
> anxious: my heart beats faster, my muscles are tighter, I'm tense, and I snap at
> people. I thought a lot of that was related to my husband's health.
>   My anxiety symptoms became worse when I started noticing that I didn't
> have any memory anymore. It was awful at work. Also, I was not able to focus
> on anything I was doing. I had a hard time concentrating and could not find my
> words or express myself. My boss almost fired me. After a while, it became re-
> ally scary. One day there was a new toaster sitting on my dryer. I called my sister
> and told her thanks for buying me this toaster, and she said, "I didn't buy it." I

had bought the toaster, but I had no memory of buying it. My daughter would tell me she told me something, and I didn't remember. It was kind of a joke. We kept it light, but I was losing my memory.

Anne's case illustrates how impairments of memory and other cognitive functions can make hypothyroid patients more anxious. Her awareness of the memory impairment and her inability to perform at work generated more worries and worsened her anxiety symptoms.

Boris Yeltsin's Underactive Thyroid

In June 1991, after the collapse of communism in the Soviet Union, Boris Yeltsin was elected the first president of the new Russia. Over the following five years, the world observed Yeltsin change from a slim and quick-thinking political leader to a slow-walking, slow-speaking president whose political career was compromised by apparently serious health problems.[14]

Toward the end of the summer of 1996, Yeltsin's health had deteriorated to such an extent that even his public appearances were curtailed. Critics and the media charged that Yeltsin was no longer in full control of his own government. In September 1996, Drs. Michael DeBakey and George Noon, cardiovascular surgeons from my institution, visited Yeltsin and recommended multiple bypass heart surgery. However, the surgical procedure was delayed by a few weeks for several reasons, including gastrointestinal bleeding, poor heart function caused by a heart attack in late June or early July, and newly diagnosed hypothyroidism, which needed to be corrected before the operation.[15]

Until September 1996, Yeltsin's hypothyroidism, which had probably affected his health for some time, was undiagnosed. Long-standing, untreated hypothyroidism increases the risk of heart attacks because it can raise cholesterol levels, which, in turn, can lead to coronary artery disease (restricted blood flow to the heart).

Before the diagnosis, Yeltsin was also described as being "slow and stiff in his gestures." His speech was said to be slurred and his behavior "peculiar," and he sometimes disappeared from public view without explanation. Rumors of heavy drinking were widespread.

Yeltsin's weight gain and puffiness developed slowly. Pictures taken of him before his heart operation confirm that his facial puffiness gradually worsened. This could be an indication that his hypothyroidism had been long-standing and went undiagnosed.

It was clear that Yeltsin's hypothyroidism caused a lingering depression, which was noticed by political critics and the news media. He had to cancel several meetings because of tiredness and became "prone to sudden mysterious absences and bouts of unusual behavior."[16] For months prior to Yeltsin's diagnosis, he withdrew from public view. In addition, his alcohol consumption increased.

We can only speculate on the extent to which Yeltsin's hypothyroidism (and quite likely the depressed mood that resulted from it) affected Russia during the years he was president. We can also only wonder whether these factors contributed to Yeltsin's loss of control of the government in the summer of 1996. It is quite possible, however, that Yeltsin's complete transformation after his bypass surgery was not due merely to the surgical correction of his heart problem. His turnaround after the treatment of his thyroid condition was spectacular and illustrates how thyroid imbalance could affect the course of history.

Physicians caring for political leaders, particularly those in high government posts, should be alert to the possibility of a thyroid imbalance anytime a change in personality, emotions, or judgment is observed and anytime a leader exhibits poorly explained symptoms.

Low-Grade Hypothyroidism

Once not discussed or even suspected, low-grade hypothyroidism and its effects on physical and mental health are increasingly pervasive. Numerous studies have now concluded that low-grade hypothyroidism can contribute to high cholesterol levels, infertility, miscarriages, tiredness, and depression. Small deficits of thyroid hormone can slow down your metabolism and the ability to burn extra fat, making you gain weight and even develop metabolic syndrome. Research has shown that correcting low-grade hypothyroidism will result in a lowering of both total cholesterol and "bad" LDL cholesterol.[17] Low-grade hypothyroidism can also cause high blood pressure and elevated triglycerides.[18] It makes the cells that cover blood vessels (endothelial cells) lose their ability to protect the blood vessels. This abnormality reverses with thyroid treatment as well; left untreated, it will make you more likely to have coronary artery disease and heart attack. A study published in the *Archives of Internal Medicine* showed that patients with low-grade hypothyroidism suffer more from coronary artery disease and cardiovascular death than people with normal thyroid function.[19] Untreated low-grade hypothyroidism can also contribute to worsening peripheral vascular disease. Research has also shown that in older people, peripheral vascular disease was present in 78 percent of those with low-grade hypothyroidism and in only 17 percent of those with normal thyroid.[20] The reason for this increased risk of vascular disease among patients with low-grade hypothyroidism stems from elevation of blood pressure caused by low thyroid, higher levels of triglycerides and cholesterol, and high homocysteine levels. Even to this day, however, many physicians continue to believe that low-grade hypothyroidism has no significance. Some will tell their patients, "The condition isn't serious enough to treat." The most common physical symptoms experienced by patients with low-grade hypothyroidism are fatigue, dry skin, hair loss, and cold intolerance. Some women may experience heavier and longer menstrual periods (menorrhagia).

In addition to having symptoms of depression or becoming vulnerable to depression (see Chapter 8), patients with low-grade hypothyroidism may experience hysteria, more frequent anxiety, and physical complaints. They may also have some impairment in memory-related abilities.[21] The memory deficit and concentration problems improve with thyroid hormone treatment. In Latin America, it was found that people who lacked iodine in their diets were more likely to have impaired cognition.[22] Too little dietary iodine often compromises the manufacture of normal amounts of thyroid hormone. Cognitive impairments in these people improved after supplementation of iodine in the diet. Another study, conducted in Sweden on older women with low-grade hypothyroidism, showed that the memory scores of 20 percent of these women improved after six months of treatment with thyroid hormone.[23] When sensitive memory tests, such as the Wechsler Memory Scale, were used, researchers have shown that more than 80 percent of people with low-grade hypothyroidism had impaired memory functions.[24] Low-grade hypothyroidism impairs both short-term memory and visual memory.

As a result of low-grade hypothyroidism, you may have difficulty remembering what you just read. You may believe that there is nothing wrong with you when in fact you have subtle deficits that can be demonstrated only by sophisticated neuropsychological testing.[25] You may also be more prone to experiencing panic attacks. If you are suffering from any of the symptoms of underactive thyroid I have described or if your cholesterol is high, have your doctor give you a TSH test. If you are a woman age thirty-five or older, have your doctor test your thyroid every five years. If you have been diagnosed with low-grade hypothyroidism, you will probably require treatment for the rest of your life. In fact, the dose of thyroid hormone required to correct your imbalance is likely to increase as time passes.

The lack of awareness that low-grade hypothyroidism may cause suffering and deficits may lead physicians to ignore subtle thyroid test abnormalities consistent with this condition. If your doctor tells you that your thyroid insufficiency isn't serious enough to warrant treatment, do not accept this. Rather, insist on seeking help from a specialist knowledgeable about thyroid disorders. I worry that many people get tested but do not receive treatment despite the fact that they clearly have low-grade hypothyroidism.

Questionnaire:
The Physical Symptoms of Hypothyroidism

As we've seen, mental suffering due to hypothyroidism is not just limited to depression. The effect of thyroid hormone deficit on anxiety levels and thinking patterns produces complex neurobehavioral changes. Physical thyroid-related symptoms can also contribute to the worsening of depression, anxiety, and feelings of inadequacy. As hypothyroidism progresses, mental symptoms intensify, job and relationships are affected, and the person feels as if he or she were drowning.

An easy way to determine the likelihood that you may be suffering from hypothyroidism is to complete the following physical-symptoms questionnaire.

Has your hair become dry, or are you losing your hair?	Yes No	___
Have your menstrual periods been heavy in recent months?	Yes No	___
Have you been suffering from joint aches and pains?	Yes No	___
Are your nails brittle?	Yes No	___
Have you been getting muscle cramps?	Yes No	___
Have you noticed a continuous weakness in your muscles?	Yes No	___
Has your skin been dry?	Yes No	___
Have your face and eyes been puffy?	Yes No	___
Have you been experiencing cold intolerance?	Yes No	___
Have you gained more than five pounds?	Yes No	___
Has your skin become coarse?	Yes No	___
Have you been constipated?	Yes No	___
Have you noticed in recent months a milky discharge from your breasts?	Yes No	___
Do you sweat less?	Yes No	___
Has your voice become hoarse?	Yes No	___
Do your fingers tingle?	Yes No	___
Has your hearing gotten worse?	Yes No	___
Has your heartbeat been slow?	Yes No	___
Have you been experiencing stiffness?	Yes No	___
Have you been fatigued?	Yes No	___
Have your eyes been dry?	Yes No	___
Have you been experiencing shortness of breath during exercise or reduced tolerance to exercise?	Yes No	___

If you answered yes to four or more of the preceding questions, you may be hypothyroid. If you answered yes to six or more of the questions, you are probably hypothyroid.

In Chapter 8, you will find questionnaires on the symptoms of depression and anxiety. Remember, even if your answers to the preceding physical-symptoms questionnaire indicate a low probability of hypothyroidism, if your answers to the Chapter 8 questionnaires indicate depression or an anxiety disorder, you still need to have your thyroid tested.

Hypothyroidism and Aging

One of my hypothyroid patients who was in her early twenties remarked that she felt as if she had begun to age at a rapid pace when her thyroid became underactive. This is quite insightful, as a number of the effects of thyroid hormone deficit are analogous to aging. As you age, your memory, concentration, and ability to process new information gradually become impaired. Hypothyroidism also causes a reduction in physical exercise, both because of direct effects on muscle function and because of how it impairs mood and emotions, in a way that mirrors how people often tend to become more sedentary with advancing years.

In fact, the normal aging process may be related to some extent to a naturally occurring decrease in thyroid hormone activity in the body. For example, the size of the thyroid gland decreases with age, and its structure and function also deteriorate gradually. The amount of the most active form of thyroid hormone (T3) in tissues decreases. This explains why the basal metabolic rate, which is highly regulated by thyroid hormone, also decreases with age. By the age of eighty-five, your basal metabolic rate has dropped to 52 percent of the level you had at age three. As a result, normal physiological responses requiring thyroid hormone become less efficient. As you get older, you may have a more difficult time regulating your body temperature during extreme heat or cold. As you age, thyroid hormone deficit in your organs also promotes a slowing of the synthesis of essential proteins in your body, a hallmark of the aging process. This natural decline in thyroid hormone activity with age could conceivably contribute to the normal aging process.[26]

Because the effects of thyroid hormone deficit are similar to the effects of aging, the physical symptoms and signs relied on to suspect hypothyroidism in younger people are less useful in the elderly. Both aging and hypothyroidism are associated with decreased mental activity, dry skin, constipation, depression, and an increased incidence of atherosclerosis and high cholesterol. Therefore, unless thyroid testing is done routinely, hypothyroidism may never be uncovered. Quite often, the symptoms of hypothyroidism are attributed to the aging process per se or to other problems.

Older people with an underactive thyroid often experience only a limited number of vague symptoms. These symptoms may be mental confusion, weight gain, poor appetite, episodes of falling, aches and pains, weakness, muscle stiffness (which may be confused with Parkinsonism), incontinence, and depression. Consequently, hypothyroidism may go unrecognized and become severe over time because of the superficial resemblance to aging itself.

As you get older, you may be more vulnerable to serious mental and emotional problems when the gland becomes minimally underactive. In addition to depression and impaired cognitive abilities, which are quite common among older people afflicted with even minor thyroid hormone deficit, a profound and severe slowing of mental activity can occur if your underactive thyroid is severe enough and is not corrected promptly. This slowing of mental activity may become extreme and lead to dementia. Dementia due to hypothyroidism is caused by disruption in the brain structures that support recent memory, concentration, and problem solving.[27]

Occasionally, family members bring a patient to the hospital or doctor's office because the person has become increasingly withdrawn and has been showing extreme slowing of mental activity. Even today, with the increased awareness of the frequency and effects of thyroid diseases, we continue to see older patients who progress to a state of dementia caused by severe hypothyroidism. Most patients with dementia are unaware of what is happening to them. Because Alzheimer's disease is one of the most common causes of dementia in older people, some patients diagnosed with dementia are thought to have Alzheimer's disease when in fact the dementia has been caused by an underactive thyroid that has not been treated for a long period of time.

The similarities between dementia caused by Alzheimer's disease and dementia caused by hypothyroidism led scientists to study whether patients with Alzheimer's disease are more likely to have a thyroid imbalance. It turned out that both patients and unaffected relatives of patients with familial Alzheimer's disease have a high frequency of Hashimoto's thyroiditis and hypothyroidism.[28] The association between Hashimoto's thyroiditis and familial Alzheimer's disease appears to be genetically mediated. Hypothyroidism may place a person with Alzheimer's disease at a high risk for having more mental and cognitive deficits. Consequently, if you are diagnosed with Alzheimer's disease, your doctor will typically test you for hypothyroidism so that thyroid hormone treatment will slow the cognitive deterioration if you turn out to be hypothyroid.

The incidence of hypothyroidism rises abruptly after menopause in women and after the age of sixty in men. Approximately 10 to 15 percent of postmenopausal women have mild, low-grade hypothyroidism, whereas in men the prevalence is 6 percent.[29] Nearly 45 percent of older people have some degree of thyroid gland inflammation characteristic of Hashimoto's thyroiditis. As noted earlier, minor thyroid imbalances often produce greater effects in the elderly than in younger people, and physicians often achieve spectacular results with adequate treatment. Thyroid hormone treatment prevents deterioration of cognition and the occurrence of depressive mood in older patients with low-grade hypothyroidism. The high frequency of hypothyroidism among older people and the similarities between symptoms of hypothyroidism and changes characteristic of the normal aging process attest to the importance of performing thyroid tests on older people who have noticeable changes in mood, emotions, or behavior.

Congenital Hypothyroidism

Nearly 20 million people worldwide suffer from brain damage caused by hypothyroidism due to iodine deficiency during the critical period of fetal development and in infancy. When iodine is insufficient in the diet (iodine being essential for the manufacture of thyroid hormone), hypothyroidism and goiter (enlargement of the thyroid) are common effects on the fetus and the newborn. It has been estimated that in areas where nutritional iodine deficiency is common, 10 percent of newborns are hypothyroid. In the United States, iodine deficiency is rarely a cause of underactive thyroid in newborns. Nevertheless, 1 in 4,000 infants is born with congenital hypothyroidism, a condition often due to the absence or incomplete development of the thyroid gland.[30] In some newborns with hypothyroidism, the gland is not in the proper place in the neck. Instead, it is somewhere between its normal location and the base of the tongue, a condition called "ectopic thyroid." Congenital hypothyroidism due to a pituitary defect causing a deficiency in the pituitary hormone TSH is much less common and occurs in 1 in 100,000 newborns. In rare instances, hypothyroidism due to a pituitary deficiency or defective TSH is a familial and genetically transmissible disorder.

Because lack of thyroid hormone during the fetal stage and from birth to age two to three results in brain damage and mental retardation, systematic screening for congenital hypothyroidism has been implemented in the United States and many other countries. Ideally, the diagnosis is made during the first few days of life. The sooner thyroid hormone treatment is initiated, the better the mental outcome for such babies. For instance, the average IQ of children who were diagnosed as hypothyroid when they were between three and six months of age is only 19. Infants who are diagnosed late experience permanent learning disabilities, poor scholastic achievement, and difficulties integrating themselves into society. However, congenitally hypothyroid children who are started on treatment early and receive adequate treatment have a normal IQ and satisfactory school performance when they are subsequently evaluated at the age of five to ten years. Ultimately, the intellectual and cognitive abilities of these children also depend on whether they take the necessary medications. If your infant suffers from congenital hypothyroidism and is taking thyroid hormone daily, you should know that soy-based formula interferes with the absorption of thyroid hormone in the intestines.[31] The dose of thyroid hormone must often be increased for infants fed with soy-based formulas.

Genetic factors seem to play a role in the occurrence of congenital hypothyroidism, with many families having had several cases. Black infants are affected less frequently than white ones. A population study in Atlanta showed that infants with Down syndrome are thirty-five times more likely to have congenital hypothyroidism than other infants.[32] According to recent research, permanent congenital hypothyroidism is also more common among twins, among female infants, and among infants who have a family history of thyroid disease or whose mother is a diabetic.[33] Also, you need to be aware of the fact that infants who are large for their gestational age are at increased risk for permanent congenital hypothyroidism. Without screening, 70 percent of infants are diagnosed within the first year, but at the cost of irreversible brain damage. One of the consequences of thyroid hormone deficit is deafness, also a symptom in patients with Pendred syndrome. Pendred syndrome is transmitted genetically and is defined by the coexistence of a genetic defect in the manufacture of thyroid hormone and deafness. This disorder accounts for nearly 7 percent of all cases of childhood deafness.

Because the symptoms of hypothyroidism in the newborn may be minimal and do not necessarily point to the thyroid, the thyroid is routinely tested in the first six days of life. The screening is done by measuring TSH and/or T4 in blood from a heel prick collected on filter paper. Although screening should ideally include both T4 and TSH, medical authorities unfortunately choose only one of the two methods because of cost. If the TSH method is used, the physician may overlook a case of hypothalamic or pituitary hypothyroidism (also known as central hypothyroidism) since, in this condition, TSH may be normal. The other important limitation of TSH screening is that some newborns with defective thyroid glands have test results that are normal at the time of screening but become abnormal weeks after birth.

If a T4 test is used as the primary screening method, central hypothyroidism is detected easily, but the pediatrician may miss low-grade hypothyroidism due to a defective thyroid. In such babies, the underactive thyroid will worsen over time and result in brain damage.

Because the T4 levels of many infants fall in the wide gray zone between low and normal that necessitates retesting, many medical centers choose TSH over T4 for screening purposes. Symptoms that should alert you that your infant might have congenital hypothyroidism include persistent neonatal jaundice, poor feeding, bluish skin color, weak muscle tone, swelling of the tongue, lethargy, constipation, and slow growth. Even if the screening

TSH level does not show hypothyroidism, if your infant is showing any unusual behavior, you need to have the pediatrician test the baby's T4 level and rerun the TSH test.

COMMON CAUSES OF CONGENITAL HYPOTHYROIDISM
- Abnormally located thyroid gland (ectopic thyroid)
- Poorly developed or undeveloped thyroid gland
- Inborn error of thyroid hormone manufacture
- Hypothalamic or pituitary deficiency
- Transient hypothyroidism of the newborn
- Ingestion by the mother of drugs that inhibit the production of fetal thyroid hormone (antithyroid drugs)
- Prematurity
- Iodine deficiency
- Iodine excess
- Antibodies from the mother crossing the placenta and affecting the fetus's thyroid

Important Points to Remember

- The most common symptom of an underactive thyroid is fatigue. This fatigue is both physical and mental and often precedes other typical symptoms of depression and physical symptoms of thyroid hormone deficit.
- Anxiety symptoms—including excessive worrying and panic attacks— are common when the thyroid is underactive. Because these symptoms are also typical of an overactive thyroid, they often give rise to confusion.
- Regardless of its severity, hypothyroidism often causes cognitive problems such as poor memory, difficulties processing information, and lack of focus. Such mental fog generates a vicious cycle of low self-esteem and increased anxiety.
- As indicated by blood test results, about 8 percent of the population has low-grade hypothyroidism. That figure might be as high as 10 percent if we include people with normal blood test results who still suffer from a thyroid deficiency.
- An underactive thyroid results in a form of accelerated aging. It can also cause brain damage and slow brain functioning.
- If a severely underactive thyroid remains untreated for a long time, the damage may be so dramatic that it can promote the occurrence of dementia in older people.
- If congenital hypothyroidism is not detected and treated early, it will lead to irreversible intellectual deficits.

6

HYPERTHYROIDISM

When the Thyroid Is Overactive

Common sense might suggest that if too little thyroid hormone can cause you to sink into a state of clinical depression and rob you of your ability to function as before, too much thyroid hormone would make you feel happy, perky, and on top of the world. This assumption, however, is only partially correct. When the brain is flooded with too much thyroid hormone, some people do experience a lasting elation. Thoughts race through the mind. Activities crowd the day.

Several years ago, my neighbor Nancy had the reputation of being overly friendly. She incessantly helped others with their chores and knew almost everyone in the condominium complex where we lived. She initiated conversations with everyone and constantly came up with new ideas and projects. It never occurred to anyone, including me, that what animated Nancy with this incredible energy and enthusiasm was an overactive thyroid.

Talking to a retired woman one day, Nancy mentioned that her electric bill was outrageous because she always felt hot and had to use air-conditioning most of the time. When I got close to Nancy, I noticed the shakiness in her hands and the stare in her eyes, symptoms of an overactive thyroid.

It turned out that Nancy's mildly manic (hypomanic) behavior was not her original nature. Nancy had, in fact, been a somewhat reserved person before she decided to move from Dallas to Houston to study and join her boyfriend. Nancy also suffered from many physical symptoms. She had lost weight despite eating more, her menstrual periods had become scanty, she had some acne on her face, her bowel movements had become increasingly frequent, she was losing some hair, and she had a rapid heartbeat— but to her all these symptoms were trivial. Her brain and body were animated by extraordinary energy and elation. Nancy did not even consider that something might be wrong with her; she simply thought that she had become happier after joining her boyfriend in Houston.

Hyperthyroid patients may have an energy, optimism, and self-confidence that are not characteristic of someone who needs medical or psychiatric help.[1] Even when these personality traits appear suddenly and unexpectedly, they are usually considered positive. The person has lost weight. He or she has a positive attitude about life, is overactive, and expends effort far beyond his or her strength. Not surprisingly, mildly manic hyperthyroid patients can go for years without being diagnosed. They may not even seek medical help unless the symptoms become severe and disturbing.

Fred, a thirty-one-year-old construction worker, was hypomanic for four years as the result of an overactive thyroid. He was viewed as a superman on the job. He told me:

> One time, three tornadoes came through, and nine thousand roofs in the area had to be redone. I was driving a truck by myself every day and throwing three hundred squares of shingles up on a roof. A square of shingles weighs 220 pounds, so that's over 6,000 pounds in a day. Several employees were hired who went out on the road with me for one day but quit. Then, after I would finish roofing, I would go work another part-time job.
>
> Later, when we bought a farm, I fenced in ten acres in about three days. Never thought twice about it.

The tremendous physical energy Fred experienced reflects only a small part of the surge in mental power. It is almost purely a case of mind over matter. The brain is set at a fast pace, similar to what happens to people taking stimulant drugs. As this extraordinary feeling of power animates the brain, hyperthyroid individuals may experience significant anxiety and frustration, primarily because they cannot do everything they considered doing. As Fred described it:

> I would ask you a question, and before you could finish answering, I could already tell what you were talking about and be going on to something else. The number of things I could keep up with at one time was phenomenal. I could watch TV, listen to a conversation, eat, and be doing half a dozen other things and keep track of them all like I was intimately involved in every single one of them.

Being hypomanic, Fred dismissed his physical symptoms as insignificant. His bowel movements had become more frequent, but a physician told him he had irritable bowel syndrome. His hands were shaking almost continuously, and he was feeling hot all the time, but he got used to it. Fred had Graves' disease, the common form of hyperthyroidism that is caused by an immune disorder. After his symptoms had continued for four years, Fred finally sought medical help—but only when he began experiencing muscle weakness and shortness of breath due to heart failure, caused by his overactive thyroid.

Symptoms of Hyperthyroidism

Too much thyroid hormone in your system can cause a wide range of effects on your body. Although a complete list of these effects would include dozens of symptoms, the following are the most common:

GENERAL
Weight loss (or, less commonly, weight gain)
Fatigue
Shakiness
Feeling hot and becoming intolerant of warm and hot temperatures
Increased thirst
Hair loss
Eye irritation

SKIN
Increased sweating
Warm, moist hands
Itching
Hives
Brittle nails

CARDIOVASCULAR
Rapid heartbeat, palpitations
Shortness of breath
High blood pressure

GASTROINTESTINAL
Trembling of the tongue
Increased hunger and food consumption
Increased frequency of bowel movements

MUSCLE
Weakness
Decreased muscle mass

REPRODUCTIVE
Irregular menstrual periods
Cessation of menstrual periods
Decreased fertility

Among the most dreaded complications of an overactive thyroid are the cardiac effects. An overactive thyroid can cause irregular heartbeat and even damage to the heart muscle—damage that, in some patients, can result in heart failure, which may improve after the overactive thyroid is diagnosed and treated. Some patients with Graves' disease may be found to have mitral valve prolapse, a slight deformity that causes a characteristic heart murmur physicians can hear through a stethoscope. Most people with mitral valve prolapse experience no symptoms, but for some, it can cause chest pain and rapid or irregular heartbeat.

An excess of thyroid hormone, regardless of its cause, makes bone lose some of its mineral content. Women, more so than men, who have had an overactive thyroid for a long time can even develop osteoporosis (thinning of the bone), which could predispose them to bone fractures. The greater vulnerability of women stems from the fact that they are more naturally prone to suffer from bone loss and osteoporosis than men. The loss of bone affects mostly the spine and typically exceeds the loss that occurs as a result of menopause. You may lose bone as a result of too much thyroid hormone even if you are not menopausal. Research has shown, however, that once the overactive thyroid is corrected, some mineral buildup occurs in bone within the next two years.[2] Nevertheless, even after the overactive thyroid is corrected, you might have lost significant bone density. To determine whether you have lost bone density as a result of thyroid hormone excess, it is wise to have your doctor order a bone density test a year or two after your overactive thyroid has been corrected.

If you have too much thyroid hormone in your system, you could also be exposed to clotting problems, as the imbalance causes high levels of von Willebrand factor and fibrinogen, which are chemicals that promote clotting.[3] The endothelial cells (cells that cover the inside of blood vessels) are also altered, promoting further clotting problems.

Breast enlargement occurs in nearly a third of men suffering from overactivity of the thyroid. This enlargement, which doctors call gynecomastia, may be minor or significant enough to be troublesome. It is the result of too much estrogen—a consequence of the overactive thyroid in men. If you are a man who has experienced weight loss, anxiety, shakiness, heat intolerance, or other symptoms of an overactive thyroid, and you begin to feel enlargement and tenderness in your breast area, you need to mention it to your doctor and have your thyroid tested.

As with hypothyroidism, the severity of physical and emotional symptoms experienced by hyperthyroid patients does not always correspond to how elevated the thyroid hormone levels are. One study that carefully measured the severity of symptoms among patients with Graves' disease found that symptoms may be mild in people whose thyroid hormone levels are high.[4] It also found that depression and anxiety can be severe in people with mild hyperthyroidism.

If an overactive thyroid remains untreated, the occurrence of severe illness can make the person slip into a thyroid storm, a dreadful condition characterized by mental deterioration, high fever, extreme agitation, and at times heart failure and jaundice.

Mental Effects of Hyperthyroidism

The mental effects of excess thyroid hormone are often described merely as *nervousness* and *hyperactivity*, terms that hide a deeper layer of mental and behavioral instability. In fact, in the mind of many physicians, the term *nervousness* connotes a physical effect (motor restlessness and the need to move around) rather than a mental effect.

Doctors frequently fail to emphasize the wide array of mental effects likely to occur in a hyperthyroid patient. The mental symptoms of hyperthyroidism may precede, or even be more prominent than, the physical symptoms. In fact, hyperthyroidism can precipitate or cause virtually any form of psychiatric condition,[5] although admittedly, psychosis triggered by Graves' disease is an exceptional occurrence nowadays. Anxiety and panicky feelings may be the earliest and most noticeable symptoms of hyperthyroidism. As time passes, the way these symptoms show up changes with the appearance of other symptoms. The most common mental effects that we see in hyperthyroid patients are:

- Social anxiety disorder
- Anxiety
- Restlessness
- Panic attacks
- Depression
- Excessive concerns about physical symptoms
- Disorganized thinking
- Guilt feelings
- Loss of emotional control
- Irritability
- Emotional swings
- Episodes of erratic behavior

- Bipolar disorder, mania, hypomania
- Paranoia
- Aggression

FROM FEELING ELATED TO LOSING TOUCH WITH REALITY

The elation experienced by Nancy and Fred is rarely a stable state characterized by self-confidence and unabated happiness. Although I have seen some patients with an overactive thyroid who stayed in a stable state of elation for months or even years without experiencing the downside of depression, the majority do experience periods of short-lived depression, such as in manicdepression. From a state of mild elation, or hypomania, patients can easily flip into an exaggerated form of elation (that is, mania) in which they lose touch with reality and begin exhibiting abnormal behavior.

Several of my patients have used the analogy that the elation of hyperthyroidism is like being on potent mind-altering drugs. Although your brain is more alert and animated by excessive thinking, your thought processes are disturbed by an inability to focus. You begin to find it hard to think something through in a way that would ultimately make any sense. Your eyes become glassy and your mind unfocused, which prevents sensible conversations. People may think that a hyperthyroid person is on cocaine. The speedy mind also becomes compromised by loss of memory. Impaired cognition coupled with rapid thinking may result in a flow of inconsistent and irrational statements and decisions.

The shift from an elated mood to the severe elation characteristic of mania brings with it confusion, poor judgment, impaired cognition, and abnormal behavior. In severe cases, hallucinations enter the picture. This is when the patient is viewed as "abnormal." The transition from hypomanic to manic behavior may be gradual or abrupt; its onset may occur soon after the beginning of hyperthyroidism or be delayed until long afterward.

Medical literature overflows with cases of acute confusion, "schizophrenialike" psychoses, and paranoia among individuals with Graves' disease. Such descriptions are reminiscent of severe cases of mania or manicdepression. In some persons, unabated, advanced mania promotes criminal or paranoid ideas, distorted thoughts, and even hallucinations and auditory delusions. In the immediately pre–World War II to post–World War II era, many people with an overactive thyroid exhibited such profound disruptions of behavior that they were considered to have severe psychiatric illnesses.

According to some old reports, up to 20 percent of patients with an overactive thyroid had psychotic symptoms.[6] Today, the increased awareness of thyroid disease and more sensitive thyroid testing have allowed earlier diagnosis. Therefore, the number of patients who reach advanced stages of psychosis has been significantly reduced. We now rarely see people becoming delirious or reaching a state in which they hear imaginary sounds, see delusionary visions, or exhibit bizarre behavior. Psychosis caused by hyperthyroidism has no unique features that will make a physician suspect that the thyroid is contributing to the mental condition.[7] It can take the form of an acute affective disorder (i.e., depression or mania) or, less frequently, a schizophreniform paranoia and delirium.

Hypomania caused by an overactive thyroid can evolve into mania and abnormal behavior. Consider Connie, a thirty-four-year-old housewife who began to exhibit mild mania three months after she gave birth. For the first eight months, she felt in full control. In fact, like Fred, her mental capabilities were enhanced to such a point that she felt no one could have known that her behavior was abnormal.

"My mind was very occupied and full all the time," she said. "I could literally go around the clock, even while I slept. I could balance my checkbook in my sleep and wake up in the morning and it would be right. I volunteered for all sorts of positions—clerk for the PTO, room mother at school, assistant at church."

Several months into her hypomanic trip, however, Connie's cognitive ability became impaired. She had difficulty focusing on any particular thought. Her memory was "halfway gone." The evident confusion that set in changed her from a self-confident person to a disorganized and anxious one. Friends began to view Connie as inefficient, disorganized, maybe even "abnormal." She said:

> After a few months, things weren't clear anymore. No longer was I getting the itemized lists in my brain where things were precise. Now they were getting confused, and I couldn't keep up with them. It got to the point where I didn't want to even look at the bills. I just avoided anything that had to do with concentration. I felt like I was losing touch with reality. I felt like a balloon that was about to pop.
>
> It was worse when I tried to sleep. My mind was so full that I had a lot of sleeping problems. I would watch TV until there was nothing else on, and then I would try to go to bed, but I wouldn't be able to fall asleep until about the time my husband would go to work, like five A.M. And then I would sleep, but it was never a comfortable sleep: it would be overwhelmed with thoughts. My mind was like a computer with no more capacity. It was like there was so much up there, I couldn't decipher one thought.
>
> The anxiety was getting worse because I wanted to hold on to reality. I didn't want to lose anything. So I tried keeping everything in my head, but I just couldn't.
>
> I came to a point where I was worrying about my kids, about my marriage, about the bills. But my worrying was abstract because, at the same time, I could not concentrate on the things I was really worried about.

As her symptoms progressed, forgetfulness, confusion, and loss of a sense of reality led to irrational behavior. Connie became unable to handle basic tasks, such as taking care of her children.

One year after the beginning of her hypomania, Connie deteriorated to such an extent that her husband became convinced she needed psychiatric help. In Connie's words:

He kept saying, "If you don't get help and find out what's wrong, you are going to have to go into a hospital. Something is wrong. This is not normal." That word *normal* came up several times. I remember getting quite upset about it. Then it came to a point where I thought getting hospitalized was a good idea. The anxiety that I had, the frustration, the way my husband saw me not knowing which end was up, whether I was coming or going, forgetting to pick up the kids, made him think I was truly becoming crazy.

Connie's self-esteem gradually slipped. She changed from having a normal amount of security and self-esteem and being able to undertake any activity to being unable to do anything right. Amazingly, it took her a year and a half to go see her husband's doctor, who diagnosed her with Graves' disease. As in most patients with Graves' disease, the nature and pattern of Connie's symptoms changed. Connie had clear-cut hypomania for the first few months, during which her mind was creative, fast, and organized. Later, she was on the verge of becoming truly psychotic. If she had not been diagnosed in time, Connie could have reached a confusional state, with delirium and hallucinations. Connie's husband was amazed when he observed his wife regaining her sanity as her overactive thyroid was treated. In most patients, the manic or abnormal behavior improves or even resolves after the imbalance is corrected.[8]

UNCONTROLLABLE ANGER

The emotional responses to what you see or experience take place in the limbic system of the brain, where thyroid hormone plays an important role in regulating the perception of your environment and the way you respond to it emotionally. Whether people exhibit mild mania, depression, or anxiety, the excess thyroid hormone reaching the brain typically causes exaggerated emotional responses to what they see and experience. These responses are expressed as emotional withdrawal (often a component of a depressive state) or, conversely, as loss of emotional control. They become impatient and may inappropriately laugh or cry about matters that would barely affect them under normal circumstances. They often become easily irritated over trivial issues, which may trigger anger or even aggression and violence.

This emotional instability makes such people feel as if they were sitting in a rocking chair on the edge of a cliff, teetering back and forth between being in control and out of control. Most individuals with an overactive thyroid feel their anger levels build up, and then they snap at anyone who comes along. It is indeed a sad place to be in. You don't understand what is making you this way, and if you don't like your behavior, you may think that you have become a bad person.

Mary Lou, a thirty-five-year-old schoolteacher, was referred to me by her gynecologist, who had diagnosed her with Graves' disease. Mary Lou no longer had menstrual periods and was suffering from heat intolerance and a rapid heartbeat, symptoms that had been attributed to early menopause. In my first encounter with Mary Lou, she described the familiar symptoms of impatience and intolerance. Later, she told me:

> Everybody and everything bothered me. I was losing my patience more easily. I had always been very good dealing with people and calming them, but after a while it was, "Mary Lou, you have to calm down. You're not handling this well." Things that would frustrate me would prompt me to react immediately. In some cases, I would have a lot of patience with people initially, and then, when they would go on and on, I would interrupt and ask them to get to the point quickly.
>
> I had a very short fuse with my children, which was odd. I was known to most people as a very patient person. I teach Sunday school, and I couldn't do that anymore. I didn't even have enough patience to read the lesson and to teach it. My co-teacher said I needed help. She told me that I had been teaching Sunday school too long and needed a break. That's the way she put it.
>
> I felt the worst about my oldest son. Being a teenager, he couldn't do anything to satisfy me. If I said, "Take out the trash," he didn't take it out fast enough. If I said, "Put away your clothes," he didn't fold them fast enough. Everything that happened was surrounded by the word *fast*. It was like my mind no longer controlled my emotions. My emotions were in total control of my mind.

Some of my patients have described the loss of control and altered behavior related to hyperthyroidism as "Graves' madness" because they felt their acts and behaviors were typical of craziness. People may become belligerent and domineering, or have spells of anger and irritability interspersed with intermittent free-floating anxiety, leading to irrational behavior and inappropriate decisions.

WAVES OF ANXIETY
Undoubtedly, the most common mental effect of an overactive thyroid is anxiety. The anxiety due to hyperthyroidism, however, is seldom a pure form of anxiety disorder. It is an exaggerated form in which the increased worrying and overall feeling of insecurity and instability are worsened by mood swings,

anger, inability to focus, and foggy memory. Often, these mental effects exacerbate each other, resulting in a tumultuous mental state. Along with the insidious intrusion of anxiety, panic attacks are another form of anxiety disorder that often appears.

The rising tide of thyroid hormone in the blood and the flooding of brain cells with thyroid hormone often produce unusual feelings. You feel as if you are going to suffocate or your soul is about to leave you. Your heart starts beating very fast. Your palms become sweaty, and you may break out in a generalized sweat. The inability to control your body takes over. You have not passed out but feel you are about to. You may get dizzy. The world around you looks strange, almost unrecognizable.

You also feel frightened—a feeling that actually begins at the peak of despair. After the sense of despair plateaus and then wanes gradually, you feel drained. Then you try to rationalize and understand what happened—to your mind and to your body. The first time this sensation strikes, you might recognize it as a panic attack. You want to pick up the phone and call a friend, your spouse, or a relative and share these feelings. Now that the anxiety attack has resolved, you are exhausted, wanting only to rest and understand what just happened to you.

A few days later, in the same unpredictable fashion as the previous time, another wave of anxiety attacks you. You panic and try to fight it. In the process, your symptoms get worse and worse. You desperately try to figure out what is wrong with you, feeling that your life is out of control and no longer your own, until finally all you feel is exhaustion. This lasts only a couple of hours, and life resumes its course.

Quite often you are embarrassed by these feelings or even frightened to discuss them with the people closest to you. Having panic attacks induces a constant fear. Because these episodes come and go unpredictably, you worry that you might experience the next one when you are closing a business deal or talking with people at a dinner party. Between these attacks, you may be seized by a chronic, constant anxiety. While you should be concentrating on a task at work, your brain goes on automatic pilot. It drifts off the task you are performing, and gradually the worries and anxiety worsen and take over your mind so your concentration is sporadic and you cannot remember what you are supposed to be doing. This irritates and upsets you. You don't understand why you are reacting this way. As anxiety builds up, you, your closest friend, or your spouse notices that you are becoming a different person.

Your moods swing and are no longer stable. In the morning, you may be happy and outgoing, making plans and excited about new projects. Two hours later, you become angry, irritable, even sad. You may be at work and this wave of sadness will drain your energy and your desire to function normally and be productive. You want to be by yourself. You have difficulty controlling your anger, and you may respond to someone in a nasty way. The waves of anxiety, constant worries, and mood swings build up, affect and reinforce one another, and slowly transform your personality.

I saw Linda for a second opinion two years after she was diagnosed with Graves' disease. She was in great despair and had almost given up on the possibility of leading a normal life again. Approximately two years before the diagnosis was made, she was thirty-six and working in a stable job as a secretary. As a result of downsizing at her company, however, her workload had doubled. She always felt behind and unable to accomplish her assigned tasks. Her stress level mounted and she began to worry about the financial repercussions if she were to lose her job. She then began noticing changes in her health.

"I started experiencing symptoms of nervousness, irritability, and increased anger," Linda said. "I was losing weight but didn't really pay attention to that. The symptoms progressed and became more intense as the months passed. I was attributing the way I was feeling to nerves, stress, and emotional reactions to things in my life, especially to my job situation."

For the first three to four months, the predominant symptoms revolved around anxiety:

> It was a disabling anxiety. I felt like I couldn't breathe, and I would become very dizzy and disoriented. The world did not look real to me any longer. It was like a disorienting feeling. I was having heart palpitations and was short of breath. It was embarrassing to be in a public place, so I would retreat somewhere to try and stop the feeling. The anxiety would occur randomly. I soon developed a fear of anticipating it happening in grocery stores, the post office, the office, in almost any setting. I had no control. I didn't know when it would happen. There was no connection or any way I could logically tie it together. The intense wave would come on maybe three or four times a day, lasting no more than ten to fifteen minutes, and wane off over an hour. Then I would be drained and exhausted. I knew it was not a realistic reaction, that I had nothing to fear. But it's hard to correlate your brain to your body.

Linda began to exhibit a fear of crowded or confined places (agoraphobia), although such circumstances had never frightened her before. People with agoraphobia have difficulty traveling away from home because unfamiliar places, which they perceive as unsafe, trigger panic attacks.

Four to five months later, Linda began to experience other symptoms in addition to her recurrent panic attacks:

> It felt like a furnace burning inside my body, and the temperature was not adjustable. No matter how cold my external environment was, I was raging inside with heat. There were days I would open the freezer door and put my head in to get relief from the heat intolerance.

I was going through a lot of symptoms that I was dismissing and trying to ignore. I was eating many times a day, and after I finished a meal, I had frequent bowel movements, almost immediately. Then I started having nausea and light-headedness. I lost hair from all over my head. I had terrible night sweats. My eyes had begun to bulge. At first, they just seemed larger. The people around me did not notice it. I had a dry, gritty feeling in my eyes. Nobody could figure it out. I went to an ophthalmologist, who didn't pick it up and attributed it to allergies.

The tremors began about the same time. I felt I was shaking all over my body, and more so in my hands. It was difficult even to squeeze toothpaste onto a toothbrush. I had to steady my arms. I would drop things. I couldn't polish my fingernails. I couldn't read my own handwriting. Anything that required any dexterity at all was lost to me. I was very short of breath. It would make me short of breath going up a short staircase. I had a lot of muscle weakness in my arms and legs. I couldn't get up from a squatting position. My legs were so weak, I had difficulty even climbing the stairs.

When I finally decided something had to happen, I was afraid I had muscular dystrophy. The muscle weakness was what made me go to the doctor.

The muscular effects of hyperthyroidism can cause weakness so severe that patients have difficulty walking, which often leads doctors to suspect a neurological condition. Some patients with muscle weakness due to hyperthyroidism may be confined to wheelchairs until the hyperthyroidism is diagnosed and treated. Linda was so disturbed by her muscle weakness that she rushed to see a physician, who referred her to a neurologist. Although extensive neurological testing was done, the results came back normal, and her Graves' disease remained undiagnosed.

In addition to Linda's anxiety feelings, which were heightened when her muscle weakness became quite pronounced, her moods changed frequently. Sometimes she was exhilarated; other times she exhibited symptoms of depression.

Finally, a chance encounter gave Linda the clue she so desperately needed:

After a full year of symptoms, I went to a party. A total stranger noted my glassy eyes and my nervousness. She asked me if I had a thyroid condition. That was the breakthrough. She told me she had Graves' disease herself and that I appeared to have the same thing. I was shocked and relieved. I knew a little bit about it because President Bush and his wife had recently been diagnosed with it. Two days later, I saw an endocrinologist who confirmed the diagnosis and started me on treatment.

DEPRESSION

The occurrence of depression in hyperthyroidism may seem paradoxical because depression has been linked primarily with an *under*active thyroid. It is rare, however, for hyperthyroidism to cause clinical depression that warrants admission to a psychiatric ward.[9] In some, antidepressants may aggravate the situation and only treatment that normalizes thyroid levels dispels the depression. People may become depressed as a result of too much thyroid hormone because of their predisposition to depression. One doctor described a patient who developed depression during both hyperthyroidism and hypothyroidism,[10] leading the doctor to conclude that the person's underlying makeup is important in determining the effect. Depressed patients suffering from hyperthyroidism tend to experience more insomnia, weight loss, agitation, anxiety, muscle pains, and fatigue than depressed patients who have a normal thyroid level.[11]

Alicia suffered from depression as a result of hyperthyroidism. She became hyperthyroid six months after she had a baby. Because her husband was a student, Alicia had to work overtime to support her family. She and her physician initially attributed her depression and anxiety to working too much. She said:

> At first, I had headaches to the point where the upper left part of my face would feel numb. My physician told me I had migraine headaches. I became withdrawn. I was tired, lost interest in everything, and started having suicidal thoughts. I felt I did too much. I would go to bed and sleep from six to ten, get up for an hour and eat dinner, and go back to sleep until the next morning and still be exhausted.
>
> I had a lot of guilt feelings and lost interest in regular activities. I could not cope with problems. If I had a problem with my husband or child, I would overreact. I would break down in tears. I was very irritable and became intolerant of my child.

Many of Alicia's symptoms satisfied the criteria for depression. Although the depression can be mild, as in Alicia's case, occasionally a hyperthyroid person may slip into a major depression. In fact, major depressive disorders accompanied by generalized anxiety disorders are much more common in patients with hyperthyroidism than in people without thyroid disease.

PHYSICAL AND MENTAL EXHAUSTION

Physicians and patients often associate fatigue with hypothyroidism and hyperactivity with hyperthyroidism. Yet in a significant number of patients suffering from thyroid hormone excess, tiredness and exhaustion may be the initial and most prominent symptoms. As in hypothyroidism, the fatigue caused by hyperthyroidism is both physical and mental.

In some patients, fatigue can be extreme. One middle-aged woman who was suffering from hyperthyroidism said, "You feel you're dragging yourself through the day. I remember standing at the supermarket waiting at the checkout counter. A friend came up behind me and carefully bumped me to get my attention. I was so exhausted that I didn't even react to it. I turned around and just looked at her."

Suzanne, a twenty-four-year-old salesperson in a clothing store who had always been energetic and enthusiastic, began complaining of fatigue and other annoying symptoms three months before her wedding date. She blamed her fatigue and symptoms on doing too much as well as stress from her wedding preparations. Her symptoms were in fact due to hyperthyroidism. She was diagnosed with Graves' disease one year after she got married.

Here's how she described the beginning of her symptoms:

I was really tired. I'd sleep ten hours a night and still be tired at work. On my days off, I would lie on the sofa. It wasn't a lack of exercise because at my job I am walking all the time. That was the most annoying thing. It wasn't like a good fatigue but just a constant irritant. Not like after you've done a hard day's work. I would wake up and feel better in the morning, and then three hours later I would be tired again. My heart rate was increasing. It was kind of scary. I would turn up the air conditioner, and my fiancé would be freezing. I was so hot. I was sweating, and I only had the sheet on me. I had hot and cold flashes. Whatever I did, it didn't really help.

When I would have headaches, I wouldn't even be able to think clearly. I wouldn't even be able to speak clearly. I felt like my vision changed. I just thought I was getting older and didn't have as much enthusiasm or energy. I started a walking program, but it did not help increase my energy. It would make me even more tired, and I couldn't understand why. That is when I would have the heart palpitations because I would push myself.

I withdrew from people. I was too tired to open my mouth and waste my breath to talk to them.

As illustrated by the cases described above, each person may experience a different pattern of mental effects besides the fatigue, although most people suffer from anxiety and intellectual deficit. These differences have to do to some extent with the differences in personality makeup. Some people with very high thyroid hormone levels experience few or no mental effects. In contrast, some people with marginal or low-grade hyperthyroidism (discussed in the next section) suffer a great deal from anxiety, tiredness, depression, and mood swings.

Low-Grade Hyperthyroidism

Recently, doctors have become more aware of the wide range of physical and mental effects of low-grade hyperthyroidism. This condition is defined as thyroid hormone excess that has not yet resulted in abnormally high thyroid hormone levels but has caused TSH levels to become low. Low-grade hyperthyroidism (called subclinical hyperthyroidism) often results from an overactive thyroid gland due to Graves' disease or to thyroid lumps that produce excessive amounts of thyroid hormone. It may also result from taking too much thyroid hormone. Low-grade hyperthyroidism due to Graves' disease may resolve spontaneously. Even if it resolves, it can recur down the road. Low-grade hyperthyroidism can progress into more severe hyperthyroidism and can exacerbate cardiac problems in patients who have heart disease.

Low-grade hyperthyroidism may induce depression, rapid heartbeat, weight loss, heat intolerance, increased appetite, increased sweating, and trembling of the fingers. It is likely to make a person more irritable and anxious.[12] This minimal thyroid hormone excess can also result in bone loss over time, particularly in postmenopausal women.[13] Although minimal thyroid hormone excess can also affect the bone density of premenopausal women, this negative effect on the bone is counterbalanced by estrogens. Low-grade hyperthyroidism may provoke heart rhythm problems in older people. In addition, it can disturb the functioning of the heart[14] and lower cardiovascular fitness.

Hyperthyroid People at Work

Job performance is frequently affected by an overactive thyroid. In extreme cases, patients can even become mentally and emotionally disabled. Often they resign from their jobs or are fired because they could not cope with the demands. When they seek other job opportunities, they are frequently unsuccessful because of their appearance, cognitive impairment, or inability to handle themselves well during interviews (displaying erratic behavior or a short temper, for example). Let's look at how the mental effects of hyperthyroidism can interfere with one's job.

At twenty-nine, Amy had been working at a paper company for five years. Although her job performance had been excellent, when Amy became hyperthyroid she got irritable and could not maintain a good working relationship with other employees. "Everything bothered me at work. I worked in the sales office, but I handled a situation on the retail floor badly, and the owner of the company heard part of the story. He came back and yelled at me in front of a whole group of people. I couldn't take it. I couldn't erase it from my mind. I wasn't getting paid enough money to deal with the public humiliation. It was so stressful, I decided to leave."

Another patient, Sabrina, who was a department store assistant manager, was terminated from her position because she couldn't cope with the demands of her work. As Sabrina put it:

My boss kept asking me, "Why aren't you working?" I was trying to express to him how sick I was. Finally, they asked me to leave. I spent several months job hunting, to no avail.

I was shaking and looking wild-eyed. I had dropped sixteen pounds. I was probably looking a little emaciated. People probably thought I was a drug addict or an alcoholic because I was antsy and nervous. I felt insult added to injury when no one hired me or called me back. I was sensitive about my nervous behavior and mannerisms. I was aware I was talking very fast. I had to be very careful and monitor how quickly I spoke. Yet I didn't realize just how fast I was talking. People couldn't even understand me.

The fact that I was not hired compounded everything. Even when I was diagnosed, I thought it was the beginning of getting out of this vicious circle. But it took some time after my thyroid was regulated to find a suitable job.

Questionnaire:
The Physical Symptoms of Hyperthyroidism

An easy way to determine the likelihood that you may be suffering from hyperthyroidism is to complete the following questionnaire.

Have your nails been brittle or separating from the nail bed?	Yes	No	___
Has your skin been unusually warm?	Yes	No	___
Have you been sweating more than usual?	Yes	No	___
Have you been experiencing hair loss?	Yes	No	___
Have you become intolerant of heat?	Yes	No	___
Have your menstrual periods become scanty?	Yes	No	___
Have you been unusually hungry?	Yes	No	___
Have you been experiencing diarrhea or increasingly frequent bowel movements?	Yes	No	___
Do your fingers shake constantly?	Yes	No	___
Has your heartbeat been rapid at rest?	Yes	No	___
Have you lost more than five pounds without changing your dietary and exercise habits?	Yes	No	___
Do you get short of breath with exertion, or has your tolerance to exercise been reduced?	Yes	No	___
Have you been experiencing generalized muscle weakness?	Yes	No	___
Are your palms sweaty?	Yes	No	___

If you answered yes to four or more of the preceding questions, you may be hyperthyroid. If you answered yes to six or more of the questions, you are probably hyperthyroid.

Other Hyperthyroid Conditions

Even though Graves' disease accounts for 70 percent of the cases of over-active thyroid that are routinely diagnosed, you need to make sure that your overactive thyroid is not the result of another thyroid disorder that can be easily confused with Graves' disease. For instance, some patients have an overactive thyroid because one or more lumps (called nodules) within the thyroid gland are autonomous and overactive. These nodules take over the function of the entire gland but produce more thyroid hormone than the body normally requires. This condition, which is common in older people, is called a simple toxic nodule or a multinodular toxic goiter, depending on whether the gland has one nodule or whether several of the hyperfunctioning nodules begin to grow independently from the rest of the gland.

To confirm these disorders, your doctor will order a nuclear thyroid scan and uptake. The nuclear medicine doctor will have you ingest a tiny amount of radioactive iodine, which will be readily picked up by the thyroid gland and can be detected when the thyroid area is scanned. Six and twenty-four hours after you ingest the radioactive iodine, a counting probe placed over your neck will detect the radioactivity present in your thyroid. High scores on this radioactive iodine uptake test tell your physician that your thyroid is overworking and producing excess levels of thyroid hormone. The pictures taken of your thyroid (scan) will show the overactive nodule(s).

Doctors can treat simple toxic nodules and multinodular goiters by administering radioactive iodine to destroy the overactive areas or by performing surgery aimed at removing the portion of the gland that contains the toxic nodules. Medications are not an option, as they are for patients with Graves' disease.

An excess of thyroid hormone may also result from silent thyroiditis and subacute thyroiditis, two conditions that cause a temporary destruction of thyroid cells that leak too much of the preformed thyroid hormone into the bloodstream while the cells are being destroyed. These conditions are easily confused with Graves' disease.

Silent thyroiditis is the result of what is believed to be a transient immune attack on the thyroid gland that produces hyperthyroidism. The hyperthyroidism is often mild and lasts only a few weeks, although in some cases it can go on for as long as three months.

After resolution of the inflammation and (temporary) damage to the thyroid gland, you may become hypothyroid for a few weeks because the damage to the thyroid renders the gland unable to meet your body's demands. After a few weeks of hypothyroidism, the thyroid repairs itself, leading to regeneration of a normally functioning gland. Your gland may not fully recover, however, and you may have residual permanent hypothyroidism. If you consult your physician during the initial period, when your thyroid levels are still high, it is sometimes difficult to tell whether you have silent thyroiditis or Graves' disease. A radioactive iodine uptake count will differentiate between the two conditions, however. Typically, a high count indicates the overactivity characteristic of Graves' disease, and a low uptake indicates the temporary destruction characteristic of silent thyroiditis.

A similar scenario occurs when the cause of your hyperthyroidism is subacute thyroiditis. This is a viral infection of the gland that results in temporary destruction followed by transient hypothyroidism and then recovery. This condition is often more easily diagnosed because you are likely to suffer from fever and pain in your neck area that may spread to one or both ears. Many viruses can cause subacute thyroiditis, including those that have been tied to the common cold, mumps, and measles. The key test to confirm that your hyperthyroidism is caused by subacute thyroiditis is the radioactive iodine uptake count, which will be low in subacute thyroiditis and high in Graves' disease.

Prior to the infection of the gland, you may experience a sore throat, pains, aches, headaches, fever, and a cough. During the hot phase, most physicians prescribe nonsteroidal anti-inflammatory drugs and a beta-blocker. One of three patients with subacute thyroiditis may need cortisone treatment because the inflammation is severe and the pain excruciating. At times, the gland may remain inflamed for several months even after thyroid levels have returned to normal. Taking cortisone may then be the solution. Even though the majority of people who experience subacute thyroiditis regain normal thyroid function down the road, some patients may remain permanently hypothyroid. One study showed that twenty-eight years after an episode of subacute thyroiditis, 15 percent of patients require thyroid hormone treatment for residual hypothyroidism.[15] Although steroids are helpful for the symptoms, they do not prevent permanent hypothyroidism. The message here is that you need to have your thyroid retested down the road to make sure that you have not become hypothyroid.

The following table summarizes the diagnostic characteristics of the most common causes of hyperthyroidism.

CAUSES OF HYPERTHYROIDISM

	TSH	Thyroid Hormone Levels	Radioactive Iodine Uptake
Graves' disease	Low	High	High
Single toxic nodule	Low	High	High
Multinodular toxic goiter	Low	High	High
Silent thyroiditis	Low	High	Low
Subacute thyroiditis (viral)	Low	High	Low
TSH excess*	Normal/high	High	High

*Such as from a tumor in the pituitary gland or a dysregulation of the pituitary cells that manufacture TSH.

Hyperthyroidism in Older People

Hyperthyroidism is quite common in older people, affecting approximately 1.5 percent of men and 1.9 percent of women older than sixty.[16] The effects of hyperthyroidism on older people are often different from those experienced by younger people. With respect to physical symptoms, thyroid enlargement, intolerance to heat, increased perspiration, and increased appetite are not as common in older people. Heart problems, however, such as atrial fibrillation, as well as weight loss and reduced appetite, increase in frequency with aging.[17] In addition, constipation (a symptom typical of hypothyroidism), depression, and decrease in muscle mass leading to weakness are quite common. Muscle weakness due to hyperthyroidism may predispose older patients to fall and further injure themselves. The falling is frequently attributed to other illnesses before the correct diagnosis is made.

Because the consequences of hyperthyroidism in older people are general and are so similar to many other health problems, even hospital physicians often diagnose the condition incorrectly. In one study of hospitalized hyperthyroid patients, the diagnosis was suspected in only one-third of the patients.[18] For those who require hospitalization, psychiatric diagnosis is the most common reason for hospital admissions. Debility and cardiac failure with atrial fibrillation also account for a large number of admissions.

The differences in symptoms are not only physical. The first adverse effects of hyperthyroidism in older people may be mental. These effects are frequently overlooked or attributed to aging. Instead of being overactive, hyperdynamic, and overwhelmed by anxiety and irritability or exhibiting mania, older people often experience withdrawal and depression. The effect of thyroid hormone excess on the minds of older people may be quite significant and manifests frequently as dementia, confusion, and apathy. They may even experience delirium. Increased nervousness, often experienced by young people, is not as common in older patients.

Older people often suffer from what doctors call "apathetic hyperthyroidism," characterized by depression, apathy, and intellectual stupor. Patients with apathetic hyperthyroidism experience exhaustion, slowing of physical and mental activity, and an expressionless face. Because this appearance and change in personality are usually ascribed to aging, the disease frequently goes undiagnosed for a long time.

Hospitals' use of imaging procedures, such as CT scans, may trigger hyperthyroidism from the iodine that is administered to provide sufficient contrast. An older person admitted to the hospital for evaluation of a cardiac or kidney condition may return home and start suffering from an altered state of mind or even delirium within a few days.

How an excess of thyroid hormone affects the brain depends on age and perhaps personality. Overactive thyroid may affect the mind in different ways. The end result is often a mixture of anxiety, emotional and behavioral changes, mood swings, anger, poor stress-coping mechanisms, impaired cognitive ability, inability to cope with job demands, and family problems. One patient described all these effects lumped together as "a monster inside me." Fortunately, you have many options at your disposal to help you tame this monster.

Important Points to Remember

- If you have been experiencing weight loss, jitteriness, tremors, increased sweating, or palpitations, you could be suffering from an overactive thyroid. But these are physical symptoms. While you are hyperthyroid, it is not unusual to become hypomanic and talkative and to feel as if you are on top of the world.
- Depression, waves of anger, anxiety, and lethargy could be symptoms of an overactive thyroid; mood swings and loss of touch with reality are also typical.
- If you are experiencing episodic panic attacks characterized by feeling out of control and a rapid heartbeat, you may have an overactive thyroid. Describe these symptoms in detail to your doctor.
- Although Graves' disease accounts for 70 percent of cases of hyperthyroidism, there are other causes, too, including transient hyperthyroidism due to temporary destruction of thyroid cells.
- As you get older, the symptoms of overactive thyroid are not necessarily the same as the symptoms typically experienced by younger people. With aging, an overactive thyroid tends to cause more depression, lethargy, muscle weakness, and heart symptoms.

7

GETTING THE
PROPER DIAGNOSIS

For years, the public has received conflicting information on how to diagnose a thyroid imbalance properly. Some holistic doctors and alternative practitioners may diagnose you as hypothyroid if you suffer from tiredness and other symptoms of low metabolism. They will use your basal (resting) temperature as an index of low thyroid and will monitor the treatment by having you check your basal temperature three to four times a day. Some doctors will treat your allergies, asthma, hair loss, dry skin, and gastrointestinal upset with thyroid hormone, believing that you have an underactive thyroid even if your blood tests are normal. They may tell you that thyroid hormone is not working well in your body and you need thyroid hormone treatment because you are hypothyroid. Many conventional doctors, in contrast, go strictly by blood tests and believe that you have a thyroid imbalance only if your blood tests are clearly out of the normal range.

Because of these differences of opinion, some people have remained undiagnosed even though they sought medical help, whereas others have been subjected to inappropriate and overzealous treatments that are damaging to their overall emotional and physical health. To avoid these pitfalls, you need to know about the most reliable tests for evaluating your thyroid and how to interpret them in light of your symptoms. That way, you won't fall through the cracks and fail to receive the help that you need from your doctor.

Before it was possible to measure blood levels of thyroid hormones, the common practice was to go by indirect clues, such as:

- Basal temperature (an indirect way of measuring a person's metabolism), which is low in patients who are hypothyroid
- Cholesterol levels, which are high in people with hypothyroidism and low in those with hyperthyroidism

- The level of iodine in the blood, which is low in hypothyroidism and high in hyperthyroidism
- Achilles reflex time (how long it takes the Achilles tendon to relax after contraction), which is slow in hypothyroidism and faster in hyperthyroidism

For years the blood levels of the hormones T4 and T3 and of the pituitary hormone TSH have been used to diagnose thyroid hormone imbalance. The pituitary is like a finely tuned sensor that detects even a subtle deficit or excess of thyroid hormone. A deficit of thyroid hormone in the blood will cause TSH to rise, and an excess of thyroid hormone will make it fall.

TSH is now recognized as the most sensitive measurement for alerting doctors to a thyroid imbalance.[1] When the levels of thyroid hormone change slightly, they will often remain within the normal range even though the TSH has already become abnormal. In fact, the majority of those who suffer from low-grade hypothyroidism or low-grade hyperthyroidism have T4 and T3 levels within the normal laboratory range. The normal range for thyroid hormone levels is very wide and is established by averaging the levels obtained from large numbers of people. Because what is a "normal" level of thyroid hormone differs from one person to the next, the normal range used in laboratories needs to be wide enough to include many people. For instance, in many laboratories, the normal levels for T4 range from 5 to 12 mcg/dL of serum, and those for T3 range from 90 to 220 ng/dL per deciliter.

Technological advances now allow doctors to measure TSH levels in a very sensitive way, both far below the lower limit and far above the upper limit of the normal range. In general, a normal TSH is between 0.4 and 4.5 mIU/L. The greater the excess of thyroid hormone, the lower the TSH below the normal range; the greater the deficit, the higher the TSH above the normal range. Now doctors can detect any minute excess or deficit of thyroid hormone resulting from an over- or underactive thyroid or from taking too much or too little thyroid hormone medication.

This sounds very straightforward. If your TSH level falls within the normal laboratory range, then your thyroid gland is viewed as working properly. If it is high, your doctor will diagnose you with an underactive thyroid; if it is low, your doctor will suspect an overactive thyroid and will measure your thyroid hormone levels, which will be expected to be high. But it is not as straightforward as it sounds. Increasingly, more and more physicians believe that you can be suffering from hypothyroidism even though your blood tests, including TSH, are in the normal laboratory range.

The Controversy Over Hypothyroidism with Normal Blood Tests

Nothing is more irritating for people suffering from tiredness, low mood, and inability to control their weight than to be told that their TSH is normal, only to be told some years later, upon being retested, that they are hypothyroid. During the intervening period, they have continued to suffer needlessly, and their thyroid gland, which was already slightly deficient, has been further damaged, resulting in an even greater thyroid deficit.

How could that be? A person might ask, "My TSH was 3 two years ago, and now it has gone up to 12. Was I hypothyroid then?" Yes, indeed, that might have been the case. The principal reason for the difficulty in detecting a low-grade underactive thyroid when doctors use this most sophisticated and sensitive thyroid test is that, as with T4 and T3, a normal laboratory reading for TSH is established based on levels measured in a large number of people. What is normal for your TSH level may differ dramatically from what is normal for mine.

Here's an example. Let's suppose that your normal TSH level is 0.6 mIU/L when your thyroid is working well. But as a result of a minimal deficit due to Hashimoto's thyroiditis, your TSH went up to 3 or 4. Your body and your pituitary gland had sensed the deficit, and the pituitary had reacted to it, raising the TSH to almost six times its original level. But a doctor may interpret a TSH level of 3 or 4 as normal and assure you that you have no thyroid problems.

In short, many people may be suffering from minute imbalances that have not yet resulted in abnormal blood tests. If we included people with low-grade hypothyroidism whose blood tests are normal, the frequency of hypothyroidism would no doubt exceed 10 percent of the population. What is of special concern, though, is that many people whose test results are dismissed as normal could continue to have symptoms of an underactive thyroid. Their moods, emotions, and overall well-being are affected by this imbalance, yet they are not receiving the care they need to get to the root of their problems.

You don't need to be a thyroid expert to realize from what I have said so far that if your TSH is close to the upper limit of the normal range set by laboratories, you have a higher risk of being low-grade hypothyroid. In fact, researchers are beginning to recognize the upper segment of the normal range as suspicious for hypothyroidism. Nearly a third of patients who are receiving thyroid hormone replacement for hypothyroidism or have a goiter and whose TSH level is in the suspicious range turn out to be hypothyroid when they are evaluated by TRH stimulation testing (a procedure that measures TSH after injection of thyrotropin-releasing hormone into the bloodstream). One study showed that more than 50 percent of women who have a positive antithyroid antibody marker for Hashimoto's thyroiditis and a TSH level ranging between 2 and 4.5 (considered normal) became clearly hypothyroid (showed a definite elevation of TSH) within ten years.[2] Even when this marker was absent, 30 percent of women with a TSH level in this high-normal range became clearly hypothyroid.

Another study also showed that LDL cholesterol, which is increased in hypothyroidism, can be lowered with fairly small doses of thyroid hormone in persons whose TSH level ranges between 2 and 4.5 mIU/L.[3] Recent research has also shown that people having a TSH level in the high-normal range are at a significantly increased risk of suffering from recurrent depression.[4] In short, many people who have a TSH level in the upper segment of the normal range may be suffering from low-grade hypothyroidism, particularly if they have the destructive disorder of Hashimoto's thyroiditis. After the publication of the first edition of *The Thyroid Solution,* medical associations such as the American Association of Clinical Endocrinologists began debating whether the upper limit of normal should be lowered. Some thyroid experts have recommended lowering the upper limit of the TSH reference range from 4.5 to 2.5 mIU/L because analysis of TSH levels in the general population has shown that the majority of people considered to be normal have a TSH less than 2.5.

In 2002, the American Association of Clinical Endocrinologists proposed that patients who have a TSH higher than 3.0 should be considered for treatment.[5] Despite this trend in thinking, there is still a great resistance among experts in the field of thyroid disease who feel that lowering the upper cutoff of the normal range to 2.5 or 3.0 could create health hazards and economic hardship on our society. They feel that many people whose TSH ranges between 3.0 and 4.5 do not have an underactive thyroid, and this is true. However, many people whose TSH is between 3 and 4.5 do have an underactive thyroid and do have symptoms. It is obvious that lowering the upper limit of the normal range to 2.5 or 3 will imply that any patient found to have a TSH higher than these levels will be treated with thyroid hormone. Based on an analysis performed by a group of thyroid experts,[6] if the upper limit of normal was lowered to 3.0, an estimate of 6.4–7.9 percent of the U.S. population older than twelve years of age (which represents 12.8 million to 16 million people) who would be viewed as having a normal thyroid by current standards would be diagnosed as having hypothyroidism. And if the upper limit is lowered to 2.5, 22 million to 28 million people who are currently considered as having normal thyroid levels will be diagnosed as having low-grade hypothyroidism. The analysis is quite correct: lowering the upper cutoff of the normal range to 2.5 or 3.0 mIU/L will promote thyroid hormone prescriptions that are not necessary, and potentially harmful, for many people. On the other hand, one of five people having a TSH between 3 and 5 have positive antithyroid antibodies. We are simply dealing with test results that

are in the gray zone that separate normal from abnormal. While I do not advocate lowering the cutoff to 2.5 mIU/L and I do not advocate automatic
thyroid treatment for anyone who has a TSH greater than 2.5, I do not advocate dismissal of those who have a TSH level in the gray zone and who have
symptoms or evidence of an autoimmune thyroid disease. It is also not uncommon to see TSH levels fluctuate, going from high normal to levels slightly
above the normal range. It is as if the pituitary were trying to adjust normal
function from one day to the next. These fluctuations often confuse doctors
and make them suspect laboratory errors. "How could a person be hypothyroid one day and normal the next?" is a lament I've heard a number of times
from other doctors. In fact, when the deficit in thyroid hormone is minimal,
the TSH level rises slightly and could be vacillating up and down across the
line marking the upper limit of the laboratory normal range, leading to confusion and misdiagnosis.

Even if the TSH level is in the lower segment of the normal range, a person may still be suffering from low-grade hypothyroidism. If you have symptoms of an underactive thyroid and a goiter, an underactive thyroid may be
uncovered by a TRH test.[7]

The wide range of normal levels for TSH is not the only reason someone
could be hypothyroid despite normal blood tests. Another possible reason
(not scientifically established yet) is that even though a person may have a
healthy thyroid gland that produces adequate amounts of thyroid hormones,
the hormones may not work efficiently in the body. Once the thyroid hormone T4 has reached cells, it is converted to T3, the most active form of
thyroid hormone. Here it interacts with genes and becomes involved in a
wide range of regulations of metabolism and a myriad of biological effects.

It turns out that the amount of the active form of thyroid hormone is
regulated locally in bodily organs as well. This regulation is the most ancient
from an evolutionary perspective, having developed much earlier than the
appearance of the pituitary gland. In primitive vertebrates such as lampreys,
the main mechanism for regulating thyroid balance is found within organs[8]
and the central mechanism of hypothalamic/pituitary control is nonexistent.
As animals evolved to rely more on the thyroid gland to manufacture thyroid
hormone, the hypothalamic/pituitary mechanism became the major system
of regulation. Local regulation in organs gradually became a secondary mechanism that controls the availability of the right amount of active thyroid hormone and its effects in target tissue.

It is conceivable that some people may have an abnormality in the process of regulation in the organs that is designed to deliver the right amount of
thyroid hormone to the metabolic machinery of the cells. People with this
type of abnormal regulation may suffer from many symptoms of low metabolism and low thyroid.

Dr. Gordon R. B. Skinner advocated in the *British Medical Journal* a trial of thyroid hormone treatment for about three months in people suffering from symptoms of hypothyroidism.[9] He believes that many people may be hypothyroid despite having normal blood tests.

The emerging evidence that one can be hypothyroid despite normal blood tests explains the common frustration among people who do not get help despite suffering from tiredness, low mood, and difficulty concentrating. It is one of the reasons why many patients turn to naturopathic doctors or other alternative practitioners after having tried to get relief from conventional physicians. A large number of naturopathic doctors prescribe thyroid hormone for symptoms of underactive thyroid in people having normal blood tests. At this time, however, there is no scientific basis for recommending thyroid hormone treatment to patients who have normal thyroid glands. If your doctor prescribes this treatment, you need to pay attention to the doses prescribed. Make sure that your thyroid levels and TSH remain normal and are monitored regularly during the treatment.

Problems with Thyroid Testing

A number of common drugs can affect TSH scores, including the following medications that tend to increase TSH:

- Amiodarone
- Haloperidol
- Metoclopramide
- Lithium
- Morphine
- Aminoglutethimide

The following drugs tend to decrease TSH:

- Cortisone and other glucocorticoids
- Dopamine
- Anabolic steroids
- Heparin
- Somatostatin analogues

If you are suffering from depression or an anxiety disorder, you may have a low TSH reading even though you do not have a thyroid disorder. Research has shown that up to 30 percent of patients suffering from major depression not due to a thyroid condition have a slightly low TSH level.[10] This is presumably caused by signals sent by the brain to the pituitary gland in response to depression. Often the TSH reading becomes normal when the depression or anxiety disorder is treated.

Beyond TSH

Once the TSH test shows evidence of a thyroid imbalance, the next step is to determine the severity of the imbalance. For an underactive thyroid, TSH is very reliable at providing your doctor with a precise measure of the severity of the deficit. The higher the TSH, the more severe the hypothyroidism. In contrast, for an overactive thyroid, TSH has little value for determining the severity of the excess of thyroid hormone in your system.

Another series of tests can be especially helpful in assessing the severity of a thyroid hormone deficit or excess. These include measurements of T4 and T3 uptake and free T4 and T3 levels. To understand these tests, let's take a look at how thyroid hormone gets around inside the body.

Thyroid hormone in the bloodstream is bound to proteins that carry it to the organs. This bloodstream hormone represents a form of reserve. One of the main carrying proteins is thyroid-binding globulin (TBG), which is produced in the liver and can be affected by illnesses, liver disease, and medications such as estrogens. The carrying proteins have bound to them more than 99 percent of the thyroid hormone found in the bloodstream. Therefore, total T4 and T3 levels can be high or low if the amount of these proteins is high or low. For example, a woman who is pregnant or takes estrogen will have high T4 levels (sometimes far above the upper limit of normal) while her thyroid system is working properly. High and low total T4 and T3 are quite common and do not necessarily reflect an imbalance. The system is set so that the levels of free thyroid hormone in the bloodstream and organs remain normal.

For this reason, your doctor will often order another test, called a T3 uptake (often confused with T3 level). T3 uptake gives an estimate of the amount of TBG. When interpreted in conjunction with total T4 or T3, it will provide a more accurate estimate of the level of true biologically active thyroid hormone in your system. For instance, a pregnant woman or a woman taking estrogens will have, in addition to a high T4 level, a low T3 uptake. This indicates that the high T4 is due to high levels of TBG. Actually, if you multiply T4 by T3 uptake, you get the free thyroxine index (FTI), a better test for assessing thyroid hormone level than T4. The free form of thyroid hormone (called simply free T4 and free T3) can also be measured in the laboratory. Free T4 often provides a more accurate picture of whether there is a deficiency or an excess of thyroid hormone in the body. A free T3 level is often requested when the gland is overactive and in some cases of thyroid overactivity during pregnancy.

Doctors use the free T4 and free T3 levels to assess the severity of thyroid hormone imbalance in the body. The higher these hormone levels, the more severe the excess. Doctors also measure these levels when they suspect a thyroid imbalance due to a disorder of the pituitary gland, even when TSH levels are normal.

Getting the Right Diagnosis

If you have decided to be screened for a thyroid imbalance, or your physician has ordered a thyroid test to determine whether you have a thyroid imbalance, make sure that the test ordered is a TSH. As the table below shows, the test will immediately tell you whether you have hypothyroidism (if the TSH level is higher than 4.5 mIU/L) or you should be further evaluated by measuring the thyroid hormones T4 and T3 if you are suspected of having an overactive thyroid (TSH is lower than 0.4). If you have symptoms of hypothyroidism and your TSH level is greater than 2, you may have low-grade hypothyroidism, particularly if you have a family history of thyroid disease.

The TRH stimulation test can help bring out any minimal excess or deficiency of thyroid hormone that has not thrown the TSH out of its normal laboratory range. The results of the test will help your doctor determine if you suffer from a minor imbalance.

HOW TO DETERMINE THYROID IMBALANCES BASED ON TSH LEVELS

Range of TSH Level (mIU/L)	Diagnosis
>20	Moderate to severe hypothyroidism
4.5–20	Low-grade hypothyroidism
2.1–4.4	Normal. Also suspicious for hypothyroidism (if there are symptoms or a goiter)
0.4–2.0	Normal
0.1–0.39	Gray zone for too much thyroid hormone or pituitary dysfunction
<0.1	Hyperthyroidism or pituitary problem

No further testing is needed if the TSH is normal and you have no symptoms. If the TSH is high or low, however, your doctor will typically measure thyroid hormone levels. T4 often remains in the normal range until the TSH level exceeds 20 mIU/L. Beyond that level, T4 will tend to fall below normal. But this is not engraved in stone. T4 may still be normal even when TSH has reached 25 or 30.

By the same token, thyroid hormone levels will be normal in low-grade hyperthyroidism. When the gland becomes clearly overactive, both T4 and T3 will exceed the upper limit of the normal range. Many people with an overactive thyroid have a normal T4 level, with their T3 being the only thyroid hormone that has risen above normal as a result of thyroid activity.

It is important to make sure that your doctor has measured your T3 level (not T3 uptake) if you are hyperthyroid. Your doctor might overlook severe hyperthyroidism if he or she orders only a T4 test.

The Thyroid Neck Check

In January 1997, during the third annual Thyroid Awareness Month, the American Association of Clinical Endocrinologists introduced the concept of the thyroid neck check.[11] This association recommends that the public learn how to do this simple self-examination for the early detection of thyroid disease.

As I've explained, whether a thyroid condition results in hypothyroidism or hyperthyroidism, it is often generated by an autoimmune disorder such as Hashimoto's thyroiditis or Graves' disease. Both of these disorders are typically associated with an enlarged thyroid, or goiter. Lumps in the thyroid that can induce hyperthyroidism and lumps that could contain cancer may also become visible. You need to pay attention to the lower part of the neck, where the thyroid gland is located. This is especially important if you have a family history of thyroid disease or symptoms of thyroid imbalance.

You can detect a bulginess or a goiter by extending your neck in front of a mirror and gently turning your head slightly to the right and then to the left. If you see that the surface of your neck area just above the sternum (which is the middle bone of the chest) is uneven or protruding even slightly, you might have a lump (nodule) or a goiter. A goiter could mean having Hashimoto's thyroiditis or Graves' disease.

Another physical sign that you can use to watch for an underactive or overactive thyroid is the pulse rate. The heart is exquisitely sensitive to changes in the levels of thyroid hormone. Excess thyroid hormone will make your heart beat faster, and low thyroid levels will cause the heart to slow down. If you know your resting heart rate and have developed symptoms of thyroid imbalance, checking your resting heart rate can alert you that your levels have become abnormal. A rapid heartbeat at rest often suggests that you have an overactive thyroid. Make sure, however, that you do not have a fever or an infection, are not dehydrated, and have not consumed caffeine— all of which can raise your resting pulse rate. Also, your pulse rate should be checked while lying down, preferably in the morning. The pulse rate is not sensitive enough to detect low-grade imbalances, however, and it is less reliable if you are older than sixty, since, with aging, thyroid hormone excess loses its ability to accelerate the heartbeat.

Having a Goiter: What Does It Mean?

In the United States, the most common causes of goiter are Hashimoto's thyroiditis, Graves' disease, and nontoxic goiters due to a wide range of growth factors. As with toxic goiters, nontoxic goiters may initially be diffuse but over time can become multinodular (containing several lumps). Studies have shown that multinodular nontoxic goiters can eventually become toxic nodular goiters that lead to an overactive thyroid (see Chapter 6).

There are no drugs that can effectively shrink a nontoxic goiter. If, after becoming multinodular, the goiter causes symptoms such as hoarseness or difficulty swallowing or breathing, however, physicians often recommend surgical removal. Several studies have shown that destruction of the goiter with high-dose radioactive iodine is safe and effective. This may be an alternative to surgery.

Although rare, it is possible for a goiter to form because the thyroid gland lacks certain enzymes that it needs to manufacture thyroid hormone. In adults, a mild deficit in these enzymes can result in a goiter even though thyroid hormone levels in the blood are normal. The goiter is the result of the pituitary hormone TSH being stimulated by a minimally defective thyroid. If several members of your family have goiters without an imbalance, it might be worthwhile to have your physician look into it. Iodine deficiency is another cause of goiter, because iodine is one of the main ingredients used by the thyroid to manufacture thyroid hormone. In the United States, goiter is rarely due to iodine deficiency. In many parts of the world, however, iodine deficiency is a common cause of goiter (see Chapter 2).

To determine the cause of your goiter, your physician may order one or several of the following tests:

- *TSH:* This test can help to determine whether the thyroid's activity is normal.
- *Antithyroid antibodies:* If TSH is normal or high and your gland is diffusely enlarged (no lumps), this test can help your doctor determine whether you have Hashimoto's thyroiditis.

- *Radioactive iodine scan and uptake:* Doctors use this test if you are suspected of having Hashimoto's thyroiditis or an enzymatic defect. They also use it to differentiate Graves' disease (high uptake) from silent thyroiditis (low uptake) and if you are suspected of having a multinodular nontoxic or toxic goiter.
- *Thyroid ultrasound:* This imaging can help doctors make the diagnosis of autoimmune thyroid disease and thyroid nodules.

Let me add a few words about thyroid tenderness. Most physicians interpret tenderness in the thyroid as a symptom of subacute thyroiditis. But Hashimoto's thyroiditis can also cause tenderness and discomfort. Even Graves' disease can cause tenderness and pain, although this is not as common. This happens when a component of Hashimoto's disease is also present in the gland. If you have Graves' disease and are suffering from a painful and tender thyroid, it may mean that Hashimoto's thyroiditis could take over and you could become hypothyroid in the near future. Rarely, Hashimoto's thyroiditis causes severe pain that would require surgical removal of the thyroid gland.

When to Measure Antithyroid Antibodies

Antithyroid antibodies are markers in the bloodstream that are released by the immune system when there is an immune attack on the thyroid gland. Although many people with no thyroid disease could have very low concentrations of these antibodies in the bloodstream, high concentrations typically indicate an autoimmune thyroid disease. The antibodies that can be readily measured by commercial laboratories for the diagnosis of Hashimoto's thyroiditis are:

- Antithyroglobulin antibody
- Antimicrosomal antibody
- Antithyroperoxidase (anti-TPO) antibody

Of the three tests, anti-TPO antibody is the most sensitive. These antibody tests, however, are not foolproof. More than 20 percent of people with Hashimoto's thyroiditis do not have high antibodies. (If Hashimoto's thyroiditis is suspected, another diagnostic test may be helpful—thyroid ultrasound. It often shows diffuse inflammation and disturbance of the architecture of the gland resulting from the autoimmune attack. Ultrasound also may help in determining whether a bulge in the thyroid represents an area of intense inflammation due to Hashimoto's thyroiditis or a distinct lump, which could raise some concern about malignancy.) Ultrasound of the thyroid also shows disturbed architecture of the thyroid gland in patients with Graves' disease. Color flow Doppler performed with ultrasound also helps evaluate the blood supply to the gland. It is useful both for making the diagnosis of Graves' disease and for evaluating whether remission is likely while the patient is treated with medication.[12]

Once antithyroid antibodies have been found to be elevated and the diagnosis of Hashimoto's thyroiditis is confirmed, do not expect your physician to monitor the levels of the antibody over time. Many people have the immune reaction in their thyroid and high levels of antithyroid antibodies for twenty years or more without problems of underactive or overactive thyroid. They may maintain normal function throughout their lives or could become thyroid-imbalanced in the future. You should also know that one or several of these antibodies may be high in Graves' disease as well.

The antibody more often released by the immune system in people with Graves' disease is thyroid-stimulating antibody (TSAb), which can be measured in the laboratory. As is the case with the other antibodies, TSAb levels may not be high in some patients with Graves' disease.

People with autoimmune thyroid disease may have high levels of antibodies used by doctors as markers for autoimmune rheumatological conditions such as lupus and rheumatoid arthritis. Some of these antibodies are ANA, anti-smooth-muscle antibody, and anti-ss-DNA. Such patients, however, may not have these conditions.[13] The high concentrations of antibodies may merely reflect a disturbed immune system mistakenly producing some of these antibodies. Also, if you are suffering from an autoimmune disorder, you are likely to have high levels of antithyroid antibodies. For instance, as many as 38 percent of children with type 1 diabetes have antithyroid antibodies.[14]

Dealing with Lumps

As I indicated in Chapter 2, thyroid nodules (lumps) are quite common and are usually detected either during an examination of your neck or through an imaging procedure such as an ultrasound. If you are diagnosed with a thyroid nodule, your doctor will want to rule out the possibility that the nodule is cancerous. However, only about 15 percent of nodules bigger than 1 cm are cancerous.

Nodules that are smaller than 1 cm are usually monitored periodically with ultrasound; generally, only if it enlarges beyond that size will additional steps be recommended. For larger nodules, usually those greater than 1 or 1.5 cm, physicians recommend a procedure known as a fine-needle aspiration biopsy. The doctor withdraws cells via a very thin needle inserted into three to five places in the nodule. The procedure is performed with the help of an ultrasound machine to make sure that the needle is in the nodule. The cells are then examined by a pathologist to determine whether the nodule is benign or cancerous. However, as many as 20 to 30 percent of biopsies are inconclusive or fail to distinguish between benign and cancerous lesions. If you have an inconclusive pathology report, there are genetic tests available that can help your doctor predict whether you have cancer or not, but they are not always foolproof.

Several factors indicate a heightened likelihood of cancer in patients diagnosed with thyroid nodules, regardless of their size:

- Nodules that grow over time
- Being male, since nodules by and large are more common in women
- Symptoms of hoarseness, difficulty swallowing, or spitting blood
- History of external radiation or exposure to radioactive fallout from nuclear accidents
- Family history of colon cancer or intestinal polyposis (genetic link)
- Family history of thyroid cancer

Many benign nodules eventually shrink without any treatment. I do not recommend thyroid hormone treatment for benign nodules. If there is cause for concern because a nodule is growing, surgery may be the best route.

The most common type of thyroid cancer is papillary cancer. This form of cancer is associated with the best outcome and accounts for 70 percent of all thyroid cancer cases. The other main type of thyroid cancer is follicular cancer, which accounts for 20 to 25 percent of all thyroid cancer cases. It is more aggressive than papillary cancer and the outcome is generally worse than that of the papillary type. In 5 percent of cases, papillary thyroid cancer runs in the family. Hurthle cell cancer is one variety of follicular cancer and accounts for 3–4 percent of thyroid cancers. Hurthle cell cancer is quite often more aggressive and spreads more rapidly. Anaplastic cancer is one of the most aggressive malignancies, but fortunately it is rare. Another uncommon form of thyroid cancer is medullary thyroid cancer.

Know Your Risk

A family history of thyroid disease may increase your risk of having an autoimmune thyroid disease such as Hashimoto's thyroiditis or Graves' disease. This increased risk is related to a genetic predisposition.[15] If you or members of your family suffer from an autoimmune condition such as insulin-dependent diabetes, lupus, or rheumatoid arthritis, you also have a much higher lifetime risk for developing an autoimmune thyroid disorder such as Hashimoto's thyroiditis or Graves' disease. One study showed that 8.2 percent of patients with autoimmune conditions such as systemic lupus erythematosus, rheumatoid arthritis, systemic sclerosis, mixed connective tissue disease, Sjögren's syndrome, and polymyositis/dermatomyositis have either Hashimoto's thyroiditis or Graves' disease.[16] The same research also showed that one of four patients with mixed connective tissue disorder and one of ten patients with Sjögren's syndrome have an autoimmune thyroid condition. The most striking finding was that 51 percent of patients with Hashimoto's thyroiditis and 16 percent of patients with Graves' disease have one or more autoimmune disorders. Because the genes that predetermine whether you will have a thyroid condition often overlap or are linked to genes that predispose you to other unrelated conditions, it is important to know that the risk for having a thyroid imbalance becomes greater if you or a family member has been diagnosed with such conditions. For example, former president John F. Kennedy had Addison's disease. His son, John F. Kennedy Jr., also suffered from Addison's disease as well as Graves' disease.[17] Some patients have two or more autoimmune disorders of the endocrine system and are considered as having polyglandular failure syndrome. A characteristic association is an autoimmune thyroid disease, Addison's disease, and insulin-dependent diabetes.

Another example is the definite increase in the frequency of vitiligo among people suffering from Graves' disease or Hashimoto's thyroiditis. Vitiligo is the presence of blanched areas on the skin due to the loss of normal pigmentation in these areas. The loss of pigment results from an immune system attack on the skin cells, called melanocytes, that maintain normal pigmentation. The loss of pigmentation may be limited to a small area or affect many areas of the skin.

One of the most overlooked autoimmune conditions that could coexist with an autoimmune thyroid disease is Sjögren's syndrome (also called sicca syndrome). Nearly half of patients with Hashimoto's thyroiditis have subtle features of Sjögren's syndrome, which can progress to cause dry mouth, dry eyes, and vaginal dryness. Clear-cut clinical symptoms of Sjögren's are seen in a third of patients with autoimmune thyroid disease. This is due to the fact that autoimmune thyroid disease and Sjögren's syndrome have a close genetic link.[18]

Other symptoms of Sjögren's syndrome are receding gums, tooth decay, and joint pains. The diagnosis is often made by a positive test for SS-A and SS-B antibodies, a high sedimentation rate, a high level of C-reactive protein, and a lip biopsy.

Sjögren's syndrome can co-occur with rheumatoid arthritis, which is another autoimmune connective tissue condition that can affect patients with autoimmune thyroid disease. Rheumatoid arthritis, whether the juvenile or adult form, tends to cause pain and swelling of the proximal joints of hands and feet, and many other joints. At times it affects only one joint. This condition tends to run in families and is diagnosed through testing of rheumatoid factor and anticyclic citrullinated peptide.

Lupus is a serious autoimmune condition that causes a typical rash and is related to inflammation of many organs in the body, including the kidneys, brain, heart, and lungs. The diagnosis is made through blood tests.

Multiple sclerosis is also an autoimmune condition closely linked genetically to autoimmune thyroid disease. Recent research has shown that patients with Graves' disease have a high susceptibility to multiple sclerosis and vice versa. The link between Hashimoto's thyroiditis and multiple sclerosis is not as strong, however.[19]

Celiac disease, a disorder of the small bowel, can also occur in patients with autoimmune thyroid disease. Celiac disease is an autoimmune disorder causing inflammation and damage to the lining of the small intestine. Approximately 2 million people in the United States have celiac disease, and nearly sixty thousand Americans are diagnosed every year.[20] One study has shown that if you suffer from celiac disease, your risk of having an autoimmune thyroid disease increases sixfold. Research has also found that 73 percent of patients suffering from celiac disease have an autoimmune thyroid disease diagnosable by ultrasound,[21] and one of five has an underactive thyroid.[22] Also, celiac antibodies, markers for celiac disease, have been detected in 14 percent of patients with Graves' disease.[23] Patients having autoimmune thyroid disorders are at a much higher risk for having celiac disease. Patients who have both celiac disease and a thyroid condition are at an increased risk of diabetes, ulcerative colitis, and dermatitis herpetiform. Also, children with Down syndrome are at risk for both celiac disease and a thyroid imbalance. The inflammation occurs when gliadin, a protein found in gluten-containing foods, such as wheat, rye, and barley, is ingested by a genetically vulnerable person. This inflammation causes malabsorption of various nutrients. For instance, vitamin D deficiency is found in at least 20 percent of patients with celiac disease, and this can promote bone loss and osteoporosis.[24] Common symptoms of celiac disease are anemia, joint pains and aches, fatigue, infertility, neuropathy, and weight loss. However, you may or may not suffer from gastrointestinal symptoms, such as abdominal pain, bloating, constipation, and diarrhea. Diagnosing celiac disease has become easy. Over half of patients with celiac disease can be diagnosed with just antibody testing. Antibody testing is most useful in patients who do not have gastrointestinal symptoms related to celiac disease.[25] The main treatment for celiac disease is adherence to a gluten-free diet.

Consult the accompanying table to learn about which conditions have been shown to increase the predisposition to autoimmune thyroid disease. This table will also help alert you to other conditions to which you may be predisposed if you have been diagnosed with an autoimmune thyroid disorder and have been or are being treated for it.

SOME AUTOIMMUNE CONDITIONS TO WATCH FOR

Condition	Cause	Symptoms
Rheumatoid arthritis	Autoimmune inflammation of one or multiple joints	Stiffness in the morning, joint pain (knuckles, wrists, elbows)
Sjögren's syndrome	Autoimmune reaction to salivary glands, tear glands, and mucus glands of the vagina	Dry eyes, dry mouth, vaginal dryness, tooth decay, joint pain (similar to rheumatoid arthritis)
Lupus	Autoimmune attack on skin and other connective tissue in various organs including the kidney, heart, and joints	Joint pain, fever, rash over the face or other skin areas, kidney damage, heart, lung, and brain damage
Ankylosing spondylitis	Inflammation and immune attacks on the joint of the spine	Pain and stiffness of the neck, back, sacroiliac joint, limitation of bending due to fusion of the spine
Scleroderma	Immune reaction causing inflammation and scarring of skin and connective tissue of many organs	Red and tight skin, stiffness and pain of fingers, Raynaud's syndrome (blanching and pain of fingers upon exposure to cold), high blood pressure, difficulty swallowing
Psoriasis/ Psoriatic arthritis	Autoimmune attack on the skin, scalp, eyes, joints, at times other organs	Psoriasis of skin, scalp, and nails, joint pain, deformity of fingers. Eye, heart, and lung inflammation
Polymyositis	Autoimmune attack and inflammation of proximal muscles	Weakness of proximal muscles, or loss of strength
Dermatomyositis	Autoimmune attack and inflammation of proximal muscles and skin	Weakness of proximal muscles, redness and inflammation of the skin
Crohn's disease	Autoimmune inflammation of any part of the small intestine and colon	Abdominal pain, diarrhea, bloody diarrhea, fever
Ulcerative colitis	Autoimmune inflammation of the colon	Abdominal pain, diarrhea, bloody diarrhea, fever
Pernicious anemia	Deficiency of vitamin B_{12} due to lack of a stomach factor essential for absorption of that vitamin	Numbness, tingling in hands and feet, loss of balance, leg weakness
Insulin-dependent diabetes	Autoimmune attack on cells in the pancreas that produce insulin	Increased frequency of urination, thirst, weight loss, blurred vision, ketoacidosis

Condition	Cause	Symptoms
Addison's disease	Autoimmune reaction to the adrenal glands (which normally produce cortisol and mineralocorticoid hormones)	Weight loss, fatigue, epigastric pain, nausea, diarrhea, vomiting, low blood pressure, fainting, dehydration, hypoglycemia, increased pigmentation of the skin
Myasthenia gravis	Autoimmune attack on acetylcholine receptors in muscle cells, essential for contraction of muscles	Muscle weakness, double vision, difficulty swallowing
Primary biliary cirrhosis	Autoimmune reaction to bile ducts in the liver causing obstruction of the ducts	Jaundice, abnormal liver function, itching
Oophoritis	Autoimmune reaction to ovaries resulting in scarring	Early menopause, loss of menstrual periods

Aside from autoimmunity, your risk of becoming hypothyroid is very high if you have received external radiation for the treatment of head and neck tumors, lymphomas, or acne. One study of eighty-one patients who were treated with external radiation for Hodgkin's disease found that up to 58 percent of them were hypothyroid when tested ten to eighteen years after the radiation treatment.[26] External radiation can also cause nodules and cancer in the thyroid gland. The same risk of underactive thyroid and thyroid nodules applies to people who have been exposed to radiation from nuclear fallout.

Radiation from nuclear fallout and nuclear reactor accidents may cause Hashimoto's thyroiditis, thyroid nodules, and cancer as well as hypothyroidism. Researchers noted that as a consequence of the 1986 Chernobyl accident near Kiev in the USSR (now Ukraine), which caused the release of radioactive material, including radioactive iodine, hypothyroidism rates increased in nearby areas. Even horses and cattle that were not evacuated from an area near Chernobyl became hypothyroid. People in parts of the western United States who were exposed to fallout from nuclear tests done in the 1950s and 1960s may be at a higher risk for having hypothyroidism as well as thyroid nodules.

In addition to autoimmune diseases and radiation, certain other conditions, discussed in the following paragraphs, might provide a clue that you or family members may be at higher risk for having a thyroid disorder.

For reasons that are unclear, the reading disability dyslexia may alert you to an increased risk for developing a thyroid imbalance. Dyslexia is characterized by a difficulty in distinguishing written symbols, and dyslexics often transpose letters and confuse right and left. Although their overall intelligence may be high, dyslexic children may perform poorly in school because of difficulties with reading and spelling. Typically, dyslexia affects males in the family. Former president George H. W. Bush indicated to me that his son Neil suffered from dyslexia when he was in his very early school years. His trouble had resolved since. Neil, however, has not had thyroid disease himself. On the other hand, President Bush's son Marvin had colitis, also genetically linked to autoimmune thyroid disorders. Marvin also has not had a thyroid problem.

Premature graying of the hair before the age of thirty may indicate that you have genes that predispose you to a thyroid disorder. Barbara Bush had premature graying of the hair, a clue that she was at risk for autoimmune thyroid disease. One small survey among patients with autoimmune thyroid disease suggested that left-handed or ambidextrous men might be at higher risk for having Graves' disease or Hashimoto's thyroiditis.

Dermatitis herpetiformis, a rare condition, may be associated with an autoimmune thyroid disease. People with this condition have fluid-filled blisters with itching and hives over their back and lower extremities. If you or a family member has been diagnosed with this condition, have your thyroid tested.

As we have seen, a thyroid imbalance can affect any organ in the body (see Chapters 2, 5, and 6). Nevertheless, there are many symptoms that doctors often fail to associate with thyroid disease. If you are experiencing any of these symptoms, discuss the possibility of thyroid disease with your doctor and have him or her test your thyroid. For instance, the red, itchy patches of hives, also known as urticaria, can occur with either hypo- or hyperthyroidism. In many patients, hives are a manifestation of an autoimmune thyroid disease. Patients with hives have a higher frequency of Hashimoto's thyroiditis.[27] In some instances, thyroid hormone treatment resolves the condition, even when thyroid hormone levels are normal. If your levels are high or low and you have hives, you may get relief from taking antihistaminic medications and from correcting the imbalance.

Easy bruising can be a sign of a thyroid imbalance. It may have something to do with a low count of blood platelets (cells that are essential in regulating clotting) or a malfunction of the platelets. Sometimes several members of the same family have a low platelet count simultaneously with Graves' disease and could experience tiny punctate bleeding spots in the skin (petechiae).[28] An often-overlooked cause of easy bruising in thyroid patients is the use of nonsteroidal anti-inflammatory drugs (NSAIDs), which doctors frequently prescribe for the aches and pains of arthritis that these patients may experience.

Hair loss has been one of the most common complaints among my thyroid patients. Hair loss occurs during both hypo- and hyperthyroidism and may persist for months even after normal blood levels of thyroid hormone have been reestablished. This symptom can be very distressing and alarming for both men and women who may also be suffering from weight problems, depression, and low self-esteem. The effect of a thyroid imbalance and immune system reactivity on the health of hair follicles can be so drastic that you may notice clumps of hair on your pillow or hairbrush. Your hair may be coming out on the brush and blocking the drain after a shower. Although you need to report this symptom to your physician, do not be alarmed. Most of the time, your hair will come back. If you continue to have hair loss for months after your blood tests become normal, it's because the hair follicles have not fully recovered from the effects of the thyroid imbalance. Although it may take six months to a year for the new, strong hair to replace the old, weak hair that resulted from an imbalance, your hair follicles will become healthy with good thyroid balance, healthy nutrition, and stress management.

If you or a family member ever suffered from the patchy hair loss of alopecia areata, you may be at higher risk for having a thyroid disorder. This condition, related to immune system reactivity and attack of hair follicles, results in bald areas in any part of the body where hair normally grows, including the scalp, beard, and pubic area. Although this condition often causes concern and worry, it may resolve spontaneously over several months. In some people, the hair loss is unfortunately permanent.

Muscle weakness is a symptom of both hyper- and hypothyroidism, but if you experience periods of paralysis after hard exercise or eating lots of sugar, it may be an indication that you are suffering from hypokalemic periodic paralysis. The paralysis is caused by low potassium levels and co-occurs with Graves' disease. It tends to afflict Asian people more frequently. Often, after you achieve a proper thyroid balance, the decline of potassium levels in your blood will no longer occur, and you will stop having the episodes of paralysis.

The following list summarizes the various conditions that should alert you to the possibility of a thyroid imbalance.

CONDITIONS THAT INCREASE THE RISK OF THYROID IMBALANCE
- Autoimmune disorder (see table, pages 125–26, listing autoimmune conditions that occur with a higher frequency in patients with autoimmune thyroid diseases)
- Dyslexia
- Premature graying of hair
- History of depression
- Manic-depression
- Dermatitis herpetiformis

- Down syndrome, Turner syndrome
- Family history of Alzheimer's disease
- History of breast cancer
- Alopecia areata
- Chronic urticaria (hives)
- Polymyalgia rheumatica
- Celiac disease

As I've mentioned throughout, older people, postmenopausal women, and women who are suffering from depression or have a history of depression, anxiety, PMS, infertility, recent miscarriage, postpartum depression, or heavy menstrual bleeding should consider thyroid disease as a possible reason for these issues.

Determining your thyroid status will, of course, alert you to whether your suffering has been caused by a thyroid imbalance. Knowing your risk can also make you pay more serious attention to this tiny gland that so intimately affects all aspects of your well-being, from mood to relationships. When you know your risk of thyroid imbalance and have become familiar with its symptoms, you will be more likely to have your physician consider thyroid imbalance early on, before the imbalance has robbed you of your overall health.

Diagnosing a thyroid condition early will also prevent many of the hidden effects that do not cause symptoms right away but could eventually come to haunt you many years later. The accompanying table lists some of the hidden physical long-term effects of hypo- and hyperthyroidism.

HIDDEN LONG-TERM EFFECTS OF THYROID IMBALANCE

Hypothyroidism	Hyperthyroidism
High total and LDL cholesterol	Cardiac rhythm problems
Coronary artery disease	Cardiomyopathy and congestive heart failure
Damage to brain structures	Damage to brain structures
High blood pressure	High blood pressure
Glucose intolerance and diabetes	Glucose intolerance and diabetes
Acceleration of aging	Acceleration of aging
	Bone loss and osteoporosis

When the Pituitary Is the Problem

Pituitary deficiency accounts for a very small percentage of the cases of underactive thyroid: as few as 5 in 100,000 people with an underactive thyroid have a pituitary or hypothalamic problem.[29] Many conditions can cause the pituitary gland to become deficient. The most common are tumors in the pituitary or hypothalamus and destruction of the pituitary as a result of poor blood supply or an infection. Destruction of the pituitary related to poor blood supply, such as can occur after delivery of a baby, can cause the person to have severe headaches and visual problems. An underactive thyroid due to an isolated deficiency of TSH is extremely rare.[30]

In hypothyroidism due to a hypothalamic or pituitary disease, the TSH level may be normal or low. The diagnosis cannot be confirmed unless the thyroid hormone level (particularly T4) is measured. In hypothyroidism due to a pituitary problem, the T4 level will be low. You need to know that you could fall through the cracks if you have a pituitary problem causing hypothyroidism but your physician has requested only a TSH test.

Important Points to Remember

- If you are suspected of having a thyroid imbalance, the first and most important thyroid test is TSH.
- You may be suffering from a "minimal thyroid deficiency" even though your TSH is normal. To uncover the imbalance, you may need TRH testing, especially if your TSH level is near the high end of the normal range.
- If you discover you have a goiter (an enlarged thyroid gland), make sure that you receive appropriate testing. If your thyroid levels are normal or if you have hypothyroidism, an antithyroid antibody test and an ultrasound of the thyroid gland will help determine whether you have Hashimoto's thyroiditis.
- If you have not been diagnosed with a thyroid disorder, learn about the conditions that may predispose you to developing a thyroid condition. These include several autoimmune diseases, premature graying of hair before age thirty, dyslexia, left-handedness in men, and familial patterns of thyroid disease.

8

THYROID IMBALANCE, DEPRESSION, ANXIETY, AND MOOD SWINGS

Your brain is unique. It creates your individual talents, perceptions, and moods. Yet its individuality presents some challenges to physicians and brain researchers when they try to figure out how the brain, body, and mind work together to generate specific mental states. For example, exact measurements or even precise definitions of what constitutes normal mental health continue to elude scientists. In the recent past, some doctors may have defined normal mental health merely as the absence of overt mental diseases such as manic-depression or schizophrenia. Today, most doctors have come to recognize that millions of people have various, more subtle forms of depression and anxiety.

More often than not, thyroid imbalance gives rise to mental and emotional symptoms of mild depression, intermittent rage disorder, mild attention deficit disorder, or other "minor syndromes"—conditions that cause suffering but are not pronounced enough to meet the psychiatric criteria of a mental condition. People with these conditions will find that their symptoms are magnified when a thyroid imbalance occurs. For a minority of patients, such magnified symptoms may cause them to slip into a more pronounced mental illness, but for most thyroid patients, the mental effects of thyroid disease—such as fatigue, low mood and mood swings, and lack of mental clarity—cause great suffering without being "psychiatric."

Just as severe hypothyroidism is much less common than low-grade hypothyroidism, low-grade and borderline depression are much more common than easily diagnosed major depression.

Low-Grade Depression: Thyroid Shadow Syndrome

It is a common misconception that depression means mere sadness. The feeling of sadness is a normal response to the occurrence of a distressing event or to a disappointment in life. Although you may feel down and sad when depressed, sadness is not always a symptom of depression. In depression, a person's feelings are disconnected from all that surrounds that person, so that he or she may be neither sad nor happy. This disconnection causes a blunting of excitement about life in general. Although when someone is asked whether he or she is depressed, the typical response is, "No, I don't feel I'm depressed. I'm not sad," this person may in fact be suffering from the characteristic symptoms of depression.

An easy way to determine the likelihood that you may be suffering from depression is to complete the following questionnaire. If you answer a question with no, proceed to the next question; if you answer with yes, score the severity of your symptoms (1 = mild, 2 = moderate, 3 = severe) before proceeding to the next question.

Are you tired all the time?	Yes No	___
Have you lost interest in activities that you used to enjoy?	Yes No	___
Are you in a sad mood more or less constantly?	Yes No	___
Are you often irritable, and do you get angry over trivial matters?	Yes No	___
Do you experience crying spells?	Yes No	___
Do you have feelings of worthlessness?	Yes No	___
Do you often experience a sense of guilt about things or have you become too critical of yourself?	Yes No	___
Has your appetite increased, and/or have you gained weight?	Yes No	___
Has your appetite decreased, and/or have you lost weight?	Yes No	___
Do you have difficulty remembering things and/or concentrating on normal activities?	Yes No	___
Do you have trouble making decisions, or do you feel inefficient?	Yes No	___
Do you have trouble sleeping through the night?	Yes No	___
Do you sleep more than eight hours (either going to bed too early or sleeping late)?	Yes No	___
Do you wish you were dead?	Yes No	___
Have you become very sensitive to criticism or rejection?	Yes No	___
TOTAL SEVERITY SCORE		___

If you answered yes to three or more of the preceding questions, you may be depressed; if you answered yes to five or more of the questions, you are probably depressed.

Now add the scores for each symptom to obtain your total severity score, the meaning of which is explained in the accompanying table. The total severity score will be useful later in assessing your response to treatment.

DEPRESSION/ANXIETY SEVERITY

Total Severity Score	Severity of Symptoms
15 or less	Mild
15–24	Moderate
25 or more	Severe

In addition to the feelings of disconnection and fatigue, the main symptoms of depression are changes in appetite, sleep disturbances, lack of interest in enjoyable activities, and problems with memory and concentration.

In general, as thyroid hormone begins to decrease, changes in a person's mental energy are barely recognizable. Gradually, subtle changes occur, and the person begins to slow down and often "loses steam" in the afternoon. The fatigue itself precipitates a growing concern that there might be something terribly wrong somewhere in the body. The lack of energy may result in a great deal of frustration, a sense of no longer being able to function as the person has done in the past. This, in turn, produces feelings of guilt, inadequacy, and lower self-esteem. Even if a hypothyroid person's symptoms do not fully satisfy the criteria for depression, he or she may be experiencing a low-grade depression (a chronic, even milder form of depression than dysthymia) that is manifested primarily as fatigue and lack of enthusiasm.

Dawn, an educational consultant who conducts seminars all over the United States, began to notice a lack of energy a year before she sought medical attention. She said:

I would hit three in the afternoon and be ready to go to bed. That was terribly frustrating, since previously I had had such a high energy level. I felt that people would think I was inadequate, that I was giving up, when it wasn't me who was giving up, it was my body. I waged a constant battle within myself to keep up with things at work and try to live a normal existence. I felt that I was dancing as fast as I could and going nowhere. At lunchtime and during afternoon breaks,

I would find a quiet place and take a quick nap to try to recoup. I would eat a piece of chocolate to give me a boost, but nothing helped.

I diagnosed Dawn with a moderately underactive thyroid. Although, when I asked, she did mention several other symptoms of hypothyroidism, what was affecting Dawn the most was the deficiency in energy. She attributed almost every other symptom that she exhibited to her tiredness, yet Dawn was suffering from borderline depression as a result of her underactive thyroid. At times, she was experiencing unexplained anger, increased appetite, and cravings. She was also deeply affected when someone was critical of her and when she perceived that someone was rejecting her.

A thirty-nine-year-old surgeon's wife, Nina, repeatedly told her busy husband, "I am tired. I feel that there must be something wrong with my body." His reply was always the same: "You are trying to do too much with all these social activities. Just slow down."

Nina didn't think it was stress or too much activity. Rather, she was convinced that something was physically wrong with her. Her energy level was low. She was sleepier than she felt she should be, and she could not control her weight gain. In her words:

> I wanted to go to sleep at seven in the evening. I was feeling down. I was not that type of person before. I could not concentrate, and I could not work. I had anxiety. Often, for no reason, when I was by myself, I would cry. Many times I was not happy even though I felt I had to be happy. I was forgetful, which would really upset me. I also had problems concentrating on things and became very bad with names. I didn't care to do much, and I withdrew.
>
> I thought to myself, what could be wrong? I knew that weight problems were related to thyroid disorders, so I went to see an experienced endocrinologist. He said, "Don't worry. This is nothing. I don't want to put you on medication."

A year later, because her symptoms had persisted, Nina came to see me. After she told me about her suffering, she said, "I know a problem exists, and there has to be a reason." I asked Nina whether she had told the first endocrinologist about all the problems besides the tiredness. "I don't think so, because he didn't ask me. I was disappointed when he said the levels were borderline normal. I didn't believe it. That's why I thought I had to see somebody else."

Nina's blood test showed low-grade hypothyroidism. She was also suffering from a case of low-grade depression. I started Nina on thyroid hormone treatment, and she showed dramatic improvement. Her tiredness and the intermittent sadness and anger went away. Nina was suffering from a "shadow syndrome" caused by a minute deficit of thyroid hormone in her system and her brain. Getting on the medicine restored Nina's energy and made her other symptoms disappear. Slowly but surely, she saw her body starting to cooperate with her again instead of being her enemy.

Many people like Dawn and Nina suffer needlessly from depressive symptoms related to low-grade hypothyroidism. Research conducted on women has shown that even those who have low-grade hypothyroidism *but no symptoms of mood disorder* show evidence of improvement in objective scores that test levels of depression, hysteria, and obsessive-compulsive behavior when they are treated with thyroid hormone.[1] This illustrates that even those who suffer from low-grade hypothyroidism may not necessarily sense the effect of the thyroid hormone deficit. They might be attributing the way they feel to just "being themselves."

Because the majority of patients with low-grade depression do not seek psychiatric help, establishing the frequency of hypothyroidism in people suffering from low-grade depression is a real challenge for researchers. I expect that a minor thyroid imbalance occurs in a significant percentage of people suffering from low-grade depression, however. In a study conducted in the German state of Bavaria, ultrasound exams showed an enlarged thyroid gland in 86 percent of patients suffering from chronic depression, but in only 25 percent of people not suffering from depression.[2]

Let's look at how even a minute thyroid hormone imbalance could be responsible for lowering mood.

Thyroid Hormone: Serotonin's Cousin

The explosive advances in the knowledge of brain chemistry and its effects on mood began in the early 1960s. Several years ago, doctors recognized that serotonin imbalance is an important factor in causing depression. Acceptance of the idea that most psychiatric conditions can be attributed to a chemical imbalance in the brain opened the door to drastic changes in the way doctors explain and treat mental disorders. This new era of biological psychiatry, or *biopsychiatry,* witnessed a convergence of psychiatry and medicine, fields previously separated by rigid boundaries. A psychiatric illness now tends to be viewed in much the same manner as a physical illness.

In the early days of biopsychiatry, neuroscientists believed that each mental disorder was associated with a corresponding brain chemical imbalance. This assumption led psychiatrists to hope that they could diagnose a psychiatric condition by measuring the levels of specific bodily chemicals or their by-products in the blood or urine. But brain chemistry is not so simple. Most often, multiple imbalances of chemicals—such as serotonin, noradrenaline, and others, including those we are concerned with here, the thyroid hormones—are responsible for mental symptoms.

Scientists now consider thyroid hormone one of the major players in brain chemistry disorders. And as with any brain chemical disorder, until treated correctly, thyroid hormone imbalance has serious effects on the patient's emotions and behavior.

Once the important thyroid hormones, T3 and T4, are released into your bloodstream, they enter cells of organs and play an important role in regulating major functions in the body. Adequate amounts of thyroid hormone are also required throughout your life if your brain is to function normally. Most of your cognitive abilities—such as concentration, memory, and attention span—as well as mood and emotions depend on normal thyroid hormone levels. Mounting evidence suggests that T3, the most potent form of thyroid hormone, is a bona fide brain chemical. It is found in the junctions of nerve cells (synapses) that allow these cells to communicate with one another.[3] This thyroid hormone also regulates the levels and actions of serotonin, noradrenaline, and GABA (gamma-aminobutyric acid), now accepted as the main chemical transmitters implicated in both depression and some anxiety disorders. Maintaining normal serotonin and noradrenaline levels in the brain depends to a great extent on whether the correct amount of T3 is available. Extensive animal and human research has led scientists to conclude that serotonin levels in the brain decrease if T3 is not delivered in the right amount.[4] Also, a deficit of T3 in the brain is likely to result in noradrenaline's working inefficiently as a chemical transmitter,[5] and noradrenaline deficiency or inefficiency is, in some people, the chemical reason for depression.[6] Thyroid hormone also regulates cholecystokinin tetrapeptide (CCK-4) in the brain. A low level of this chemical caused by an underactive thyroid promotes inner tension, a quite common symptom of hypothyroidism.[7]

Findings that T3 is very highly concentrated near the junctions between brain cells strongly support the concept of T3 as a brain chemical transmitter that is essential for maintaining normal mood and behavior. This is the location where chemical transmitters such as noradrenaline are released to relay messages from one brain cell to another. The potent thyroid hormone T3 is found in greater quantities in the limbic system, a region of the brain that regulates mood, emotions, and perception of happy and sad events. The resemblance of thyroid hormone to other important brain chemicals is also striking: the amino acid tyrosine is an essential constituent both of thyroid hormone and of the brain chemicals noradrenaline and dopamine.

Beating the Blues

My wife and I once attended the symphony with a colleague, Jim, and his wife, Lorraine, whom I hadn't seen in several years. Upon being reintroduced to Lorraine, I was surprised to see that she now had a slightly enlarged thyroid gland, or goiter. Even though she used to be an avid devotee of the symphony, she was clearly not enjoying herself that evening. She had a hard time smiling and appeared isolated, disconnected from her husband, hardly paying attention to our conversations or the music. During the intermission, when my wife and Lorraine went off by themselves, I mentioned to Jim that I was surprised to see how much Lorraine had changed. I also suggested that she appeared to have thyroid disease.

Jim seemed relieved at the opportunity to talk to someone and confessed that his wife had completely changed three or four years earlier. She gained weight, was often very tired and sleepy, and became overly sensitive to criticism. Lorraine didn't seem to enjoy many things that used to bring her great pleasure, such as cooking and the symphony. Her relationships with Jim and their children were really suffering. She had undergone counseling for six or eight months, thinking her problems were psychological, but no real changes resulted. Several physicians said she was simply "stressed" and told her to learn to relax. A holistic doctor administered herbs, which, like everything else, did not seem to help. Obviously, these physicians had failed to pay attention to Lorraine's enlarged thyroid gland. Lorraine became pretty discouraged about going to doctors for help and seemed resigned to this as her new way of life.

A week later, Jim convinced Lorraine to try one more time. She came in to see me and tested positive for hypothyroidism and Hashimoto's thyroiditis. After three months of treatment, Lorraine dramatically improved. She started to enjoy life again and regained control over her weight. In retrospect, Lorraine was suffering from a case of hypothyroidism with symptoms of atypical depression that resolved with thyroid hormone treatment.

Atypical depression is a common form of chronic depression experienced by people with an underactive thyroid. Such patients can be cheered up temporarily by positive events, but the recovery tends to be brief. The patients often slip back into a depressive state a few hours or days later. The symptoms may be mild to severe. In this type of depression, the patients become sensitive to rejection and criticism and develop a tendency to overeat, especially carbohydrates, and to oversleep. Overeating and oversleeping are important characteristics of atypical depression. They help psychiatrists distinguish this quite common type of depression from other types of depression such as major depression, which causes the person to suffer from insomnia and loss of appetite.[8] Some patients with atypical depression experience anxiety attacks and severe lethargy, which may impede their normal functioning. The depression and fatigue are frequently worse in the evening. The patients may appear introverted and gloomy.

People with atypical depression often remain undiagnosed because their suffering rarely reaches the severity of major depression and is easier to hide.

They may not consider themselves depressed; at times they may not realize that anything is wrong with them; and suicidal thoughts are unusual.

Hypothyroidism can also cause the person to suffer from dysthymic depression, or "chronic blues," another common form of chronic depression. It is perhaps also the most common type of depression experienced by people with normal thyroid function. It affects at least 6 percent of the general population during their lifetimes. Patients afflicted with dysthymia are depressed more often than not. They feel down but are able to function. People with this form of chronic depression also tend to oversleep; their appetite may be either increased or decreased, however. They frequently become used to the way they feel and may not even recognize that they have a problem. Dysthymic people do not go through well-defined periods of depression but remain more or less depressed constantly: it is a lingering type of depression.

The accepted diagnostic criterion for dysthymia requires that at least two symptoms—change in appetite, insomnia, fatigue, low self-esteem, poor concentration, indecision, and feelings of hopelessness—in conjunction with depressed mood be present for most of the time over at least two years.[9] Although two years of suffering may be acceptable as a psychiatric criterion, that doesn't mean you should suffer unnecessarily for two years before being diagnosed and treated. This is especially true if the cause of your depression is a thyroid imbalance.

As you can see, atypical depression and dysthymia share many features. They are chronic, lingering forms of depression that do not lead to suicidal thoughts. The fatigue in atypical depression, however, is in general much more severe. Further, although overeating is characteristic of atypical depression, loss of appetite can be seen in many patients suffering from dysthymia.

Erica, a forty-year-old teacher, suffered from dysthymia along with other physical symptoms of hypothyroidism for two years. She said:

> I became so tired. I would lie down and sleep for hours just to get my energy back. I would take naps in the afternoon after school. I would go to bed early. It was like a stress relief. I loved to sleep. I never got enough.
>
> I wasn't suicidal, but I was very depressed. I took one day at a time. I didn't talk to anyone. I kept to myself. I rarely visited family. When I came home from work, I immediately went to sleep. I lost my appetite and kept losing weight. I worried about paying bills. I always had to write things down or I would forget.
>
> I wondered where my life was going. I was afraid of the future. Urged by my sister, I began to see a psychologist, but this was not helping.

One day, Erica saw her general practitioner for a sore throat. The doctor noticed a goiter and suspected hypothyroidism. Erica tested positive for hypothyroidism, and her depression completely resolved with thyroid hormone treatment. A few months later, Erica said, "Thyroid treatment has helped me cope with the depression and stress. I am more alert. I am not as depressed. I am able to really talk to my therapist frankly and follow her suggestions."

Erica's dysthymia was partially caused by an underactive thyroid. People with thyroid imbalance who suffer from dysthymia often continue to try to function despite their tiredness and other symptoms and attribute the tiredness to stress, work, or too many activities. Gradually, they feel overwhelmed and start perceiving that what they are doing is more than they can handle. Yet this can be corrected, and they can feel like their old selves again if treated promptly and properly. The key is to think thyroid and to have your doctor order the appropriate thyroid test.

Major Depression and Thyroid Imbalance

Hypothyroidism also makes patients at a higher risk for slipping into major depression—the most extreme and most dreaded form of depression. Recent research has shown that patients admitted to the hospital with hypothyroidism have a much greater risk of readmission with depression.[10] A minimal thyroid imbalance is enough to trigger a vicious cycle that ultimately leads to major depression. When hypothyroidism is not immediately addressed and lingers untreated for years, minor depression can evolve into major depression, which can lead to a severe feeling of disconnection and even suicidal thoughts. In such patients, the extreme tiredness associated with hypothyroidism and depression is part of a never-ending vicious cycle that drains them and ultimately leads to deeper depression.

Christina, a thirty-four-year-old receptionist, suffered from gradually worsening depression. She described her two years of suffering before doctors diagnosed her with hypothyroidism: "I would come home from work really, really tired. I didn't want to do anything. I had no motivation to go out and spend time with my friends. It was a struggle to work around the yard and to do all the daily chores like cooking and taxiing kids. For the past two years, I have gone to bed by nine or nine-thirty. It is a joke in my family that the kids stay up later than I do."

As the months passed, Christina felt as if she had become disconnected from the world and was no longer able to sleep. She quit her job and one day tried to kill herself by taking an overdose of painkillers. "I just wanted to escape and die," she said.

Before she became severely depressed, Christina had been in a state of minor, lingering depression. Because doctors failed to diagnose and treat her hypothyroidism, however, she progressed from minor depression to full-blown major depression. Her struggle with the extreme tiredness was a signal that more serious depression was evolving.

In major depression, a patient becomes quite disconnected from his or her surroundings and meets whatever happens with extreme indifference. The feelings of disconnection and tiredness are worse in the morning. The person typically suffers from insomnia and may wake up several hours early and have difficulty falling back to sleep. Other characteristics are loss of appetite, disinterest in eating, weight loss, and difficulty concentrating. People suffering from major depression often have the feeling that life is not worth living. They blame themselves and feel that they do not deserve help. Often they begin to think about death and suicide. Major depression can occur unexpectedly at any age and gradually worsens over a period of months. In some cases, the patient may be out of touch with reality and have hallucinations (major depression with psychotic features).

Researchers who screened severely depressed patients for thyroid disease found that up to 15 percent of them have an underactive thyroid.[11] But the striking finding was that their underactive thyroid was often low-grade rather than severe.

A study also demonstrated that nearly 20 percent of patients hospitalized because of severe depression had Hashimoto's thyroiditis.[12] The fact that a significant number of people, particularly women, being treated for major depression have low-grade hypothyroidism is best explained by the fact that a minor deficiency of thyroid hormone in the brain makes the person more vulnerable to slipping into major depression. In fact, women with low-grade hypothyroidism who are not currently suffering from major depression often experienced one or more episodes of depression in the preceding years.

In one study that compared the psychiatric history of sixteen women who had low-grade hypothyroidism to the psychiatric history of fifteen women with normal thyroid function, none of the women in either group was suffering from major depression at the time of the study.[13] The researchers found, however, that 56 percent of the women with low-grade hypothyroidism had a major depression episode at least once in their lives, compared to only 20 percent in the group with normal thyroid function. The study also showed that most episodes of depression had occurred in the preceding five years in the patients with low-grade hypothyroidism. This illustrates that low-grade hypothyroidism may make a woman more vulnerable to major depression when stresses occur in her life. Correcting low-grade hypothyroidism in such women should be viewed as a way to prevent the occurrence of major depression.

Scientists have been intrigued for years by the fact that a tiny thyroid hormone deficit in the brain (such as results from a minimally failing thyroid gland) can precipitate major depression. Stress, depressing events, and threats to livelihood are perceived and integrated in the brain, and messages are immediately transmitted to the thyroid gland so that the gland can adjust its function and increase the production of thyroid hormone.[14] The increased production of thyroid hormone triggered by these threatening events will help maintain an adequate brain chemistry that allows you to deal better with the stress, depressing event, or threat to your livelihood.

Even in low-grade depression, serotonin levels in the brain tend to decrease. The brain transmits the decrease in serotonin levels, however, to the pituitary. The message prompts the pituitary to produce more TSH, so the thyroid gland manufactures and releases more thyroid hormone. This thyroid adjustment works to bring serotonin levels back to normal so that mood does not deteriorate further. Thyroid hormone in the brain has the ability to enhance the production of serotonin in brain cells (see the accompanying diagram illustrating the role of thyroid hormones in preventing depression). But if the thyroid is failing and is unable to rescue brain chemistry or provide the extra thyroid hormone needed, serotonin levels will continue to fall, and depression escalates. This explains how a dysfunctioning gland could deprive a person of a primary defense mechanism against major depression. The increased vulnerability to major depression in patients with a previous history of major depression was elegantly illustrated in a study that assessed the severity of mood disturbances occurring in people who became hypothyroid after the surgical removal of their thyroid gland. The study showed that patients who previously suffered from major depression had the most severe symptoms when they became hypothyroid.[15]

THE ROLE OF THYROID HORMONES IN THE PREVENTION OF DEPRESSION

Brain	Low serotonin	Increased serotonin
	↓ (+)	↑
Hypothalamus	TRH		
	↓ (+)		
Pituitary gland	TSH	(+)
	↓ (+)		
Thyroid gland	Thyroid hormones	

Consider the case of Sara, age twenty-nine. She had been engaged for six months, was extremely happy and excited, and had just begun preparing for her wedding. She was a sales manager in a big department store, and the demands of her job were overwhelming because the Christmas season was approaching. She began feeling tired in the afternoon. When she went home, all she wanted to do was to sit down, watch TV, and then go to bed.

Sara also began to lose interest in going out with her fiancé. As the stress of preparing for the wedding and the demands of her job increased, she became easily irritated, had crying spells, and became angry about trivial matters. Gradually, the relationship deteriorated, and ultimately, the wedding was canceled. She attributed all of this to stress, the demands of her job, and her inability to cope with all these things at the same time. Over a few weeks, Sara slipped into a state of major depression.

Sara tried several antidepressants, but none of them seemed to work. Unable to function any longer, she stopped eating, lost a lot of weight, and was nearly fired from her job.

"I had problems with memory," she said. "I could not remember orders or where I placed papers. I would not return phone calls to customers." This made Sara feel even worse, and she started having suicidal thoughts. When finally a psychiatrist tested her thyroid, she was found to have low-grade hypothyroidism. As a result of thyroid hormone treatment added to the antidepressant, her memory improved, and she began eating again. Her original perky, happy personality reemerged. Her energy level increased, her performance at work improved, and her moodiness and anger disappeared.

In Sara's case, the job- or wedding-related stress and a genetic predisposition toward depression could have been what originally triggered the depression. But hypothyroidism made her more vulnerable to slipping into a state of major depression. When her brain needed a little extra T3 to prevent serotonin from falling further during the stress of the approaching Christmas season and her wedding, her thyroid gland was unable to do its job, and a complex sequence of brain chemistry imbalance led to major depression.

Diagnosing and treating a thyroid hormone imbalance may help prevent you from slipping into major depression. But if you are already suffering from depression, as in Sara's case, you must have your thyroid hormone imbalance diagnosed and treated. If the thyroid imbalance is not corrected, the depression will not be helped by conventional antidepressants. Research has shown that 52 percent of patients who suffer from major depression and do not respond to antidepressants have hypothyroidism.[16] Once doctors add thyroid hormone treatment to the antidepressant, the depression often resolves. Hypothyroidism also accounts for nonresponse to antidepressants in a significant percentage of people suffering from chronic minor depression. If you are suffering from depression or have recently experienced depression, you should be tested for a thyroid imbalance.

Clearing the Depression

If you are suffering from depression and test positive for hypothyroidism, in general you can expect the depression to clear once you correct the thyroid imbalance. The depression, in some cases, may not fully respond to thyroid hormone treatment alone. The depression may have taken on a life of its own and require additional treatment, particularly if the underactive thyroid had been undiagnosed for a long time.

Generally speaking, if you have a dysthymia, an atypical depression, or a low-grade lingering type of depression and your doctor diagnoses an underactive thyroid, your doctor should treat the underactive thyroid first for at least three months. The depressive symptoms are more likely to improve or resolve if you are treated with medications that combine T4 and T3 (see Chapter 20). If the depression does not fully resolve despite adequate thyroid hormone treatment, your doctor will add an antidepressant, such as a selective serotonin reuptake inhibitor (SSRI). However, if you have major depression and hypothyroidism, you must immediately begin treatment with both thyroid hormone and an antidepressant.

After your thyroid is well regulated and the depression has fully resolved, your doctor will probably consider stopping the conventional antidepressant after twelve months. If, despite normal thyroid levels, depression recurs after you stop the antidepressant, then antidepressant treatment should be resumed. (See Chapter 18 for information on antidepressants.)

Anxiety Disorders and Thyroid Imbalance

As is the case with depression, anxiety disorders can be triggered or worsened by your thyroid condition. According to a survey by the National Institute of Mental Health, 10 percent of the adult American population suffered from an anxiety disorder in the preceding six months.[17] It is estimated that 27 percent of adults suffer from an anxiety disorder during their lifetime. At any one time, nearly 15 million Americans suffer from an anxiety disorder. Undoubtedly, thyroid imbalance accounts for some of this anguish. One study even demonstrated that thyroid disorders are very common among family members of patients suffering from an anxiety disorder.[18] Also, in some people anxiety seems to predispose them to the occurrence of an overactive thyroid.[19]

Two types of anxiety disorders often occur as a result of a thyroid imbalance:

1. Generalized anxiety disorder, defined as excessive, exaggerated, and unrealistic worrying about trivial matters for at least six months

2. Panic disorders, characterized by attacks of abnormal physiological responses accompanied by extreme fear, causing physical symptoms

Less common anxiety disorders that have been noted to occur as a result of thyroid imbalance include:

• Social phobias
• Specific phobias
• Obsessive-compulsive disorder
• Post-traumatic stress syndrome (see Chapter 4)

In addition to excessive and unrealistic worrying, the most typical symptoms of a generalized anxiety disorder are restlessness, feeling superalert and on edge, fatigue, difficulty concentrating (which may be expressed in extreme cases as an inability to think or process information), irritability, muscle tension, and difficulty falling or staying asleep.

As is the case with depression, the severity of anxiety disorders varies. Many people with mild, generalized anxiety disorders become used to the way they feel: the mental and emotional struggles can become a way of life, and they may not even suspect that something is wrong. Other people, in contrast, are overwhelmed by the symptoms. Many seek medical help and may go from physician to physician trying to find a reason for their suffering.

Although, as noted earlier, it is commonly assumed that anxiety accompanies an overactive thyroid and depression accompanies an underactive thyroid, in fact, hypothyroidism frequently causes significant anxiety and even panic attacks. Abnormal noradrenaline levels in the brain may be the basis not only for depression but also for anxiety disorders such as panic attacks. A decrease in serotonin and an increase in noradrenaline activity in certain parts of the brain, coupled with an increase in the activity or the sensitivity of the body's respiratory center, cause the mental and physical symptoms of panic disorders.[20] Noradrenaline firing in the midbrain is the main reason for the physical effects on the heart and respiratory system experienced during a panic attack. The physiological responses accompanying a panic attack are real and are generated by the autonomic nervous system. An overactive thyroid causes noradrenaline activity to increase, which results in symptoms of anxiety and panic attacks. An underactive thyroid is likely to cause the levels of GABA, an antianxiety brain chemical, to decrease. This also contributes to the occurrence of anxiety during hypothyroidism-caused depression.

Panic Attacks

As explained in Chapter 1, the physical symptoms of a thyroid imbalance are similar to those resulting from an anxiety attack. Thus, a physician evaluating a patient with a thyroid disorder may believe that what the patient is experiencing results from an anxiety disorder rather than a thyroid imbalance.

Among the most common symptoms of a panic attack are:

- Pounding heart
- Accelerated heart rate
- Sweating
- Trembling or shaking
- Sensation of shortness of breath
- Feeling of choking
- Chest pain or discomfort
- Nausea
- Feeling of dizziness, light-headedness, unsteadiness, or faintness
- Feeling of unreality or feeling disconnected from oneself
- Fear of losing control
- Fear of dying
- Numbness or tingling sensation
- Chills or hot flashes

When patients experience their first panic attack, they often go to a hospital emergency room. Because the rapid heartbeat, difficulty breathing, dizziness, and other symptoms may resemble a heart attack or other heart problem, people suffering from panic attacks, including those with a thyroid imbalance, may undergo repeated and costly cardiac and neurological evaluations. Whether a person needs to have more than one panic attack to fulfill the criteria for a panic disorder is debatable. A person who has had only one panic attack will fear having another one. It has been estimated that nearly 30 percent of the American population experience at least one panic attack in their lifetime.[21]

Too often, doctors imply that a patient's symptoms are not real or are "in your head." For someone who has just experienced a rapidly beating heart, tingling in the hands and feet, and dizziness or nausea, this is not helpful.

When panic attacks recur, people enter a vicious cycle of anticipatory anxiety—excessive worrying about when the next attack will occur. They may also become afraid to be in a place or situation from which they cannot exit quickly because of the fear that a medical catastrophe or death might happen at any time. The vicious cycle of attacks and fear of attacks becomes debilitating and leads sufferers to see physician after physician, specialist after specialist. They continue to receive the same answer: "There's nothing physically wrong with you!"—which further perplexes the patients, who know their symptoms are real.

An easy way to determine the likelihood that you may be suffering from an anxiety disorder is to complete the following questionnaire. If you answer a question with no, proceed to the next question; if you answer with yes, score the severity of your symptoms (1 = mild, 2 = moderate, 3 = severe) before proceeding to the next question.

Have you intermittently been having difficulty breathing calmly?	Yes No	___
Do you experience feelings that something bad is going to happen?	Yes No	___
Do you feel tense all the time?	Yes No	___
Do you feel at times as if your arms and legs shake for no obvious reason?	Yes No	___
Do you often feel restless and unable to sit still?	Yes No	___
Have you had trouble falling asleep, or have you been waking up restless in the middle of the night?	Yes No	___
Have you been worrying excessively over trivial matters?	Yes No	___
Do you often feel as if you have to do things right now?	Yes No	___
Have you been experiencing spells of pounding heart, rapid heartbeat, and sweating?	Yes No	___
Have you been experiencing spells of shakiness, shortness of breath, and feelings of choking?	Yes No	___
Have you been experiencing spells of chest pain, nausea, light-headedness, and unsteadiness?	Yes No	___
Have you been experiencing spells when the world feels unreal?	Yes No	___
Have you been excessively afraid of dying?	Yes No	___
Have you been getting unexplained numbness, tingling, chills, or hot flashes?	Yes No	___
TOTAL SEVERITY SCORE		___

If you answered yes to three or more of the preceding questions, you may be suffering from an anxiety disorder. If you answered yes to five or more of the questions, you are probably suffering from an anxiety disorder.

Now add the scores for each symptom to obtain your total severity score, the meaning of which was explained earlier in the chapter, in the "Depression/Anxiety Severity" table (see page 133). The total severity score will be useful later in assessing your response to treatment.

Mood Swing Disorders and Thyroid Imbalance

From birth, all human beings have mood swings that occur during the day as well as over periods of weeks and months. These swings, however, are confined to a normal range, and we adjust to them. In the normal upswing, trivial news or events may make you unusually happy. If the same events or news occurred in the normal downswing, you would experience much less happiness. Similarly, bad news or a minimal disenchantment could make you very sad if it happened during the normal downswing but might not have much effect during the normal upswing. These are healthy mood swings.

With mood, as with most biological variables, there is a gray zone between normal and abnormal. Biopsychiatrists see abnormal mood swings as being due to defects in regulatory biochemical mechanisms that normally maintain mood swings within an acceptable range. The confinement of mood within what is considered to be a normal range is tightly regulated by several brain chemicals, including serotonin and noradrenaline. If, however, you suffer from clear-cut symptoms of depression in the downswings and symptoms of hypomania or mania in the upswings (even if the symptoms are mild), you will be considered as suffering from a mood swing disorder.

In many people with minor forms of mood swings, the symptoms are not disturbing enough to be noticed. Family members and friends may regard such people as being somewhat different, sensitive, or emotional, or as having an "unstable personality."

Because the severity of mood swings varies from one person to another, often only severely disturbing up- or downswings are noticed and lead to a psychiatric evaluation. Based on the rigid criteria used by psychiatrists, a bipolar disorder in its severe form (bipolar depression) affects nearly 1 percent of the population. Minor forms of mood swings, however, affect 5 to 8 percent of us and either remain undiagnosed for a long time or are not properly diagnosed.[22] Bipolar disorder is actually often mistaken for a straightforward case of depression. The reason is that manic-depressive patients often suffer primarily from recurrent depressive episodes.[23] Some patients experience very few intermittent manic or hypomanic episodes. The misdiagnosis is more common in women, notably because they tend to have more depressive symptoms but also because their upswing is often in the form of hypomania.

When manic-depressive people go through the mild upswing of hypomania, they are charming and successful in business or any other undertaking. They appear to be very organized, efficient, and able to achieve more than normal people. Hypomanic people have much more energy than usual and are very creative. They may exhibit impulsive behaviors, consume unusual amounts of alcohol (dipsomania), and engage in impulsive buying and excessive gambling. In fact, all this is typically overlooked and the family notices that there is something wrong with them only during the depressive period. When depressed, they tend to become lethargic and sleep all the time.

This explains why many patients diagnosed with "depression," even in a mild form, actually suffer from an undiagnosed bipolar disorder and are not properly treated. When such patients are prescribed an antidepressant such as an SSRI, they may flip into mania.[24]

Stress has a major effect on your symptoms and on whether you experience elation or depression. Unhappy life events in life will tend to trigger depression, while trying hard to reach a specific goal often triggers elation or even a manic episode. Manic-depression can be rapid-cycling, in which the swings may last hours or days, or it may follow the typical bipolar disorder pattern of no more than three or four cycles per year.

In many patients with a typical bipolar disorder, periods of abnormal mood are separated by periods of normal mood lasting months or years. Mood swing disorders often begin earlier in life (typically in the early twenties) than major depression. If you have been diagnosed with "depression," your physician should reconsider the diagnosis if your first episode of depression occurred at an early age (adolescence or early adulthood), if you have a family history of bipolar disorder, or if you had an episode of mania in the past.

Bipolar patients frequently suffer from a coexisting anxiety disorder. Research has shown that patients with generalized anxiety syndrome have an increased genetic predisposition to suffer from a bipolar disorder. One study reported that 24 percent of patients with bipolar disorder experience an anxiety disorder, and 16 percent of them have a panic disorder.[25] Anxiety can make bipolar disorder worse and makes the mood swings more frequent. In many, anxiety precedes the beginning of the bipolar condition and can also contribute to misdiagnosis.

A balance of thyroid hormone in the brain is crucial for maintaining mood stability. If you suffer from a deficit or an excess of thyroid hormone you may even experience clear-cut mood swing disorder. Severe hypothyroidism has even been blamed for causing manic-depression, with poor judgment and hallucinations. Doctors always wonder, however, whether such patients might not have preexisting minor forms of manic-depression, which have become more severe as a result of the thyroid imbalance.

Hyperthyroidism can also cause mood swings in a person who does not have a preexisting mood disorder. In some people, an overactive thyroid can result in an elated mood called "hypomania" or "mania," depending on whether the elation is moderate (hypomania involves no major behavioral disturbances) or severe (mania is associated with irrational behavior). In some patients, the thyroid condition may not be diagnosed until several years after the onset of the mood swing disorder that it caused.

By and large, if you are suffering from manic-depression, you have a much higher chance of having a thyroid disorder. Psychiatrists have recognized for quite a few years that hypothyroidism is much more common in patients with manic-depression than in the general population.[26] Although the reason for this higher frequency is not entirely clear, one factor is that patients suffering from manic-depression are often treated with the chemical element lithium. One of the first substances recognized as a mood stabilizer, lithium has since been shown to decrease thyroid activity. Hypothyroidism is ten times more common in bipolar patients treated with lithium than in patients not receiving lithium. Recent research, in fact, has shown that 30 percent of bipolar patients treated with lithium have an underactive thyroid, compared to 6 to 11 percent of patients not receiving lithium.[27]

One study conducted on a large number of psychiatric patients in the Netherlands showed a clear association between rapid-cycling bipolar (mood swing) disorder and autoimmune thyroid disease.[28] Women seem predisposed to mood swing disorders and depression when they suffer from an immune attack on the thyroid even when they are not treated with lithium. Is the immune system in these patients producing substances that affect the limbic system and alter mood and emotions, or do some thyroid antibodies cross the blood-brain barrier and affect the limbic system? It is likely that, in addition to thyroid imbalance, inflammation chemicals produced by the immune system contribute to the manic-depression.

Doctors diagnose many patients with mood swing disorders only when the thyroid condition is recognized because of how the superimposed thyroid imbalance affects mood swings. Low thyroid promotes a longer duration of the bipolar disorder, causes more frequent mood changes, and makes manic episodes more severe. Psychiatrists and thyroid specialists who fail to consider these effects may find it difficult to obtain optimal results treating their patients.

The most common reshaping of a mood swing disorder resulting from hypothyroidism is the precipitation of severe depression and the blunting of the upswings. When hypothyroidism is superimposed on top of a mood swing disorder, the person's depression may be more pronounced and he or she may simultaneously lose touch with reality. This is frequently the point at which the individual or his or her family seeks help from a psychiatrist.

Thyroid imbalances have another important effect on the kind of mood swings a patient has. Approximately 10 to 15 percent of persons suffering from manic-depression have rapid cycling, in which episodes of depression alternating with mania occur rather frequently—more than four cycles per year. Patients whose manic-depression involves infrequent swings may change to a rapid-cycling pattern when they become hypothyroid. Although mood swing disorders occur about equally often in men and women, rapid cycling is more common in women. This is related to some extent to the co-existence of hypothyroidism. In fact, about half of the patients with rapid cycling who fail to respond to conventional treatment for bipolar disorder are hypothyroid. Some patients with mild mood swing disorders, in whom the elation and the depression are not drastic enough to be noticed when their thyroid function is normal, become more manic-depressive (having a clear-cut bipolar disorder) when they have a severe thyroid imbalance.

BEWARE OF TEENAGE BEHAVIOR

Frequently, manic-depression starts at a young age, as do Hashimoto's thyroiditis and hypothyroidism. A teenager who begins to show mood instability leading to behavioral changes may frequently be thought to have "age-related issues" or be suspected of having drug problems. Leslie, the daughter of a woman afflicted with manic-depression and hypothyroidism, exhibited drastic changes in behavior. Her mother explained:

> When everything started showing up, it showed up as attitude problems. Until it got severe, being twelve, starting her periods, and going into the teenage years were the ways it was explained. A teenager with manic-depression may be sleeping a lot, but so do many teenagers. She was being a problem in school. The teachers sent notes that she was having outbursts and that this was totally out of character.
>
> It was like an alien had entered her body. She cried every day. She started doing irrational things that she would never have done in the past. She took acid. I could see her—if it continued—reaching suicide before she reached health.

With thyroid hormone treatment and lithium, Leslie experienced a major improvement in her energy level, attitude, and concentration. Her mood stabilized. Since then, her mother made sure she took the thyroid medication every day, and she became compulsive about testing Leslie's thyroid quite often (maybe too often), fearing that a thyroid imbalance would trigger the rapid cycling again.

THYROID IMBALANCE AND THE MILD MOOD SWINGS OF CYCLOTHYMIA

Cyclothymia, a long-standing condition characterized by periods of mild depression alternating with periods of slightly elated mood, often begins in late adolescence. In some people, the change in mood may be quite rapid, involving a shift from an upswing to a downswing every few days. At times, one type of mood lasts longer than the other. Frequently, the more noticeable swings are the downswings, which may be described by some as intermittently depressive moods. If you are suffering from cyclothymia, an underactive thyroid may make you experience a blunting of the upswings that results in chronic low-grade depression. Or it may make you shift continually from a happy mood to a depressed one.

An overactive thyroid could also make the swings in mood more apparent and more severe. Even if you have never suffered from cyclothymia, thyroid imbalance can cause patterns of mood swings similar to those of cyclothymia.

Evelyn, age thirty-seven, had been diagnosed with hypothyroidism fifteen years previously. She had been doing well on a stable dose of thyroid hormone and never had mood problems in the past. Then, two years ago, her general practitioner inadvertently reduced her thyroid hormone dose by half. As a result, she became hypothyroid. She also began experiencing noticeable mood swings, similar to the pattern of cyclothymia. As Evelyn described it:

> For three or four days, I could make decisions quickly. The self-confidence was there. I didn't let anybody else tell me I couldn't do something. I felt like I was on top of the world. I'd do various creative projects and activities.
>
> Three days of that, then I didn't want to do anything. I'd find it very difficult to come up with an idea for what to make for dinner. When I played bridge, I couldn't concentrate and my play would slip.

Three months after Evelyn's thyroid treatment was adjusted, her mood swings went away.

For most patients with mood swing disorders, treatments to stabilize mood do not work well when the brain is not receiving normal levels of thyroid hormones. Therefore, a mood swing patient who is also hypothyroid may be more difficult to treat. This may be due to depression causing the patient to neglect to take his or her medications. Family members of mood swing patients ought to make sure that thyroid medications are taken regularly to avoid difficult cycles. During depression, alcohol abuse may add to the pattern of self-neglect. To make matters worse, alcohol has a greater effect on a hypothyroid brain.

An End to Needless Suffering

In this chapter, we've seen how new discoveries are helping us understand thyroid disease better—especially how thyroid hormone balance affects the brain. As a result of these advances, endocrinologists and neuroscientists are focusing more on thyroid hormone because it is such an important component of brain chemistry. Unfortunately, because thyroid imbalances can go unrecognized, people experiencing psychiatric problems may not be receiving the appropriate treatment.

Physicians stand on the verge of a breakthrough to a more complete understanding of the processes that thyroid hormones set in motion. Psychopharmacology and endocrinology are drawing closer together as disciplines, and nowhere is this more important than in the treatment of the thyroid, our annex to the brain. Thyroid hormone may even be the serotonin of the new millennium.

Important Points to Remember

- The mental and emotional consequences of a thyroid imbalance may include serious conditions such as manic-depression. More often than not, however, the symptoms are more subtle and typical of borderline or shadow syndromes, such as mild depression.
- Thyroid imbalance magnifies the symptoms of people with mild mood disorders and emotional problems.
- Even if a hypothyroid person's symptoms do not satisfy the full criteria for depression, he or she may be experiencing borderline depression that is manifested primarily as fatigue.
- Women who have low-grade hypothyroidism, even without obvious symptoms of depression, may achieve mood benefits from taking thyroid hormone.
- Scientists now recognize thyroid hormone as a major brain biochemical that, like serotonin, has prominent effects on moods, emotions, and behavior.
- If you are suffering from depression or have had depression in the recent past, you should be tested for a thyroid imbalance, especially if you are currently experiencing other symptoms of thyroid imbalance.

9

MEDICINE FROM THE BODY

Thyroid Hormone as an Antidepressant

Biopsychiatrists often say that the first drugs shown to alleviate depression by altering brain chemistry were lithium and imipramine, the first tricyclic antidepressant. (Developed in the mid-1950s, tricyclics were hailed for being able to "normalize" mood without causing euphoria.) In a way, however, thyroid hormone pills are one of the oldest medications known to treat depression.

In 1890, Spanish doctors implanted a sheep's thyroid gland beneath the skin of a thirty-six-year-old woman suffering from severe hypothyroidism. They noted an immediate improvement in her symptoms and appearance. This experiment inspired Dr. George Murray to extract a fluid from sheep thyroid glands the following year. He achieved spectacular results by injecting this fluid into a severely hypothyroid patient.[1]

The discovery that extracts of animal thyroid could reverse the physical and mental effects of an underactive thyroid was the first major breakthrough in the history of thyroid disease. Patients who had been institutionalized due to extreme symptoms, such as a form of madness from severe hypothyroidism, regained their sanity when they took extracts. Suddenly, underactive thyroid—once a fatal condition—became controllable, allowing afflicted people to lead normal lives.

Subsequently, the production of desiccated (dried) extract of thyroid in the form of tablets provided a more standardized form of thyroid hormone replacement for hypothyroid patients. Desiccated thyroid, commercialized as Armour Thyroid, is obtained from animal thyroids. It contains both thyroxine (T4) and its by-product triiodothyronine (T3). Until the early 1970s, Armour Thyroid was the most widely used thyroid hormone pill.

Even though many doctors continue to prescribe the natural Armour Thyroid (primarily because it contains the two principal forms of the hormone, T4 and T3), most doctors treat an underactive thyroid with just a synthetic form of T4 (thyroxine).[2] This form of the hormone stays active longer in the body, which converts a portion of T4 into the more potent T3. Although synthetic T3 became available in the 1950s, doctors did not find it useful in treating hypothyroidism because T3 caused blood levels of thyroid hormone to fluctuate too much, and it was active in the system for a much shorter period than the synthetic thyroxine pills.

Over the years, however, many psychiatrists have used T3 in conjunction with conventional antidepressants to treat patients with major depression who failed to respond well to the antidepressants alone.[3] Even depressed patients treated with electroshock therapy benefit from taking T3. When given T3, these patients need fewer electroshock sessions, thus helping to avoid the cognitive impairment that may result from this treatment.

Norma was among the first of my patients to find in T3 the solution for depression. A forty-five-year-old lawyer, Norma is divorced and shares custody of two adolescent boys. According to Norma, when she first became ill, her boys were the only reason she got out of bed at all. Norma had changed from an expansive, high-energy woman with a vibrant intellect into a listless and somewhat desperate person. Three years before I met her, Norma had gone into severe clinical depression with no apparent precipitating incident. Although her psychiatrist had treated her with conventional antidepressants, she was still exhausted and suffering from mental anguish.

Norma's relentless search for a way to get back to normal led her to insist that she be tested for a thyroid imbalance. Norma was convinced that her thyroid was the key to her illness. A well-read woman, she was familiar with the similarities between a thyroid imbalance and the symptoms of fatigue and lack of joy that plagued her. But thyroid hormone testing showed that her thyroid gland was in working order and was not at the root of her persistent symptoms.

Despite the fact that Norma's blood tests were normal, I prescribed synthetic T3 (Cytomel) in addition to Prozac, which she had been taking for the past six months. For the first time in three years, Norma regained her former sense of self. The helpless feelings, exhaustion, and sense of isolation resolved.

There was nothing wrong with Norma's endocrine system. Her symptoms were due to a mix-up in her brain's use of such biochemicals as serotonin, noradrenaline, and also thyroid hormone. Although Norma's thyroid was fine, the mechanism that distributes the hormone through her brain and transports it to where it is needed was deficient. That's why she required chemical assistance with thyroid medication.

Thyroid Hormone's Role in ADHD and Depression

Thyroxine (T4), the main thyroid hormone produced by the thyroid, is a small molecule that contains four iodine atoms. In the cells of many organs (including the brain), a well-regulated process causes thyroxine to lose iodine, generating the much more potent thyroid hormone T3. In the brain, probably more so than in any other organ, T3 rather than T4 appears to be the critical form of the hormone that regulates cell functions. Because the amount of T3 present in the brain must remain in an optimal range to keep the mind functioning properly, fluctuations in the crucial process of converting T4 to T3 will inevitably affect the mind.

The thyroid system is one of the body's most tightly and precisely regulated systems. Minute changes in the way thyroid hormone is delivered to or dispersed in the brain can have drastic effects on mood, emotions, attention, and thinking. A problem with the delivery of T3 can cause disorders ranging from depression to attention deficit in people with normally functioning thyroids. Neuroscientists are teaching us the wide range of ways in which T3 regulates brain function and the brain chemistry syndromes that are likely to result from the alteration of thyroid hormone levels in the brains of people with normally functioning thyroid glands.

For instance, researchers recently discovered a connection between addiction to alcohol and thyroid imbalance in the brain. Free University of Berlin researcher Andreas Baumgartner conducted an experiment involving rats and alcohol.[4] He found that the animals that had slower inactivation of T3 in the amygdala—an area of the brain that plays a major role in emotions, sensory perceptions, and "reward memory"—exhibited greater behavioral dependence on alcohol. In essence, it is possible that, like rats, humans are more prone to alcoholism if that region of the brain produces more T3 from T4. High levels of T3 in some regions of the brain induced by chronic alcoholism could be part of the reason for the psychological and physical symptoms that chronic alcoholics often experience, such as irritability, aggression, sweating, and trembling. In the field of psychothyroidology, another breakthrough is the discovery that an imbalance of thyroid hormone in the brain can be responsible for attention deficit hyperactivity disorder (ADHD).

Cynthia, twenty-five years old, was referred to me by a family practitioner because of elevated thyroid hormone levels and a slightly high TSH. She had been changing jobs on a regular basis because she was never able to concentrate well enough or stay still while working.

Cynthia had been suffering from attention deficit hyperactivity disorder since childhood, but doctors never made the connection between her attention deficit and the thyroid. She told me:

When I was younger, the teacher would be talking, and I would be off looking at the acoustic ceiling and getting totally lost. Then I would go back, and everybody would be flipping the page, and I would be trying to catch up. In class, I tried to listen to the teacher, but I couldn't understand why I didn't get it. I understood what she was saying, but I couldn't catch on. We had a comprehensive exam in English, and I tested low even though I read pretty well.

Even now, I read two paragraphs and may not even remember what I read because I would be thinking of something else simultaneously. I cannot concentrate on what happens at work or what I'm going to fix for dinner. I'll be driving and not remember having driven to a certain point. I'm aware of the cars around me, but I'm not really thinking about my surroundings. At the same time I feel hyper. I can't keep my feet still. I have a lot of energy. All up and about.

Cynthia's condition turned out to be related to a familial, genetically mediated brain thyroid hormone imbalance called "syndrome of thyroid hormone resistance." In these patients, a genetic defect causes thyroid hormone to work less efficiently in the brain, pituitary, and other organs.[5] Therefore, despite high blood levels of thyroid hormone, the brain may in fact be deficient in the hormone, resulting in attention deficit.

Relatives of children with ADHD seem to be at much higher risk for having the disorder as well. Some relatives have been noted to be antisocial or depressed, perhaps as a result of how inefficiently T3 works in their brains. Adults afflicted with this condition tend to have high anxiety levels and often become drug addicts.

Because the pituitary becomes less sensitive to thyroid hormone (does not sense correctly the amount of thyroid hormone in the bloodstream), higher TSH levels result, causing the thyroid gland to produce more thyroid hormone. Paradoxically, despite high levels of thyroid hormone, many of these patients exhibit symptoms of underactive thyroid function and frequently experience hyperactivity as well.

In patients suffering from generalized resistance to thyroid hormone, thyroid hormone levels could affect other chemical transmitters such as noradrenaline, which is considered to be one of the culprits in ADHD. In such patients, the behavioral symptoms, such as distractibility and restlessness, may improve with T3 treatment. Thyroid hormone treatment could be used alone or in conjunction with other medications to regulate the noradrenaline levels in the brain.

In Chapter 3 we saw that thyroid hormone is essential for the chemical noradrenaline to work as a transmitter and perform its function in the brain. In fact, the highest levels of T3 produced in the brain are present in areas that are richest in noradrenaline.[6] This striking overlap in brain regions between thyroid hormone and noradrenaline explains why, if the body is not producing enough T3 or if it is not delivering it to the brain in the right amount, you require supplemental T3 in order for noradrenaline to work effectively.

In many patients suffering from depression, the root of the problem may be a low level or abnormal distribution of T3 in the brain even though the thyroid gland produces adequate amounts of thyroid hormone. The reason for this may be a lower conversion of T4 to T3 or an inability of T3 to produce its effects on brain functions efficiently. Research has also concluded that some depressed patients have reduced levels of a protein called transthyretin, which normally carries T4 from the bloodstream into the brain.[7] Transthyretin regulates noradrenaline in the brain and plays a major role in behavior. It also carries vitamin A in the brain and therefore has a protective effect against degenerative diseases of the brain.[8] Depressed patients whose depression is caused by low transthyretin are less likely to improve with conventional antidepressants.[9] Treatment with T3 in addition to the antidepressant can circumvent these delivery and conversion problems to enhance brain T3 content and thus resolve depression.

This is probably what happened to Anita. She is one of many patients I've treated who did not respond to a conventional antidepressant at first but then showed an almost miraculous response when T3 was added. A few months later, when her depression had resolved, I stopped her Zoloft but continued the T3 treatment. Her depression did not return while she was taking T3 medication alone. In her case, which is not necessarily the case of everyone suffering from depression, the primary source of the depression was probably an inability to generate sufficient amounts of T3. For this reason, T3 by itself eventually led to a long-term stability in mood.

Even if the primary brain chemistry problem is decreased noradrenaline or serotonin levels rather than T3, T3 levels in the brain decline as well, due to complex brain chemistry interactions. Therefore, depressed people with low noradrenaline or serotonin levels also have a low T3 content in certain regions of the brain. In essence, patients suffering from depression due to either low noradrenaline or low serotonin levels in brain cells have brain hypothyroidism even though blood thyroid hormone levels are normal. To some extent, the depression caused by low serotonin or low adrenaline could be at least partly the result of low T3 levels in brain cells. In fact, antidepressants work to some extent by restoring normal T3 levels in the brain.[10]

For instance, the SSRI fluoxetine (Prozac) increases the conversion of T4 to T3 in brain cells and therefore ensures the availability of T3 in the brain. This, in turn, will raise serotonin. Other pharmaceutical treatments of depression (lithium, carbamazepine, and desipramine), and even some non-pharmaceutical ones such as sleep deprivation, seem to produce some of their effects by increasing T3 levels in the brain and restoring normal serotonin levels.

The accompanying diagram illustrates the role of T3 in the maintenance of normal brain chemistry and shows how T3 treatment can help antidepressants become fully effective.

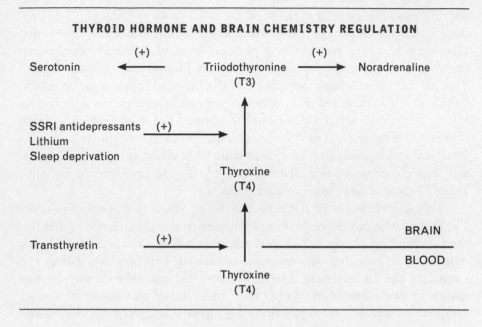

THYROID HORMONE AND BRAIN CHEMISTRY REGULATION

Research suggests that those patients with slightly higher T4 and lower TSH levels are more likely to respond to the addition of T3 to an antidepressant.[11] These changes are consistent with some deficit of T3 in the brain. In Chapter 8, we saw how depression, whether due to low serotonin or decreased manufacture of T3, will cause the hypothalamus and pituitary to stimulate the thyroid to produce more hormone. Decreased availability of T3 in the brain causes an activation of the thyroid system, which is designed to correct the deficit of T3. But often this activation is not sufficient, and T3 levels in the brain remain low. Once a patient receives T3, the symptoms of depression resolve, T4 goes back down, and TSH goes back up to normal.

Consider the case of Melissa. She tried several antidepressants, but none of them cured her depression. It was only when T3 was added to her treatment that the depression resolved. Most likely this resistance to the antidepressant medication was caused by the persistence of low T3 levels in the brain. After she divorced her husband, Melissa said:

My mind had a dullness. I didn't really experience life. I was dealing with the children and the tremendous amount of financial worries. I went into a depression. Sometimes I couldn't get out of bed. I went to counseling. But gradually I was not able to cope with anything. I tried to commit suicide.

They first put me on Prozac, which gave me relief for a few weeks. It took a lot of inhibitions away. The second month, I started noticing the depression coming back. Then the psychiatrist thought I would do well on the tricyclic antidepressant Anafranil, and in some ways that drug was very pleasant. Things weren't quite as stressful. All the sexual function was back. I ate slower. Then the depression came back.

Melissa's depression improved and temporarily resolved in the first few months of Anafranil treatment. But the symptoms returned, possibly because of the persistence of low T3 levels. When a T3 medication was added, at 5 mcg three times a day, Melissa's depression went away.

"The thyroid pill was a miracle for me," she said. "Now I am like a new person. When I started on thyroid hormone, I started having energy. In the mornings, I would feel good when I got up. A lot of my self-esteem came back. I was sleeping better. The anxiety went down. The mood swings were better."

The Best Way to Use T3 in Treating Depression

Norma and Melissa are among the millions of patients suffering either clinical depression or mood swing disorders who can benefit from treatment with thyroid hormone. Research has shown that antidepressants do not work in 40 percent of patients diagnosed with depression, even when high doses of antidepressants are used.[12] Half of those who fail to respond to tricyclic antidepressants, for instance, improve when the potent thyroid hormone T3 is added to the antidepressant medication.

Augmenting or potentiating the action of antidepressants is not the only way T3 can be useful. Thyroid hormone treatment also accelerates the action of antidepressants. In most patients, it takes several weeks for an antidepressant to begin showing an effect on the depression. When T3 is added to the antidepressant from the outset, the antidepressant may begin to relieve the symptoms sooner. An analysis of research published in the *American Journal of Psychiatry* showed that in five of six studies, T3 is much more effective than placebo in speeding up the response to the antidepressant.[13] The speeding-up effect is more obvious in women than in men. We don't know why this accelerating effect of T3 is seen mostly in women.

T3's effectiveness in boosting the efficacy of antidepressants in controlling depression is similar to that of lithium.[14] The patient's symptoms often respond to the addition of a T3 medication within a few weeks. Therefore, if no beneficial effect has been noted within three to four weeks, T3 treatment should be stopped.

Taking T3 along with the more modern antidepressant drugs—such as the SSRIs fluoxetine, sertraline, paroxetine, and citalopram—seems to benefit patients who have failed to respond using these medications alone. A study published in the *Journal of Affective Disorders* showed that the addition of T3 to an SSRI antidepressant causes a significant improvement in depressive symptoms and even remission of depression in 42 percent of patients who failed to respond to an SSRI alone.[15] Another study showed that the addition of T3 to fluoxetine was effective in 62.5 percent of patients.[16]

Taking T3 along with an antidepressant does not work for all patients, however. One of the reasons may be the way psychiatrists administer T3 treatment, both in their clinical practices and in their research in this field.

In contrast to T4, T3 (Cytomel) stays in your system for a much shorter period. Cytomel comes in 5-, 25-, and 50-mcg tablets. Taking a single dose of 25 mcg of T3 in the morning, for instance, causes T3 levels to increase above the normal range for a few hours. High amounts of T3 not only may not help but can cause adverse effects, both physical and mental.

A marked drop follows by midafternoon, resulting in wide fluctuations of T3 in your system. Since fluctuating T3 levels may reduce the effectiveness of this medication, I recommended that psychiatrists divide the total dose into two or three small doses, which is more effective and safer. A better regimen is 2.5 to 5 mcg three times a day, to be taken five hours apart (7:00 A.M., noon, and 5:00 P.M.). Using T3 treatment in this fashion, I have observed beneficial effects in many patients who had not responded to antidepressants or had responded only marginally. Perhaps the secret is to provide steady levels of T3 without the major fluctuations that inevitably result from the high conventional doses given once a day by psychiatrists.

The dose that helps one person may not help another. For this reason, I also use compounded T3 in conjunction with antidepressants. This way you can have the dose adjusted according to your needs. You can use as little as 3 mcg of T3 to help your depression. Compounded T3 will give you flexibility with respect to the dose, but also compounded T3 stays in your system longer than the synthetic Cytomel. Patients who suffer from significant anxiety often prefer the compounded T3 over the synthetic T3, Cytomel.

T3 alone prescribed in the way I just described may have great potential as an effective medication to help treat depression, but it has not been tried frequently enough to advocate its use as a sole treatment at this time. It would theoretically work as the only medication in some depressed patients whose primary chemical imbalance is a low level of T3 in the brain. But research is needed in this field. It surprised me to see that one of the first two studies examining the use of synthetic T3 as an antidepressant assessed patients who were not taking antidepressants.[17] T3 used alone was effective in treating the depression in those studies.

Note that not much research has been conducted on the use of T3 in combination with the atypical antidepressants, the newer serotonin-norepinephrine reuptake inhibitors (SNRIs), and the noradrenaline reuptake inhibitors. I have found, however, that T3 in the right amount does work with all newer antidepressants.

Treating Manic-Depression with Thyroid Hormone

The discovery in the 1940s that lithium could control manic-depression marked a watershed moment in psychiatry. Until that time, doctors believed that only psychotherapy could help manic-depressive patients. Now the options available to treat mood swing disorders have been expanded to include thyroid hormone treatment.

Treatment of bipolar disorder can be quite challenging to your doctor. In severe cases of bipolar disorder, the mood swings and the recurrent depression can affect the person at all levels and can lead to a wide range of health and social issues.

Bipolar patients are more likely to suffer from alcohol and substance abuse, eating disorder, obesity, insulin resistance, polycystic ovary syndrome, and non-insulin-dependent diabetes mellitus.[18] The social stigma of having a bipolar disorder and the physical and mental suffering impair patients' social functioning and their performance at work. For this reason, you will need a tremendous amount of help not only from your doctor but also from your family. You should also learn to recognize the early symptoms of recurrence and seek help right away. You should learn to improve compliance, accept the illness, manage your social life better at both the professional and emotional levels, and learn to deal with stress that could trigger a depressive episode.

In recent years, several new medications have become available that are quite effective in stabilizing your mood and in preventing recurrent mood swings. A well-balanced treatment can make your mood more even and will enable you to prevent the occurrence of health issues associated with bipolar disorder. But you need to keep in mind that the thyroid could be part of the problem and the solution for this condition. In Chapter 8, I detailed how a thyroid imbalance can promote a bona fide mood swing disorder or reshape and exacerbate a preexisting mood disorder.

Even if your thyroid gland is perfectly normal, a thyroid imbalance in the brain may be contributing to your mood swing disorder, and thyroid hormone treatment could greatly enhance the effectiveness of the medication you are receiving for your condition.

There is now increasing evidence that, in some people, a thyroid hormone imbalance localized in the brain, or an inability of thyroid hormone to work efficiently in certain regions of the brain, may contribute to the disorder. In such patients, the thyroid gland is functioning properly and producing adequate amounts of thyroid hormone, but the abnormality is in the brain. Correcting this abnormality by thyroid hormone treatment can lead to resolution of the mood swings.

As mood varies during the day, the amount of T3 produced in the brain by conversion from T4 also changes. Dr. Angel Campos-Barros, a researcher at the Free University of Berlin, has shown that the activity of the enzyme in the brain that converts T4 to T3 is subject to variations during the day.[19] This leads to fluctuations in T3 levels in certain regions of the brain. The increase in conversion of T4 to T3 in brain cells corresponds to periods of increased activity in animals. The normal fluctuations of T3 levels in the brain during the day and at night could be playing an important role in normal mood swings. Body temperature also fluctuates during the day. The same variations in T3 levels could be related to these temperature fluctuations. People suffering from a bipolar disorder tend to have lower temperatures during the day and higher readings at night,[20] possibly as a result of more ample changes in the levels of T3 in the brain.

If you are suffering from a mood swing disturbance called seasonal affective disorder (SAD), you may also be having a problem with the delivery of adequate amounts of thyroid hormone in your brain. Like thyroid disease, SAD affects more women than men. It is estimated that 80 percent of patients with SAD are women.[21] For some patients, SAD of the depressive type occurs annually, usually in winter or early spring. Research suggests that persons with SAD lack thyroid reserve[22]—a shortage that becomes more pronounced in winter and spring. The seasonal variation in thyroid hormone levels (higher in winter than in summer) suggests a need for more thyroid hormone in the wintertime, when your body tends to generate more heat. People unable to meet these demands may have a seasonal deficit in thyroid hormone in the brain that could account for seasonal mood abnormalities. With that in mind, and in light of the fact that patients with mood swing disorders may have a thyroid hormone abnormality in the brain, it is not surprising that thyroid hormone treatment is effective in the treatment of mood swing disorders.

Researchers have been able to successfully treat patients suffering from manic-depression with high doses of thyroid hormones. This treatment added to lithium, for example, eliminates the wide mood swings. Lithium may not be effective when used alone.[23]

Thyroid hormone also enhances the benefits of other mood stabilizers that are typically used for the treatment of bipolar disorder. A mood stabilizer is a medication that is effective in treating acute manic and depressive symptoms, and at the same time is useful in preventing the occurrence of manic or depressive episodes down the road. If you are taking an antidepressant without a mood stabilizer, you may easily flip into mania.

Newer medications are often used instead of or in conjunction with lithium to treat and prevent mood episodes. The current trend, in fact, is to use a combination of at least two medications for optimal mood stabilization and prevention of major mood swings, simply because no medication used alone can provide perfect mood stabilization. When added to antiseizure medication and atypical antipsychotics, thyroid hormone will enhance their effectiveness in patients with bipolar disorder.

The atypical antipsychotics are medications that stabilize mood and prevent depression and anxiety symptoms. They act through dopamine and other transmitters in the brain. The most-used atypical antipsychotics are olanzapine, risperidone, quetiapine, ziprasidone, and aripiprazole. A combination of an atypical antipsychotic and lithium is well tolerated and should be the first way to treat patients with severe mania.

Anticonvulsants and some other novel treatments have more pronounced antimanic effects than antidepressant effects. Lamotrigine works very well in treating acute mania, preventing bipolar depression and recurrence of mania. Research published in the *Journal of Affective Disorders* showed that lamotrigine is also effective in patients with mixed cyclothymic-dysthymic temperament.[24] In fact, it is effective in all forms of mood swing disorders and can be used in conjunction with thyroid hormone. The other antiseizure medications (e.g., valproate and divalproex) are also effective in preventing mood episodes and can be used instead of lithium. If you suffer from anxiety as well, you will be less likely to respond to antiseizure medications. Low-dose risperidone will better help your anxiety symptoms.[25]

You need to know that valproate can cause menstrual abnormalities and an excess of male hormones. It can also promote insulin resistance, metabolic problems, and even polycystic ovary syndrome.

The addition of an antidepressant such as an SSRI to mood stabilizers is often done to prevent depressive episodes. How long you need the antidepressant, however, depends on your clinical situation. Thyroid hormone is likely to have effects similar to those of an SSRI when used in conjunction with a mood stabilizer. Thyroid hormone also can help patients with rapid-cycling bipolar disorder, reducing the number of mood episodes. This suggests that mood swing disorders can be caused at least partly by a low thyroid hormone level in the brain or an inability of thyroid hormone to work efficiently in certain parts of the brain.

Research conducted at the University of California in Los Angeles also showed that addition of thyroid hormone in patients who failed to improve with medications resulted in either a total or partial response in all patients. The researchers also measured brain activity with positron emission tomography (PET) before and during treatment and found that the improvement in the bipolar condition correlated with an increase in activity in certain regions of the brain (the prefrontal and limbic regions) that are involved in mood disorders.[26]

As I explain in Chapter 8, thyroid hormone imbalance plays such a significant role in the brains of patients with manic-depression that when their thyroid gland starts to fail, leading to a minimal shortage of thyroid hormone, they begin to experience a worsening of the manic-depressive seesawing.

Many physicians and patients have wondered, however, whether high doses of thyroid hormone would have harmful effects on other organs, particularly the heart and bones. A study assessed bone density in ten premenopausal women receiving high doses of levothyroxine for the treatment of manic-depression.[27] The patients exhibited no significant bone loss compared to control subjects and seemed to experience no adverse effects when given high doses of thyroid hormone.

More recent research has shown that patients with mood disorders do not experience side effects from too much thyroid hormone when compared with healthy people.[28] This implies that patients with mood swing disorders are somewhat resistant to thyroid hormone. However, despite this, I do not advocate high doses of thyroid hormone. If you have been prescribed high doses of thyroid hormone, you need to be monitored carefully for potential side effects.

It is clear that T3 should not be administered in doses higher than 10 to 15 mcg a day. If higher doses are given, there is a risk of having too much thyroid hormone in your system.

Let me give a quick example of how T3 can help a patient with manic-depression. Priscilla, age forty-eight, had been diagnosed with manic-depression five years previously. She had tried several medications but in recent months had been taking valproic acid, an anticonvulsant medication also effective in treating manic-depression. Despite maximum doses of the drug, however, she had continued to relapse frequently into depression.

Priscilla's condition had been noticeable as far back as her teens. She had a tremendous drive and desire to do wonderful things. Her creativity flowed constantly. She had great ideas and liked to accomplish things. Her inability to bring some of these ideas to fruition was due to the fact that she would intermittently get into a depressed state and become unable to carry out her plans. Priscilla, like many bipolar patients, struggled with this discontinuity, in which periods of creativity and artistic sensitivity are typically interrupted by depressive episodes.

Priscilla described the struggle she had been enduring most of her life:

During the depressive period, I would become more withdrawn and agitated at the same time. The depression came about very insidiously. Unless you know that you have a bipolar disorder, which I did not know most of my life, you are ignorant about what is going on. It is slow and sneaky, and before you know it, you are overwhelmed with anxiety and depression and a feeling of hopelessness.

Her sister said, "It was absolutely tragic to see what happened to Priscilla. There came a point in time when I simply said to my family that I couldn't stand by and watch Priscilla live like this. She was deteriorating in front of our eyes, and if we didn't intervene and do something to help her, we were going to lose her."

Priscilla's treatment with valproic acid helped somewhat, but the dreadful depressive periods, albeit of shorter duration, continued to haunt her. It was not until she started taking T3 5 mcg daily that Priscilla's mood became more stable and she felt better than ever. Priscilla has now been receiving thyroid hormone for three years, during which time she has not experienced a single relapse of severe depression.

If you have suffered from rapid-cycling manic-depression and have not improved with conventional medications such as lithium, anticonvulsants, and atypical antidepressants, discuss with your psychiatrist the addition of a gentle and safe dose of T3 medication. It may reduce the frequency of your mood cycles and stabilize your mood for a long period of time.

Monitoring T3 Treatment Is Crucial

The dose of T3 used to treat depression varies considerably from one psychiatrist to another. Regardless of the dose used, careful follow-up and regular thyroid testing are important to avoid the serious physical and mental effects of thyroid hormone excess. Such thyroid monitoring, however, is not always done.

If a high dose of thyroid hormone is given to a patient with a psychiatric condition, hyperthyroidism may occur. Not only does the depression fail to improve, but further mental suffering is likely. The following example is of a manic-depressive patient who was followed by her psychiatrist for two years, during which she experienced tremendous mental suffering as a result of an unchecked thyroid hormone excess—an excess that her psychiatrist virtually ignored.

Natalie was thirty-seven when I first saw her for her thyroid condition. She had been diagnosed with manic-depression three years earlier, was treated with lithium, and was then prescribed T3 (Cytomel) at a dose of 50 mcg daily. Her psychiatrist failed to do a regular follow-up, however. The excess thyroid hormone resulting from the Cytomel led to hyperthyroidism, which, in turn, caused Natalie's manic-depression to deteriorate significantly.

During her first visit to my office, Natalie said, "Initially, I noticed an increase in my energy level, but only for a short time. Then I reached a plateau. Later, the Cytomel made me progressively more sick. It was masked by the exaggerated symptoms that happen to someone on lithium, so it was deceptive and insidious. I developed such a sense of hopelessness."

When I tested Natalie, I found that her thyroid levels were very high. After she stopped the Cytomel, her thyroid levels returned to normal. She said, "It took me sixteen weeks to reach a point where I was beginning to get my thoughts back together—to be able to assess my situation rationally and reasonably. For the first time, I looked at things in terms of how I was going to make things better. That was monumental."

Endocrinology's impressive progress in finding remedies for mental suffering is overshadowed by the use—and perhaps the overuse—of antidepressants as primary solutions to brain chemistry imbalances. Yet the science of endocrinology is reaching a promising new frontier, one that begins at the border where we can resolve mental anguish with thyroid hormone treatment. In this chapter, I have shown how thyroid hormone can be used as part of the treatment of both depression and mood swing disorders in patients with normal thyroid glands.

Important Points to Remember

- If you are suffering from depression, mood swing disorders, alcoholism, or attention deficit disorder, the root of the problem may be a thyroid hormone imbalance or a disturbance in the way thyroid hormone works in some parts of your brain.
- Increasing evidence indicates that T3, the most active form of thyroid hormone, is an effective antidepressant when used in conjunction with a conventional antidepressant.
- If you have been suffering from depression but your antidepressant has not fully worked for you, adding 5 mcg of synthetic T3 three times a day may resolve the depression.
- If you are about to start taking an antidepressant, you may want to consider adding 5 or 10 mcg of T3 three times a day. This is likely to speed up the effects of the antidepressant. Remember that it usually takes two to three weeks for an antidepressant to start working on the symptoms of depression.
- If you have been combining an antidepressant with T3 and have done very well, discuss with your psychiatrist the possibility of decreasing the dose of the antidepressant.
- If you have a mood swing disorder such as a bipolar disorder, thyroid hormone can help your condition when used in conjunction with a mood stabilizer, even if your thyroid gland is perfectly normal.

PART II

NO, YOU ARE NOT MAKING IT UP

Common Emotional and Physical Interactions

10

THE STRUGGLE WITH WEIGHT GAIN
AND SLUGGISH METABOLISM

Melinda, a thirty-three-year-old tax attorney, came to see me after having struggled with fatigue, mood swings, lack of motivation, and gradual weight gain for roughly three years. Prior to this problem, she had been a cheerful, outgoing person. I diagnosed Melinda with Hashimoto's thyroiditis and low-grade hypothyroidism. As a result of her thyroid condition, Melinda had gained thirty-five pounds and became mildly depressed. Her weight issue had further affected her mood and self-esteem. She had tried losing weight by following the Paleo diet and then tried Weight Watchers, but neither was successful. This further affected her depression and motivation. She also became a victim of food cravings, overeating unhealthy and fattening foods. She told me, "I ate virtually nothing for six months and was very strict with what I was eating, yet I started gaining weight. Despite my low energy levels, I forced myself to exercise five days a week, but that didn't help either. After giving up on dieting and exercise, here I am, thirty-five pounds fatter. I feel like a fat seventy-year-old lady and that my life is turning upside down."

Melinda's struggle is typical of the vicious cycle of thyroid imbalance, weight problems, and emotional conflicts. Her example serves to demonstrate the intricacies of the relationship between the brain, immune system, and thyroid function. As for most thyroid patients, Melinda's weight gain issue resulted from at least five factors:

- A slowing of metabolism (the ability of the body to break down fat to generate heat) due to her low thyroid
- An agitated immune system producing inflammation chemicals that cause general body inflammation
- Significant free radical buildup in cells caused by the thyroid imbalance, making metabolism-boosting hormones less efficient at burning fat

- Increased appetite and food cravings related to depression, anxiety, and the effects of thyroid imbalance and inflammation chemicals on the brain, compounded by low self-esteem and loss of willpower
- Reduced physical activity because of the fatigue and exhaustion from thyroid disease

These five interrelated factors typically result in significant weight gain among thyroid patients. Melinda blamed her depression and reduced self-esteem on her weight problem, when in fact the root of the problem was a thyroid imbalance caused by thyroid autoimmunity. When I treated Melinda's hypothyroid condition with the right thyroid medication and addressed her body inflammation and immune system reactivity, she began to lose weight, her confidence returned, and her outlook brightened. Once again she became more physically active. She also followed my comprehensive weight loss program, paid attention to food sensitivities, took natural supplements to reduce body inflammation and support the immune system, and was able to regain her energy and self-esteem and rid herself of her food cravings. In a six-month period, she was able to lose all the extra weight she had gained over the preceding three years.

Although, as we'll see, not all weight problems can be blamed on thyroid-related conditions, Melinda's battle with weight gain is one faced by many people, women in particular. Weight gain issues, including obesity, are becoming a worldwide epidemic, particularly in Western societies.[1] They are also at the root of a wide range of debilitating health conditions such as diabetes, high blood pressure, heart disease, sleep apnea, cancer, and osteoarthritis. At the present time, two-thirds of American adults have some sort of weight problem. Because we know that autoimmune thyroid disease and thyroid imbalances are highly prevalent in the United States, it is not surprising that thyroid disease contributes to some extent to the rising incidence of weight problems.[2] The connection between weight problems and thyroid disease is further enhanced by the fact that when you gain weight or become obese, you become more likely to be affected by thyroid autoimmunity, which in turn can make your weight problem worse.

The social and cultural challenges faced by overweight people, especially women, can be tremendous, due to the social pressure of feeling the need to be slim. Many women claim that they eat virtually nothing and exercise but still have weight problems. The reason is most likely a slow metabolism. The growing awareness that an underactive thyroid can result in a slow metabolism has led many people whose weight won't drop despite countless efforts to seek medical help and insist that their thyroids be tested.

Thyroid hormone is one of the most important body chemicals that regulates your weight and body composition.[3] It is part of a powerful hormonal system working in harmony to regulate and determine how much fat you should have in your body.[4] This powerful system has a say in what and how much you eat, and how much fat you burn, including at rest.[5] Even a minute thyroid hormone imbalance can lead to a slowing of metabolism and other effects that cause gradual weight gain.[6] Many women with a subclinical thyroid condition continue to struggle with weight gain but have not been diagnosed as having an underlying thyroid disease. The weight problems in these women cannot be corrected without appropriate treatment of their thyroid condition. Equally important for weight loss success is the need to reduce body inflammation to support the immune system and address mood and emotional issues.

The Hormonal System That Regulates Your Metabolism and Eating Behavior

To understand the weight issues that you may be facing, you need to have a basic understanding of how hormones regulate your weight, appetite, and metabolism. Even though the amount of food we eat differs from one day to the next, we manage to maintain a fairly stable body weight because our food consumption matches the calories that we burn at all times. This regulation comes from the interplay of several chemical signals that regulate energy stores. The three leading hormones that work together at maintaining your energy balance at all times are leptin, ghrelin, and thyroid hormone.

Leptin: The Metabolism-Boosting Hormone

Leptin is a hormone produced by fat cells that has the ability to reduce appetite and enhance metabolism. The name is derived from the Greek *lepto*, which means "thin." The amount of leptin in your system depends on the amount of body fat you have. Because women often have more body fat than men, their leptin levels are usually higher than those of men. When you reduce your food intake and lose weight, leptin levels go down, which makes your brain sense the need to eat in order to compensate for the weight loss you have just experienced. At the same time, because your leptin levels have become lower, your body will burn less fat, because your metabolism has slowed down in an attempt to conserve your energy stores and keep you from losing more weight. When you gain weight, your leptin levels go up, sending a signal to the brain that will make you want to eat less; at the same time, those high leptin levels will normally make you burn more fat. As you can see, leptin has two functions: making your body burn fat and lowering your appetite.

The effect of leptin on the hypothalamic centers that regulate appetite, food choices, and food impulses is quite dramatic. Leptin works on a wide range of chemicals in the hypothalamus that regulate satiety (feeling full), such as neuropeptide Y. These hypothalamic chemicals interpret and process all information concerning the energy situation in your body.

You may have adequate leptin levels yet still experience weight gain if leptin has become inefficient at performing its functions in the hypothalamus and/or in other parts of the body, resulting in a situation similar to having low leptin levels. The issue of leptin inefficiency is the central problem of most people who have a weight issue, be it related to a thyroid condition or not. Obesity is in part due to the inability of leptin to carry out its job properly both in the brain and as a regulator of metabolism. As you gain weight, inflammation occurs in both the hypothalamic center, damaging the cells that regulate your energy balance, and the body parts that burn fat, making leptin less efficient. As you gain more, leptin levels rise (because there is more fat that produces leptin). However, the increased body inflammation caused by the weight gain makes leptin less able to help you control your appetite and burn fat. This situation is called leptin resistance. The efficiency of leptin is also to some extent determined by genetic factors. That is why, for instance, you may eat the same amounts and kinds of foods as another person but your body composition and weight will be different. If you have genes that make leptin less efficient, any minor deviation from a good diet will worsen leptin inefficiency, making you gain more weight. One of the most important causes of leptin resistance is eating meals rich in fat and/or simple sugars, because of the inflammation induced by these nutrients in the body and in the hypothalamus. For leptin to work efficiently in your body, it requires perfect levels of thyroid hormone. Low thyroid levels will impair the ability of leptin to make you burn fat.

The efficiency of leptin at speeding up your metabolism goes hand in hand with the efficiency of insulin at regulating sugar and fat metabolism. Insulin is a hormone produced by the pancreas in response to consuming simple sugars. When you digest sugars or carbohydrates, your pancreas releases insulin, which has the ability to make glucose enter the cells and be processed through metabolic reactions. Insulin also enables your fat cells to convert excess glucose into fat. But when cells damaged by inflammation stop responding to insulin in the same way they did before, insulin becomes less effective in some body parts; this is called insulin resistance. The more fat you gain, the more insulin resistance you have, causing more inflammation and putting you at a higher risk for developing metabolic syndrome. Metabolic syndrome is defined as having too much abdominal fat (an "apple" body shape) and increased cholesterol and triglyceride levels, increasing the risk of narrowing of the arteries, heart disease, high blood pressure, and non-insulin-dependent diabetes.

Ghrelin: The Hormone That Slows
Your Metabolism and Makes You Eat More

Eating behavior and satiety are also regulated by chemical signals produced by the gastrointestinal tract. The gastrointestinal system and brain communicate at all times to regulate how much and what you eat. The amount and type of chemical signals triggered by a meal depend to a great extent on the amount and type of foods you eat. One of the signals produced by the gastrointestinal tract that regulates your satiety level is the hormone ghrelin. When you do not eat for a few hours, ghrelin levels go up. Ghrelin's function is opposite to that of leptin—instead of suppressing your appetite, it makes you want to eat more.[7] It is the normal rise of ghrelin in the morning, at lunchtime, and at dinnertime that tells your body it is time to eat; when you eat enough, your ghrelin levels go back down, making you less hungry.

Ghrelin also has the opposite effect of leptin on metabolism in the sense that it slows metabolism down and makes you burn less fat.[8] As you gain weight, ghrelin levels become higher than normal, perpetuating increased hunger and cravings. Research has shown that when you eat too much fat, your ghrelin levels remain high, making you feel hungry despite having consumed a large number of calories. When you eat a high-protein meal, ghrelin levels go down, making you want to eat less. If you are successful at losing weight, your ghrelin levels improve, reducing your overall hunger levels. When you lose weight, you are less likely to be hungry. In essence, excess weight brings in hunger, and hunger brings in excess weight. In addition to being a potent stimulator of appetite, ghrelin helps your fat cells hold on to fat, creating a slowdown of the fat-burning process at the cellular level. In essence, ghrelin is a weight-gain-promoting hormone.

Thyroid Hormone: The Cornerstone of Metabolism Regulation

The two extremely powerful metabolism-energizing hormones that make the body able to burn extra fat and convert it into heat are leptin and thyroid hormone. These two hormones work in concert at almost every single level in the body to regulate energy balance.[9] I view thyroid hormone as the executive hormone that fine-tunes energy balance, eating behavior, and metabolism. It works in conjunction with leptin to control both appetite and fat burning. Optimal thyroid hormone levels are essential for leptin to work optimally. Thyroid hormone also regulates the amount of leptin produced.[10] Too much thyroid hormone in your system will make your leptin levels go down, and this will contribute to the excessive hunger that hyperthyroid patients constantly experience.

Low thyroid levels make leptin less efficient, so your cravings increase and your metabolism slows; the result is weight gain and an inability to lose weight by dieting. Inefficiency of leptin, in turn, will make thyroid hormone inefficient at speeding up metabolism. This explains why a deficiency of thyroid hormone, even minute, can engender a self-perpetuating cycle of leptin and thyroid hormone inefficiency, which can lead to a significant drop in metabolism, weight gain, and resistance to weight loss.

Another way thyroid hormone influences your weight is through its effect on neurotransmitters. Some of the chemical transmitters in the brain that regulate emotions, mood, and perception of stress, such as serotonin, noradrenaline, GABA, and beta-endorphin, are the same chemicals implicated in the complex interactions regulating satiety, food selection, and even taste. For example, when you eat, serotonin rises in the brain; at a certain point, it causes the hypothalamus to sense a feeling of satiety, making you eat less or stop eating altogether. Noradrenaline increases the desire to eat fats and carbohydrates, while serotonin decreases that desire. An excess or deficiency of thyroid hormone alters the levels of these chemicals and will change your eating behavior.[11] Thyroid hormone also has direct effects on brain appetite centers.

When a thyroid imbalance both lowers your serotonin and affects your mood, you are likely to crave fats and carbohydrates and to consume larger food portions. Too much thyroid hormone in the brain causes a person to eat more often and select carbohydrates over other foods. A patient with a thyroid imbalance who is depressed experiences more impulses to overeat, because these impulses are triggered when serotonin levels are low, in an attempt to ease or relieve low mood and anxiety. Typically, people suffering from serotonin deficiency report an improvement in their mood after consuming carbohydrates.

For thyroid hormone to fulfill its function as a metabolism-boosting hormone, it is crucial that the mitochondria, the organelles inside the cell where chemical reactions take place to create energy, are healthy and not overburdened by oxidative stress from free radicals. Toxins, lack of essential micronutrients, inflammation, and free radical buildup can all damage cells. If the cells in your body are unhealthy, it won't matter if your hormone levels are perfectly normal, because the efficiency of leptin and thyroid hormone will be impaired (for example, cells will not be able to convert T4 to T3 efficiently), and you will end up having significant thyroid hormone inefficiency, leading to slow metabolism.

Often people who are hypothyroid lose control of their eating patterns and end up not following the nutritional and lifestyle guidelines necessary to reduce caloric intake and boost mood. They may no longer be able to schedule meals and snacks or choose mood-enhancing foods. The increased caloric intake coupled with low metabolism may result in significant weight gain.

Hypothyroid women who gain weight are often more aware of their weight gain than non-hypothyroid women because of their hypothyroidism-related anxiety and depression, which in turn are exacerbated by weight gain. In yet another vicious cycle, hypothyroidism frequently leads people to stop exercising because of tiredness, muscle weakness, shortness of breath, and depression, even if they used to exercise routinely before. The lack of exercise coupled with an increased appetite may result in rapid and significant weight gain, potentially causing profound depression.

Candace is an attractive young woman who had been married for two years when I first saw her as a patient. She used to be health-conscious and physically fit; going to the gym was a part of her daily routine. Her lifestyle gradually began to change when she started feeling tired, slept more, and experienced other symptoms of hypothyroidism. When she became hypothyroid, keeping her weight down was a struggle. This is what she told me:

> When I started to gain weight, I didn't want to be around any of my friends, nor did I want to do anything that involved being social because I was so self-conscious about the way I looked after gaining so much weight. I also became generally less active as a result of my unexplained fatigue. I increasingly ate nutritionally poor foods, especially in the afternoon; the chips and chocolates just felt like the best thing to look forward to during the day. It would get to a point where I would start off every day being careful with what I ate until the afternoon came and exhaustion and fatigue would hit me like a train. I quickly lost all motivation to exercise and began eating more. As I gained weight, I became more irritable, and as a result of that irritability ate more and gained more weight. I would crash on my bed after work, lying there doing nothing for hours until my cravings made me order pizza for dinner, convincing myself that it would be the last time. This pattern took complete control of my life and I continued following it until I had gained thirty pounds in total.

Motivational coaching or lectures have no effect on people like Candace; their willpower is crushed by something they don't understand, and it is not their fault. Candace's mother told me, "We went on Jenny Craig together. The diet worked for me, but not for her. She didn't have the willpower to do it and kept cheating. She became very depressed and cried all the time."

Candace's case illustrates the vicious cycle frequently generated in hypothyroid people, where hypothyroidism triggers depression, low self-esteem, and changes in metabolism. The depression substantially contributes to the weight gain, which in turn exacerbates the depression. Weight gain and depression make exercise less likely, leading to more weight gain. In this setting, when doctors diagnose hypothyroidism and administer appropriate treatments, people typically lose weight and experience an alleviation of their depressive symptoms. The point is that the vicious circle can be broken in two ways—by enhancing metabolism and by alleviating depression.

Low-Grade Hypothyroidism: A Relentless Cause
of Slow Metabolism and Weight Gain

Like its negative impacts on energy and quality of life, the effects of low-grade hypothyroidism on metabolism and weight have been trivialized, ignored, and even denied by the medical community. Yet, as we have seen, having an autoimmune thyroid disease and a small deficit of thyroid hormone can trigger a wide range of hormonal changes in your body that affect the efficiency of leptin and thyroid hormone, impair fat-burning processes in the cells, and lead to a cascade of changes in your body including inflammation and gradual weight gain, which in turn can lead to metabolic syndrome.[12] The long-term metabolic effects of untreated low-grade hypothyroidism include body inflammation, leptin resistance, insulin resistance, and cardiovascular damage.

Weight Struggle May Persist Even After
Your Low Thyroid Is Corrected with Medication

Most patients believe that once their hypothyroidism has been corrected with thyroid medications, their weight issue will disappear. Unfortunately, often this is not the case. Many patients are disappointed by their lack of weight loss after beginning medication; some may actually continue to gain weight. This is a typical dead end faced by many thyroid patients, who may think that their thyroid is still poorly regulated and responsible for their weight problem.

Part of the problem is that balancing thyroid hormone levels doesn't always completely reverse the inefficiency of metabolism-boosting hormones that had been triggered by the low thyroid and associated autoimmunity. If you are treated with a T4-only medication, you may be missing the right amount of T3, which can slow your metabolism.[13] Also, low T3 makes leptin less efficient at regulating satiety and making you burn fat. So in addition to working on your overall thyroid hormone levels, you may need a change in your medication regimen that includes the right amounts of T4 and T3. Another important reason for having a hard time losing weight is the body inflammation caused by an immune system that continues to be agitated and reactive.

If your low thyroid condition is caused by Hashimoto's thyroiditis, be aware that the thyroid medication you are taking may actually be contributing to your slow metabolism. In addition to the active thyroid hormone ingredient, T4, T3, or both, thyroid medications may also contain some inactive ingredients, such as silicon, soy, and gluten. If your immune system is sensitive to one of the inactive ingredients in your tablet or capsule, the medication can trigger the release of even more inflammation chemicals that promote leptin and thyroid hormone inefficiency, making you experience weight gain and difficulties losing weight.

Persistent mood issues and anxiety can be another factor in remaining overweight. When you suffer from lingering low mood, you are more likely to continue to suffer from food cravings even after you correct your low thyroid with the right thyroid medication. And unless you provide your body with healthy nutrition and antioxidant supplementation, your body will continue to suffer from a buildup of free radicals. As I explained in Chapter 2, free radical buildup impairs T4 to T3 conversion, causes cellular thyroid hormone imbalance and inefficiency, and slows all the biochemical reactions that help you burn fat.

If you are still overweight despite adequate thyroid hormone treatment, you need to follow a strict diet and regular exercise program. The exercise program should focus not only on burning extra calories but also on building the muscle mass that was lost during the imbalance. At least now the medication will have eliminated your cravings and fatigue, a barrier that had prevented you from losing weight before the diagnosis of an underactive thyroid. It is equally important to address all the issues that may be contributing to your weight gain, including food sensitivities, sleep problems, and stress. (See Chapter 21 for details of the ThyroLife Diet and my weight loss program.)

When Your Thyroid Gland Is Overactive

Many people with an overactive thyroid, especially women, are pleased with the weight loss resulting from their condition. The weight gain that they experience when they begin taking a medication to correct the overactive thyroid can be a disappointment. I have seen women who purposely stopped taking their thyroid medication—if the other symptoms of hyperthyroidism are not so severe, they prefer to continue putting up with them if it means not regaining the weight. This is something I try to discourage. If left untreated, excess thyroid hormone in your system can lead to heart problems, bone loss, and osteoporosis, among other debilitating conditions.

Audrey, age thirty-two, struggled with being overweight most of her life but became slim when she became hyperthyroid. I started her on antithyroid medication and asked her to return for a follow-up and repeat thyroid testing. Displeased with the weight gain after only three weeks of treatment, Audrey stopped taking the medication and returned to see me eight months later, still hyperthyroid.

When I asked her why she had not followed through with her treatment,

Audrey replied honestly: "I didn't feel that bad, so I figured I would just stop taking the medication since it started making me regain the lost weight. When we went on vacation, I purposely left it at home. My husband found out and made me go to a pharmacy that was able to fill the prescription. I still didn't take it for the subsequent two weeks we were there. I was finally wearing a smaller bikini that made me feel good about myself and I thought, 'There is no way I'm going to take this medication and gain weight while I'm down here.' Even after the vacation, I kept off the medication so I could keep myself slim." I explained to Audrey that correcting her overactive thyroid was a priority and that the longer she remained hyperthyroid the more she would struggle with weight issues down the road, when her thyroid levels become normal with treatment. She complied with the treatment, her thyroid hormone levels balanced, and she followed my weight management program, which helped her avoid the weight gain she feared.

Note that an overactive thyroid does not always result in weight loss. In fact, some people with an overactive thyroid gland gain weight instead of lose it. What happens in these patients is that the increase in body metabolism, which tends to reduce fat storage, is coupled with increased caloric intake. Hyperthyroid patients often crave higher than normal amounts of fattening food and tend to overeat. The increased caloric intake is probably a defense mechanism designed to preserve the body's energy when it is flooded with thyroid hormone. So when you consume more calories than the calories burned, you will end up gaining weight even though you are hyperthyroid.

Weight Gain Struggle After Hyperthyroidism

Hyperthyroid patients tend to gain a significant amount of weight after their excess of thyroid hormone has been corrected with treatment.[14] Nearly half of women treated for hyperthyroidism experience a significant weight gain after their thyroid function becomes normal. Research has shown that the weight gain experienced by patients treated for Graves' disease was the same whether the patients were treated with radioactive iodine or surgery. This suggests that the weight gain issue they experience is a real aftermath of the hyperthyroidism. Although many patients believe that their thyroid has become underactive and is therefore responsible for the weight gain, that may not necessarily be the case. These are the four main reasons hyperthyroid patients experience weight gain and weight loss resistance after their thyroid hormones are brought into balance:

1. When your body is exposed to too much thyroid hormone, your metabolism shifts to a high level, possibly leading to weight loss. After normal thyroid function is restored, your metabolism becomes slower

than normal for some time as a result of leptin inefficiency. In addition, leptin and even growth hormone levels may remain suppressed for some time.

2. Excess thyroid hormone in your system often disturbs the appetite center, and this disturbance may persist for a long time after the excess of thyroid hormone has been corrected. This could lead to uncontrollable hunger and increased caloric intake.

3. Hyperthyroidism causes muscle breakdown. Many hyperthyroid patients experience some loss of muscle mass, especially in the quadriceps and biceps, as a result of too much thyroid hormone.[15] Once thyroid levels have become normal, the compensatory rebound of building up energy stores will be directed at building up fat rather than muscle. One study showed that after correction of hyperthyroidism, muscle strength remains lower than normal for a long time. For this reason, a well-balanced exercise program aimed at building muscle mass, such as my 20/10 exercise protocol, will enhance your metabolism and help you overcome the weight loss resistance.

4. Excess thyroid hormone causes a major depletion of antioxidants, which leads to free radical buildup; that, in turn, causes inflammation, making the metabolism-boosting hormones less inefficient. This results in the slowing of metabolism and worsening insulin resistance.

If you suffer from excess thyroid hormone, you need to be proactive and implement a weight management program as soon as your thyroid levels become normal with treatment (see Chapter 21). You need to be patient and persevere. As time goes by, you will find it easier to control your weight as long as you keep your thyroid well regulated and adhere to the weight management guidelines I recommend in my program.

Do You Also Have Growth Hormone Deficiency?

Despite perfect thyroid hormone balance with medication and embracing my entire mind-body program, some of my patients continue to struggle with the inability to lose weight and may also continue suffering from fatigue and low mood. This could be caused by a problem with the pituitary gland, resulting in growth hormone deficiency.[16] Growth hormone is a metabolism-boosting hormone, like leptin. It contributes to the regulation of fat burning and is produced in higher amounts at night when you sleep. In humans, the purpose of growth hormone is not only to promote normal growth when you are a child; it also has many metabolic effects and regulates mood, emotions, bone growth and maintenance, and muscle function. If you have an autoimmune thyroid condition, your immune system could be attacking your pituitary (a condition called autoimmune hypophysitis), leading to impaired production of growth hormone. Research has shown that 5 percent of patients with Hashimoto's thyroiditis have growth hormone deficiency. The most common symptoms of growth hormone deficiency are weight gain, fat accumulation around the waist, depression, mood swings, anxiety, fatigue, muscle weakness, and sleep problems. Although autoimmune hypophysitis is the most common cause of growth hormone deficiency in patients suffering from autoimmune thyroid disease, growth hormone deficiency can also be the result of pituitary gland damage from a tumor or other inflammatory conditions.

The Foods That Add to Your Weight Gain Struggle

As I explained in Chapter 3, sensitivities to certain foods can make the immune system produce inflammation chemicals that can affect your energy, mood, and mental capabilities. These nonspecific inflammation chemicals also promote inflammation in the body. Roughly half of the population has some sort of food sensitivity; this may or may not have any impact on well-being and systemic inflammation.[17] If you are suffering from an autoimmune thyroid disease that has resulted in a thyroid hormone imbalance, your chances of having more significant sensitivities to foods become remarkably higher simply because autoimmunity makes your immune system more reactive.

Eating foods you are sensitive to creates a chronic challenge to the immune system, which inevitably responds by generating inflammation. As we have seen, that inflammation will result in insulin resistance, leptin resistance, and thyroid hormone inefficiency, causing slowing of metabolism as well as increased hunger. The inflammation caused by immune system chemicals is widespread, but in particular it affects food appetite centers in the hypothalamus and the health of the cell mitochondria where fat burning takes place.

By and large, thyroid patients tend to suffer from sensitivities to foods containing gluten and to dairy products, particularly those made from cow's milk. Eggs, especially egg yolk, are also very immunogenic and are often responsible for fatigue, inflammation, and weight loss resistance. Addressing food sensitivities is of extreme importance to thyroid patients, not only to feel well again but also to overcome the struggle that many experience with weight gain and slow metabolism.

The foods that your immune system is reactive to may not be the only ones that can alter the efficiency of the metabolism-boosting hormones leptin, thyroid hormone, and growth hormone. Eating meals loaded with carbohydrates, and in particular simple sugars, will make your blood sugar levels rise more significantly, causing higher insulin spikes in your bloodstream. Eating high-glycemic-index foods promotes weight gain, insulin resistance, inflammation, and free radical buildup in your body, affecting most organs, including the brain centers that regulate satiety and food choices. This explains why eating high amounts of carbs makes you want to eat even more carbs. The inflammation also targets the immune system, making it more unstable and reactive, generating more inflammation chemicals. Eating too many carbs at night will have even more detrimental effects on your metabolism because high insulin levels at night impair the efficiency of growth hormone at burning fat while you sleep.

Fructose is a simple sugar found mostly in fruits. When it is consumed in high amounts, it has damaging effects on your metabolism, because it is directly converted into glucose, making blood sugar levels rise even higher and promoting more inflammation and insulin resistance. In fact, high levels of fructose consumption, whether from fruits or from foods containing high-fructose corn syrup, have been strongly linked to metabolic syndrome. The fruits with the highest fructose content include dates, bananas, pineapples, kiwi, and oranges.

Saturated fats and trans fatty acids also promote general body inflammation and free radical buildup, making leptin and thyroid hormone inefficient at burning fat.[18] They inflame the appetite and hunger centers, making you want to eat inappropriate quantities of foods that aren't good for you.[19] They are also strong agitators of the immune system and powerful contributors to autoimmunity. As a result, they make your immune system produce more antibodies that target your thyroid gland as well as nonspecific systemic inflammation chemicals that generate more inflammation in your body, further slowing your metabolism and perpetuating weight gain. Foods rich in saturated fat include red meats and dairy products such as cheese. Therefore, select low-fat or nonfat dairy products if you are not sensitive to dairy. Foods that contain high amounts of trans fats include fried food, fast food, chips, and pastries.

How Stress and Depression Make
Thyroid-Related Weight Problems Worse

In Chapter 4 I detailed how stress can make the immune system more agitated and prone to attacking the thyroid gland, causing autoimmune thyroid diseases such as Graves' disease and Hashimoto's thyroiditis. I also detailed the escalation cycles in which stress brings in thyroid imbalance and immune system reactivity, making your perception of stress amplified, which in turn makes your immune system more reactive. Stress can promote weight gain, body inflammation, and inefficiency of the metabolism-boosting hormones leptin and thyroid hormone, whether you have a thyroid condition or not. If, however, you suffer from an autoimmune thyroid disease, the impact of stress and your perception of stress is even worse, primarily because your immune system is much more likely to produce large amounts of the nonspecific inflammation chemicals that affect your mood, emotions, appetite, and metabolism.

Chronic stress will make your adrenal glands produce more cortisol, the stress hormone, which causes fat accumulation around the waist. Too much cortisol makes leptin and thyroid hormone less efficient at burning fat, consequently making you crave more fattening foods. High cortisol levels have the ability to impair the conversion of T4 to T3 in the cells, making you hypothyroid-like even when your blood thyroid hormone levels are normal. The ultimate consequence is a further slowing of metabolism. Cortisol also alters the activity of brain neurotransmitters such as noradrenaline, serotonin, and dopamine, explaining why stress makes you crave sugary foods and foods rich in saturated fats and trans fats[20]—these food choices are linked to the sensation of pleasure and comfort.

Continuous stress, as you can see, will generate a cycle of bad food choices, higher caloric intake, more inflammation, and more metabolism slowing, all leading to a weight gain trend accelerated by the effects of an agitated immune system. As reiterated throughout the book, one of the main consequences of thyroid disease is depression, which can trigger and perpetuate autoimmune thyroid disease. Being overweight can also make you become depressed and vice versa. If you are a thyroid patient struggling with weight gain issues and thyroid-related depression, understand that your depression can significantly exacerbate your weight gain problem and make you struggle with weight loss resistance. Depression, like stress, can affect your food choices and your willpower, and cause your immune system to be more reactive.

Sleep Problems: A Hidden Cause
of Weight Gain and Weight Loss Resistance

The hormonal regulation of energy balance and of how much fat your body contains can be seriously damaged if you do not get enough good-quality sleep. When you sleep, your body repairs damage that occurred when you were active and awake. It is also during sleep that your metabolism adjusts to keeping your weight and fat storage stable from one day to the next. For example, leptin, the metabolism-boosting hormone, rises significantly when you are asleep, in order to suppress your appetite and make you burn more fat. Growth hormone is also produced in high pulses when you are asleep, further contributing to fat burn. In essence, it is during sleep that your body gets rid of the unnecessary calories you have consumed during the day through activation and efficiency of the hormones that make the body burn fat. Amazingly, it is also during sleep that the hormones that make you store fat, such as insulin and cortisol, are at their lowest levels. This explains why insomnia, sleep interruptions, or any form of sleep deprivation will have a serious negative impact on your metabolism, which can lead to more weight gain and to an inability to lose weight even with dieting and exercise.[21]

You may be suffering from a sleep disturbance caused by your thyroid disease. Common sleep problems that occur in thyroid patients are insomnia, waking up from anxiety, and sleep apnea. These sleep disturbances are even more common in menopausal women and women going through the menopausal transition. You are more likely to have a sleep issue if you are also dealing with depression, stress, or fibromyalgia. Not getting at least seven hours of sleep will make you crave fattening foods and increase your hunger levels during the day.

The functioning of your immune system also depends on good-quality sleep. Being sleep deprived or having sleep interruptions will make your immune system more agitated and more likely to produce higher amounts of inflammation chemicals and antibodies. These can affect your thyroid function and promote inflammation in the body's tissues, which in turn slows down your ability to burn fat.

If you have difficulty falling asleep or if you wake up in the middle of the night, consider using a melatonin supplement (1 mg before going to bed). Melatonin is a hormone produced by the pineal gland that naturally helps you fall asleep. It also has beneficial antioxidant and anti-inflammatory properties. It can also help you with your weight loss efforts because it lowers inflammation and reduces insulin resistance; for that reason, it can be beneficial for people suffering from metabolic syndrome.[22]

Other than melatonin, I often recommend two natural supplements, GABA (500 mg) and L-theanine (200 mg) at bedtime, to my thyroid patients who suffer from anxiety and difficulties falling asleep.

Thyroid patients are more vulnerable to sleep apnea, the periodic cessation of normal breathing during sleep. The most common cause of sleep apnea is the collapse of soft tissue in the throat, blocking the airway, and that tends to occur more often in overweight people. It also is seen more often in women going through the menopausal transition, because of how changes in sex hormone levels affect muscle tone in the neck. Sleep apnea can make your weight gain worse and can ultimately make you become obese and suffer from metabolic syndrome and diabetes. The interruption of airflow, even for a few seconds, disturbs sleep and causes a drop in blood oxygen levels. This affects the efficiency of your fat-burning hormones. The drop in oxygen also promotes the buildup of free radicals in your body and in the immune system; the result is a cascade of cytokines and other chemicals that escalate inflammation, increase leptin and thyroid hormone inefficiency, and cause more weight gain. Thyroid patients already burdened by inflammation and hormonal imbalance will have a hard time losing any extra pounds if they do not get the right diagnosis and treatment for sleep apnea. The two most popular forms of treatment of sleep apnea are continuous positive airway pressure (CPAP) machines and mouth appliances. Both help to restore adequate airflow through the upper airways while you sleep.

Sleep apnea, in addition to slowing your metabolism, can add more symptoms such as cognitive changes, attention deficit, fatigue, headaches, high blood pressure, worsening anxiety and depression, neck pain, and sexual dysfunction.

The Sex Hormone Factor in Your Weight Struggle

For thyroid patients, having well-balanced sex hormone levels is crucial because of their effect on metabolism and inflammation. The main sex hormones that influence metabolism and fat balance are estradiol (the main estrogen hormone), progesterone, testosterone, and DHEA. For women, the wide fluctuations in sex hormones and the drop in estradiol that occur around the transition to menopause can have a wide range of mental effects, including anxiety, irritability, and depression. There are also significant metabolic effects, including the slowing of metabolism and a shift in body fat distribution from the buttocks and thighs to the abdomen, with a concurrent loss of fat underneath the skin (this has to do with the greater number of estrogen receptors in the buttocks, thighs, and subcutaneous fat tissue than in the abdomen). Low estrogen levels engender insulin resistance and leptin inefficiency as well, making your body less able to burn the extra fat you don't need.[23] With the drop in estrogen, menopausal women typically see their LDL cholesterol levels rise and a gradual increase in their weight.

As I explain in Chapter 3, the hormone changes that occur during menopause are associated with the flare-up of autoimmunity,[24] making the immune system more reactive and likely to attack other body parts in addition to the thyroid, potentially initiating other autoimmune conditions. The immune system also generates more inflammation chemicals and responds more forcefully to any additional challenger such as stress, depression, environmental toxic chemicals, and foods. To rebalance estrogen levels, I recommend that menopausal women take estradiol replacement therapy in the form of a patch, gel, or sublingually. The dose of estrogen has to be tailored to your needs, as for thyroid hormone, and monitored with blood testing, since excessively elevated estrogen levels are as detrimental to metabolism as excessively low levels are. As estradiol level falls, women produce less growth hormone, which in turn makes them lose more muscle. For menopausal women who still have a uterus, I recommend that you also take progesterone in the right amount.

For women who have decided to take testosterone replacement for the purpose of improving libido, I cannot emphasize how important it is that the dose be as low as possible. Testosterone receptors are quite prevalent in abdominal fat, and taking inappropriately high amounts of testosterone may counteract the beneficial effects of estradiol on body fat distribution.

Polycystic Ovary Syndrome: A Common Sex Hormone Imbalance in Overweight Thyroid Patients

Women who have an autoimmune thyroid condition and are struggling with a weight issue may have polycystic ovary syndrome (PCOS). PCOS is a common hormonal disorder that is three to five times more prevalent in patients with Hashimoto's thyroiditis.[25] Additionally, low-grade hypothyroidism is five times more common in patients with PCOS. PCOS affects 5 to 10 percent of women. (An equivalent syndrome occurs in men, causing them to suffer from hair loss before the age of thirty, as well as insulin resistance and being more prone to becoming diabetic down the road.)[26]

This condition often begins around puberty and continues even after menopause. In PCOS, imbalanced sex hormone levels can disrupt ovulation, cause infertility, and result in excess hair growth and irregular menstrual periods or loss of menstrual periods.[27] Even after menopause, testosterone may remain high,[28] which can promote fat accumulation around the abdomen, cardiovascular disease, and endometrial cancer.

Moreover, PCOS patients often have insulin resistance and typically high fasting insulin levels. If you have PCOS, the more weight you gain, the more insulin resistance you have. Research has shown that the weight gain associated with PCOS is fundamentally due to an inefficiency of leptin in controlling your hunger and speeding up metabolism, making you eat more food while burning fewer calories. If you have an underactive thyroid and PCOS at the same time, and the root of your low thyroid is autoimmunity, the weight problem is drastically worsened. The reason is that the immune system increases body inflammation, causing more leptin and thyroid hormone inefficiency and further slowing your ability to burn fat, even at rest. The insulin inefficiency will increase your risk of becoming diabetic.[29] It has been estimated that 45 percent of women with PCOS have glucose intolerance, and 10 percent have type 2 diabetes.

The cause of PCOS is not quite clear, but it seems to be related to a dysregulation of chemicals in the hypothalamus that affect satiety, metabolism, and the signals that regulate the ovaries. Your genes have a say in whether you will be affected by PCOS[30]; in fact, research has shown that sisters of PCOS patients who do not themselves have the syndrome still tend to have higher levels of androgens. Moreover, the genetic predisposition explains why thyroid patients are more affected by PCOS than are people without thyroid issues.

If you have PCOS, you are also genetically predisposed to depression or bipolar disorder.[31] Research has shown that 28 percent of patients with PCOS also suffer from bipolar disorder. As explained in Chapter 8, if you have bipolar disorder, you may already be struggling with weight gain as a result of how much and what you eat, and the medications you take for the mood disorder can promote weight gain as well. You can imagine the consequences for your weight if you are suffering from the triple threat of thyroid imbalance, PCOS, and bipolar disorder.

Losing weight is the most important component in the treatment of polycystic ovary syndrome. When you lose weight, your periods may become regular, your excess hair growth may go away, and infertility problems may disappear. You need to adhere to the weight management program that I recommend for thyroid patients. The low-glycemic-index diet will both help you lose weight and treat all the symptoms of PCOS listed above. Reducing simple sugars in your diet is one of the most important ways to deal with polycystic ovary syndrome. This program will also prevent you from having type 2 diabetes down the road.

You may need to supplement your diet with chromium at a dose of 200 mcg a day in order to improve insulin resistance, and you should take adequate amounts of vitamins and antioxidants to speed up weight loss and keep that weight off. Birth control pills will help regulate your menstrual cycle. Yasmin, a low-estrogen birth control pill, has become quite popular for the treatment of PCOS. It will improve acne and help reduce the level of male hormones.

Metformin, a medication used for diabetes, improves insulin efficiency and will make leptin levels go down, indicating that leptin has become more efficient.[32] It will also normalize menstrual irregularities and promote normal ovulation, possibly restoring fertility. Metformin, at a dose of 500 mg three times daily, improves growth hormone secretion, which may be impaired in PCOS patients (possibly as a result of the excess weight). Other drugs that improve insulin efficiency, such as rosiglitazone or troglitazone, can be useful in regulating menstrual cycles and ovulation but have less of a beneficial effect on male hormone levels.

Controlling Your Weight

Many people are haunted by the metabolic and inflammation consequences related to thyroid imbalance, immune system reactivity, sleep issues, sex hormone imbalance, stress, and mood problems. If you are among them, then to counteract the weight gain trend you need to embrace a comprehensive thyroid and immune system wellness program while paying attention to the factors that can slow your metabolism and make your weight loss goals difficult to achieve. These are some steps that you need to take in order to succeed in your weight loss efforts:

1. Keep your thyroid hormone levels perfectly well balanced at all times with a thyroid medication treatment tailored to your needs (preferably a combination of T4 and T3 in the right amounts).

2. Follow the right eating plan. To lose weight in a healthy way and to keep the weight off, you need to follow a well-balanced eating plan while reducing your daily caloric intake. Follow a balanced-deficit diet, which takes into account roughly how many calories you burn in a day and gives you somewhat fewer calories than you would require to maintain your current weight. Do not opt for a very-low-calorie diet (less than 800 calories a day), such as Optifast or Medifast, as this will not give you the long-term weight loss that you desire. Low-calorie diets (800–1,200 calories a day), such as Slim-Fast, Jenny Craig, or Nutrisystem, will obviously make you lose weight initially but will not work for thyroid patients on a long-term basis. In Chapter 21 I provide details on the ThyroLife eating plan, which will help you lose weight and keep it off. This diet takes into account the fact that you have an autoimmune thyroid problem, and it addresses what the metabolism-boosting hormones leptin, thyroid hormone, and growth hormone require to perform optimally. This eating plan will provide you with low-glycemic-index meals to combat insulin resistance and make your metabolism faster. Finally, it is aimed at keeping your body inflammation levels as low as possible in order to maximize feelings of wellness, thyroid hormone efficiency, and speedy metabolism.

3. Avoid foods that your immune system is reactive to, in order to reduce inflammation chemicals that have detrimental effects on your metabolism and cravings.

4. Make sure you get adequate, good-quality sleep. Address any sleep disturbances, and consider the possibility of sleep apnea if you have symptoms such as snoring, waking up at night for no apparent reason, waking up tired despite sleeping eight hours or more, or having persistent fatigue and mental fog.

5. Learn how to manage stress and practice relaxation techniques (see Chapter 4).

6. Rebalance your sex hormones. If you are a perimenopausal or menopausal woman, discuss the benefits and the potential negative effects of hormone replacement therapy with your doctor. If you have PCOS, be

scrupulous about following my eating plan and consider, with your doctor, the use of medications to reduce insulin resistance.

7. Reduce the inflammation and free radical burden in your body and immune system by taking the right antioxidants and vitamins in the proper amount. In Chapter 21 I provide more details on my entire weight loss program. This comprehensive program will give you all the necessary tools to succeed in your weight-loss goals. It includes a diet that has helped thousands of patients suffering from thyroid disease efficiently lose weight and keep the weight off.

Important Points to Remember

- Thyroid hormones and leptin are the two most powerful metabolism-boosting hormones that make your body burn fat, even at rest.
- Hypothyroidism, even low-grade, can slow down metabolism and make you gain weight over time.
- Although hyperthyroidism typically causes weight loss, in some people it may cause weight gain by affecting the appetite center in your brain.
- Any thyroid hormone imbalance can affect your eating behavior and exacerbate stress-related cravings.
- After thyroid imbalance has been corrected, you may continue to struggle with weight problems. It is important to follow a healthy, high-protein, high-fiber, low-glycemic-index, low-saturated-fat diet and to engage in a well-balanced exercise program.
- For successful weight loss, you need to rebalance thyroid hormone levels. You also need to address other factors such as sleep problems, stress, and sex hormone imbalance. You also need to take the right amounts of vitamins and antioxidants that will help you with your weight loss efforts.

11

HORMONES OF DESIRE

The Thyroid and Your Sex Life

When I began my career in the thyroid field, it never crossed my mind that I would play the role of marriage counselor. Most of the time when patients have marital or sexual difficulties as a result of a thyroid imbalance, I refer them to a couples therapist or a sex therapist. Yet sex therapy or couples therapy may not be successful unless I take the initiative to counsel the patient and explain the effects of thyroid imbalance on sexual function.

Both hypothyroid and hyperthyroid patients experience changes in their sexuality. Some of the examples discussed in this chapter can shed light on important aspects of how the thyroid affects sexual desire and activity.

Beatrice and Leonard had been married for almost fifteen years and had a daughter. The CEO of a large company, Leonard was quite successful, and the family was wealthy. During most of their marriage, they had a happy, stable relationship. All this changed rather suddenly.

Beatrice's gynecologist referred her to me because he had noted a goiter and a tremor in her hands. In my first encounter with Beatrice, I established that she had an overactive thyroid due to Graves' disease, and I started her on treatment. A few days later, I received a call from Leonard, who wanted to discuss some issues with me. He told me his wife had been unfaithful in recent months, and because of this, he was planning to divorce her. He was wondering if by any chance there was a connection between her thyroid condition, hormones, and the changes in personality and sexual desire his wife had experienced during the past year.

At her husband's request, Beatrice returned to my office to explain the situation from her viewpoint. She said:

> We got married when I was twenty-five years old. I loved Leonard and was attracted to him, but from the very beginning, I was not all that interested in sex.

Even before the marriage, I never really understood what the big deal was about sex. In fact, if I had any problem with my husband, it was because for years I was not very interested in sex. I'm sure that after our child was born, what little of me had been there for him was probably totally taken away. I had a lot of guilt feelings about not being a good wife sexually all the time.

Beatrice recalled that the previous summer she had started losing weight, feeling hot, sweating, and at times feeling shaky. Then, gradually, she became more and more interested in having sex with her husband. She said:

Definitely once in the morning, definitely at night before bed, and almost always in the middle of the night. At least three times a day and, if the opportunity arose, four times a day. This was in addition to when I was by myself. It became a constant thing on my mind.

I began to log on to our computer and go into chat rooms on the Internet. At that point, I wasn't thinking I was going to get involved with somebody or experience sexual fantasies, but later I was totally consumed by the possibility of sex. It got to the point where I couldn't wait for my husband to leave the house so I could get on the computer. It would annoy me when he wouldn't leave when he was supposed to.

I was sexually stimulated most of the time. This happened when I was on-line pretty much throughout the day. Most definitely when I was with my husband it happened. I masturbated while talking with people on the computer. In turn, they masturbated when I was talking to them. That whole sick thing went on for a few months.

During the same period of time that all this was going on, my husband and I were partying, drinking, and dancing all the time. I just had energy constantly. I started becoming more aware of myself, more aware of everybody else, and wanting to get out and do things. I was paying less attention to my daughter.

The constant sexual obsessions and the manic behavior led Beatrice to have an affair that almost destroyed her family. One of the men to whom she had been talking on the computer decided to meet her. She described the encounter as follows:

I had talked to him for a number of months on the computer and also on the phone. I told Leonard I was going to spend the night with my cousin. The affair lasted one night, but Leonard found out almost immediately. How come other people can have affairs their whole lives and never get caught while I'm good as gold for fifteen years and get caught from having a one-night stand? Probably Leonard was already suspicious because of my behavior over a period of time. He confronted me about the episode, and I couldn't lie. I said yes, and everything went downhill from there.

Leonard became totally depressed and unsure of himself. Our relationship became like a roller coaster. We'd be okay for a day or two, and then he'd give me a zinger or we'd get into an argument. We started seeing a counselor, but that didn't seem to be helping at all.

After my interview with Beatrice, Leonard called me on the phone. He confirmed that his wife's infidelity had affected him tremendously, and he was having difficulty coping with it. I explained to Leonard that what he and his wife had experienced could be the result of hyperthyroidism's effect on the functioning of the brain. The total transformation of Beatrice's personality—from a fairly nonsexual, stable, supportive, and loving wife and mother to a self-centered person obsessed with sexual thoughts—was due to chemical changes in the brain that were making her a different person.

Although he found my explanations comforting, Leonard remained somewhat skeptical. His doubts persisted even though Beatrice returned to her previous self two to three months later when medication helped correct her hyperthyroidism. She stopped having the sexual fantasies and chatting with strangers on the computer. Beatrice herself could hardly believe that she had really been doing these things. In a subsequent conversation with Leonard, I dissuaded him from thinking that hyperthyroidism had unmasked Beatrice's "true" personality. Hyperthyroidism did not unmask hidden desires and hidden personality. It triggered and changed feelings, drives, and perceptions. Thyroid dysfunction altered the most intimate aspects of Beatrice's life, as it has with many other people.

Thyroid disease can precipitate or contribute to significant sexual problems, which are often a source of frustration between couples and can lead to the deterioration of relationships. Such problems aggravate the emotional chaos that both partners feel when one suffers from a thyroid condition.

Most patients with thyroid disease do not discuss their most intimate acts with their physicians and seldom bring up sexual disturbances, except sometimes to refer vaguely to "changes in my sex life." Sexual issues remain hidden and unexplained, yet they can be responsible for distancing and significant marital problems. Physicians seldom inquire about the sexual difficulties that thyroid patients may be experiencing, nor do they provide explanations or counseling. People who experience sexual difficulties often hide them and do not attribute them to the thyroid disease. In extreme cases, when sexual dysfunction weighs on the relationship and becomes a source of conflict between two partners, the couple may seek psychological counseling. Some people may even seek help from a sex therapist. Yet, for the majority of thyroid patients who experience sexual dysfunction, neither psychotherapy nor sex therapy will help unless the thyroid imbalance has been corrected and both the therapist and the partner have a good understanding of the thyroid disorder and its effects.

How Thyroid Function Governs Sexuality

In the sex act, there are four steps or stages that normally lead to sexual fulfillment or orgasm, each of which is affected by thyroid function. A sexual thought, a touch, or a signal that our brain interprets as erotic causes certain parts of the brain to emit chemical transmitters. These transmitters generate a surge of sexual interest and fantasies, making us willing to become intimate. Brain chemistry stimulates the autonomic nervous system, which will make us experience a range of physical responses: the skin becomes more sensitive, breathing and heart rate become more rapid, blood rushes to the genital organs, and so forth. This phase of excitement (or readiness) varies in duration from one person to another. As stimulation continues, the physical responses generated by the autonomic nervous system intensify, causing lubrication and engorgement of the external genital organs in women. The vaginal opening narrows, the labia swell, and the clitoris pulls in and becomes close to the pubic bone. In men, the autonomic responses cause an erection due to engorgement of the penis with blood.

The brain chemistry involved in sexual arousal and excitement is affected by the level of thyroid hormones. They promote the pleasurable body-mind response that culminates in orgasm. At the time of climax, the brain increases the release into the bloodstream of the hormone oxytocin, which causes the involuntary rhythmic contractions of muscles in the genitals, anus, and uterus. These orgasmic contractions depend on normal thyroid hormone levels. After we reach orgasm, we experience a period of relaxation. In women, the resolution of the lubrication and engorgement may take several hours, whereas in men, the resolution of the engorgement and return of the penis to a flaccid condition occurs almost immediately after ejaculation.

Women tend to suffer from sexual dysfunction more often than men. Research has shown that 40–45 percent of women and 20–30 percent of men suffer from sexual dysfunction.[1] Low libido (lack of desire and loss of sexual fantasies), called hypoactive sexual desire syndrome, is the most common form of sexual dysfunction among women. According to a study conducted in Switzerland, one of two women suffering from sexual dysfunction has lack or loss of sexual desire, and one of ten has an issue with reaching an orgasm.[2] Sexual dysfunction causes significant personal distress and promotes major interpersonal problems. Any kind of sexual dysfunction among women has several roots and includes both physiological and psychological reasons.[3] You are more likely to suffer from hypoactive sexual desire syndrome if you are not satisfied at work, if you have relationship problems, if you have a medical condition, or if you feel that your partner has low libido and does not reach a climax. You may also suffer from hypoactive sexual desire syndrome because of abnormal hormone levels or as a result of taking certain medications.[4]

Women's sexual problems often arise from the differences that exist between men and women with respect to thinking and feeling.[5] Generally speaking, men focus on sexual intercourse, but women can be satisfied with just the emotional affection associated with sex. Typically, when a woman loses interest and desire in sex, the couple often stops having intercourse. A woman also does not want to have sex if she suffers from pain during intercourse. Wanting to have intercourse, for women, is more linked to the affection that she has for her partner and to the anticipated physical and—equally important—mental and emotional satisfaction experienced during intercourse. In essence, men and women have different ways of thinking about sex.

Because of this high vulnerability to sexual dysfunction, women's sexuality becomes easily impaired at all levels if they have a thyroid imbalance. In patients with this condition, depression makes sexual dysfunction worse. This often explains why women with thyroid imbalance may continue to suffer sexual difficulties even after the imbalance has been corrected with treatment. Another reason why a woman may continue to have low libido is hyperprolactinemia—an excess of prolactin, the pituitary hormone that regulates lactation. High prolactin can be caused by an underactive thyroid, by medications, or by a pituitary dysfunction. Recent research has shown that 88 percent of patients with hyperprolactinemia have sexual dysfunction. High prolactin level in women impairs all phases of female sexual function, including libido and orgasm.[6] Women with high prolactin also have problems with arousal, lubrication, and satisfaction with sex. The higher the prolactin level, the more severe the dysfunctions.

Thyroid hormone not only has a direct effect on the brain chemistry interactions that lead to the autonomic nervous responses of sexual arousal and fulfillment; it also has an effect on the levels of sex hormones. In women, hypothyroidism lowers estrogen and progesterone levels and can contribute to a cessation of ovulation.[7] The lack of estrogen has significant peripheral effects, not only on the brain but also on the lubrication of genital organs.[8] Low thyroid makes the ovaries produce less testosterone as well. In a hyperthyroid woman, testosterone levels are higher, and estrogen levels may remain normal or decrease.[9] Thyroid hormone excess may enhance libido in some women because of the increase in androgen levels coupled with the direct effects on brain chemistry. In fact, this same increase in androgen can cause acne, growth of facial hair, and loss of scalp hair due to a shortening of the life of the hair follicle.[10] In men, hypothyroidism often causes a decrease in the testosterone level.[11] Treatment with radioactive iodine in men is another cause of lower testosterone levels. Low testosterone in men causes the levels of some forms of female hormone to become higher than normal.[12]

The various effects of thyroid hormone on the brain, on the autonomic nervous system, and on sex hormone levels account for the multiple sexual disturbances that thyroid patients often experience. Because thyroid imbalance is much more common in women than men, and its effects on sexual function are quite often more complex, I will focus primarily on women's sexual problems in this chapter.

Hypothyroidism and Low Sexual Energy

When a woman becomes hypothyroid, the decrease in estrogen levels and the effect on the brain of low thyroid hormone levels often lead to lack of interest in sex. Desire gradually declines and may ultimately vanish. The healthy fantasies that existed prior to the occurrence of hypothyroidism occur less and less often. Most hypothyroid women have a tendency to masturbate less than they used to, again reflecting the evaporation of the sex drive. A woman may not wish to be intimate with her partner or with anyone else.

The frustrations related to sexual dysfunction that hypothyroid women experience stem from an inability to cope with the changes. The effect on self-esteem and the fact that the women may not understand the reason for the changes tend to exacerbate these frustrations. An additional frustration, which may preoccupy women more than the dysfunction itself, is the need to deal with unsatisfied partners. Whereas one male partner may feel rejected and no longer desired, another may be understanding (or at least give the impression that he is). The woman may reassure him that her problem "has nothing to do with him" and that she "is working on it." The hypothyroid woman who describes this situation to her gynecologist may be given estrogen to improve the sexual dysfunction, often to no avail. A friend may advise the woman that, to reduce the conflict with her partner, she should just have sex when her partner wants, regardless of whether she is in the mood. Often, however, if a woman isn't aroused, she simply doesn't want to bother with sex.

A good example of this problem is Olivia, who was hypothyroid for at least a couple of years. She told me, "When I was hypothyroid, I didn't want anybody near me." Another hypothyroid woman said, "You need more sleep, your hair is falling out, and you have no sexual drive, which is abnormal for a young married woman. Watching something erotic on TV doesn't do anything for you. You know something is wrong. You don't want to be bothered or touched. You may think to yourself, 'I know it's my problem. I don't want to tell him no. That's not right for him.' "

Another factor contributing to sexual problems is that a hypothyroid woman often suffers from fatigue. As soon as she comes home from work, she wants to rest and sleep. "I feel miserable," said Anne, who had just been diagnosed with hypothyroidism. "I'm tired. I don't feel good. My body aches. Being intimate is the last thing in the world I want. I want somebody to give me a massage and let me sleep."

Weight gain may lead to a decline in self-esteem and distorted perceptions of body image, further contributing to marked decreases in sexual activity. Melanie had been married for only two years when, as a result of hypothyroidism, she reached the point of seeking excuses not to have sex with her husband. She was quite affected, as are many hypothyroid patients, by her physical appearance. She said, "It is hard to feel sexy about yourself when you look like a toad, you gain all this weight, and you are all bloated. The physical part of it is very detrimental to your psyche. It gets in the way of even being able to enjoy yourself or put yourself in that position."

When a hypothyroid woman engages in a sex act just because she wants to please her partner, some sexual arousal may occur, but she may have difficulty reaching a normal state of sexual excitement. A woman who, during foreplay, normally reaches an excitement plateau within ten to twenty minutes may not reach that level when she is hypothyroid even after an hour of foreplay. Many hypothyroid women will continue to work at it, but because they are exhausted and have not reached an adequate level of arousal after such a long period of foreplay, they often give up and interrupt the sex act.

Nicole, who was suffering symptoms of hypothyroidism when she first came to my office, described this problem to me in the following way:

> I have never been a really highly sexed person: sex once every week or two was fine with me. In the early years of marriage, we engaged in sex more. Then it was kids and mellowing, so it was probably about once a week. In the last year, I have had no interest. I don't really miss it or need it. We probably have sex maybe once every two months. It has taken longer to stimulate me. Sometimes I even think, "Are you up for all this?" It takes longer, and it's more work.

Because thyroid hormones are crucial for the response that women need in order to achieve engorgement of the clitoris and lubrication of the vagina, they may not achieve this state in a normal sex act. The vaginal dryness in particular may cause women to experience pain during sexual intercourse. So in addition to the lack of desire, the pain then becomes another reason for avoiding sex. Fear of pain may also become a source of anxiety, which prevents the woman from relaxing enough to enjoy sex. The pain and the lack of pleasure during intercourse become a significant burden in the mind of a hypothyroid woman, and she often prefers to avoid sexual contact. Women who continue to be sexually active at the insistence of their partners often fail to achieve an orgasm, and if they do, it is short-lived. Multiple orgasms are unlikely, even if they were common before hypothyroidism.

According to a young woman being treated for an underactive thyroid:

> Sex is not enjoyable any longer. The dryness in the vagina and the severe pain during intercourse make it a horrible experience. When my thyroid has been

under control, I have felt sexier. I have actually desired sex. The pain during intercourse disappeared. When my thyroid is not under control, when it is too low, that is the last thing on my mind. Then sex is like work, and it causes great discomfort.

Many couples face similar problems. Painful intercourse can be a frustrating barrier to a gratifying sex life. Surveys have shown that 15 to 30 percent of all women experience physical discomfort or pain when they engage in sex.[13] Causes may include superabsorbent tampons, allergic reactions to contraceptive foams or creams, and vaginal infections. Often when a gynecologist finds no obvious vaginal or abdominal abnormality, he or she may merely suggest psychotherapy. Yet the problem has several possible causes, including thyroid imbalance leading to inadequate arousal and lubrication.

Pain or discomfort during intercourse may also be due to lichen sclerosus, an inflammation of the genital skin that can cause extreme itchiness. One doctor reported that nearly 50 percent of women suffering from this skin condition have a thyroid disorder.[14] Lichen sclerosus is treated with hydrocortisone ointment or 2 percent testosterone ointment twice a day for two to three months.

Lichen sclerosus appears as a patchy white lesion on the labial skin (outside the vagina). This lesion at times extends to the area between the legs and up to the anus. If you continue to have discomfort and pain during intercourse after your thyroid imbalance has been corrected with treatment, have your gynecologist look for lichen sclerosus. Another often overlooked reason for the dryness is Sjögren's syndrome, an autoimmune condition that occurs in a large number of thyroid patients, resulting in dryness of the eyes, mouth, and vagina (see Chapter 7).

When Depression Aggravates the Problem

When women are depressed and hypothyroid, they lose any interest in sex and may even develop an aversion to it. Although these women may experience an improvement in many of their symptoms with thyroid hormone treatment, the lack of sexual desire may persist. One patient who continued to have residual depression after correction of hypothyroidism told me, "Since I increased the dose, I don't think I have more arousal. I'm more energetic and less tired. I sleep less. The PMS symptoms are less. I feel less impatient. But when it comes to desiring sex, this has not changed. I still don't have any interest." When a lack of sexual desire persists, it may be due to depression or to a distancing that has developed between the two partners over a period of time.

Dana, age twenty-eight, who has suffered lingering effects of thyroid imbalance, told me, "Before all this, I remember having the desire to have sex,
and we were very active sexually. Now the desire has pretty much gone away,
even when I am on the thyroid medication. I do have desire, but it's very
seldom and not like it used to be. I like to be with my husband and talk to
him. Mainly I want *just* to be close to him without the sex."

The struggle to maintain a loving, caring relationship is common among
patients suffering from hypothyroidism. The husband may not understand
that although his wife has lost her desire to engage in sex, she still loves him.
If her husband is supportive, the woman may attempt to please him, quite
often to no avail. Relationships can be seriously disturbed, however, by the
sexual dysfunction resulting from thyroid-related lingering depression.

Raging Libido and Other
Sexual Problems of Hyperthyroid Women

The effects of hyperthyroidism on sex life are more complex and varied.
Many hyperthyroid women respond in the same manner as hypothyroid
women: they gradually lose interest in sex, both because they are overwhelmed by their chaotic thoughts and because of the indifference to
pleasure so characteristic of depression. Some hyperthyroid women may experience greater depression, and the accompanying physical exhaustion and
tiredness may cause them to lose interest in sex.

I saw Robin for the first time when she was referred to me for hyperthyroidism. She had been married for three years and had just recently become
separated from her husband, who had filed for a divorce. She said:

> I had noticed a loss in my sex drive. That was the first thing that happened to
> me. We had been married for six months, and it was just great. We had great
> sex. Then, all of a sudden, I had no interest. It took forever to excite me. I
> would still be able to get excited once I had allowed myself to relax completely.
> My husband thought that I didn't love him anymore! I tried to explain it wasn't
> that. I told him I wasn't interested in anybody else. I just had lost the desire. He
> couldn't understand why, and I couldn't tell him why.

Her husband hired a private investigator, who followed Robin for a
month. When the investigator came up with nothing, Robin's husband gave
up. Then he met a woman who could give him what he wanted. For months,
Robin continued to feel guilty that she hadn't been able to control what was
happening to her sexually. Later, when Robin's overactive thyroid was corrected, it took months of counseling and psychotherapy for her to regain a
normal sex life.

Julia, another young woman who became hyperthyroid in her first year of marriage, said:

I think my lack of interest in sex was tied in with the exhaustion. The sexual interest started going when I began having many other symptoms of hyperthyroidism. I would have liked to have somebody else to talk to, especially some other person who had gone through it. When I was diagnosed, my doctor was quite open with me and told me everything that could possibly go wrong except for the sexual effects.

The increased anxiety and mood swings of a hyperthyroid woman often create a distance between her and her partner, and this may cause her to avoid intimacy. Her moodiness and self-esteem problems make communication and focus difficult. She may think about sex and be interested, and she may experience a burst of fantasies and sexual desire, but these feelings can dissipate quickly in a wave of anxiety.

Many hyperthyroid women, however, do not lose their sex drive. Their excitement period is unaffected or may even be shortened. It takes less time for them to achieve a state of lubrication and engorgement, but during sexual intercourse, they may experience tremendous pain, similar to what hypothyroid women would experience. At times, the pain is caused by an involuntary spasm of the outer part of the vagina (vaginismus). The fear of having pain during sexual intercourse may create significant anxiety in hyperthyroid women, who may then attempt to avoid sexual intercourse altogether.

Some women with an overactive thyroid experience too much vaginal lubrication, even before they start showing symptoms of hypomania and raging libido. This happened to Alexandra, who could not understand why she was experiencing excessive lubrication, even during the day, and initially thought she had a yeast infection. She said:

I called my gynecologist and told him that I had an excessive amount of mucus, even in the daytime, and I didn't understand it. He did a Pap smear and said everything was clear. I was worried about infections, and he said because it was a clear mucus, nothing was wrong. At that time, I became wet very quickly. To reach an orgasm, however, it took longer. It was fine for me, but it was very stressful for my husband.

Thyroid hormone excess may have a direct effect on the brain chemicals that regulate sexual interest. As I illustrated at the start of the chapter, hyperthyroidism can cause a hypomanic state and increased sexuality in women. Karen, a thirty-eight-year-old housewife who experienced a sudden surge in her sexual interest and fantasies after several years of marriage, told me:

I became extremely involved in my appearance. I was overweight at that point. I began having sexual fantasies. I started reading books that were more erotic. It seemed to happen rather suddenly. I spent hours reading erotic books and lying down fantasizing. My fantasies didn't involve my husband and not even any men I knew, really, just fantasy people—strangers.

At that time, I was home and not working. I engaged in masturbation several times a day. I started having dreams that I was developing relationships with men that I saw on talk shows on TV. I was also experiencing other symptoms of hyperthyroidism. I had a rapid heartbeat, I was feeling hot, and at times, I was shaky. I was talking faster and definitely talking louder.

This hypomanic state induced by thyroid hormone excess is similar to what can be seen in manic-depressive disorders during the elated phase, when a woman may typically seek more sex and become obsessed with sexual thoughts. Increased sexuality rarely occurs without other manifestations of elation. Women become more interested in their bodies and appearance. They may spend unusual amounts of money on new, extravagant clothes and often plan or even decide to have plastic surgery.

Sexual Problems in Men

As I said at the start of the chapter, thyroid imbalance is much more common in women than in men, and its effect on women's sexual function is quite often more complex. Yet men suffering from thyroid imbalance may also experience drastic changes in sexual activity. Hypothyroid men often experience a lack of desire and a blunting of fantasies. Even if they are excited or stimulated, erection may not occur. If the hypothyroidism is severe, the erection may be transient, causing an interruption of the sex act. As in women, the tiredness and depression make men disinterested in sex and unable to fulfill their partner's sexual needs.

A hyperthyroid man loses the patience to engage in foreplay to excite his partner. He may become obsessed with the physical act and may not allow his partner to reach an adequate level of excitement before intercourse. One wife of a hyperthyroid man complained:

It was boom, and it was over with. Before, we would engage in a lot of foreplay, and afterward we'd sit in bed and talk for hours. Then, for several months when John was hyperthyroid, he wanted to have sex almost every day. After maybe one or two minutes of kissing, he would just like to have intercourse. I was not ready. It was frustrating, and I could not refuse. I got angry so quickly.

Hyperthyroid men may also lose the emotional aspect of making love. Sex becomes just a physical activity. Both Richard and his wife noticed a change in his sexuality. Richard said:

At the beginning, sex was something very important—and it wasn't just sex, it was making love, and there is a difference! Then later, sex became just sex. There was a period when we just stopped. Before, we would have sex two or three times a week, and it got to maybe once every three weeks. Later on, the desire just went away. The amazing thing about Graves' disease is that it makes you emotionally bland to everything around you. You have so much energy that you feel you need to be doing something physical all the time.

Other men become sexually interested in the morning, but in the evening, they are physically exhausted and have neither the desire nor the physical strength to perform sexually. As one man said, "In the morning, I would be Superman. By the time I get to bed, I am so tired!"

Hyperthyroid men also lose their normal orgasms. One hyperthyroid man said:

Before, sex lasted a lot longer and maybe even more than one time. Now it is only one time and sometimes not even that. With Graves' disease, you're going at 100 percent of what you should be, and all of a sudden, you're at minus 20 percent. You're so exhausted. Anytime between eight and ten in the evening, you crash. It is like you expended all the energy you had, and then you are left with nothing.

Toward a Better Sex Life

Theoretically, once a woman's thyroid imbalance is corrected, her lack of interest in sex and avoidance of it should subside and her fantasies and usual drive should return. Unfortunately, this may not always be the case. Patients may believe that the change in their sex life is due to reasons other than the thyroid. Some attribute it to age, and others remain perplexed by their loss of sexual interest. As I noted in Chapter 4, a thyroid imbalance can be a significant stressful condition. Some women may continue to suffer from depression or post-traumatic stress syndrome after the imbalance is corrected. Depression and post-traumatic stress syndrome could in themselves cause a lack of sexual interest. Once distance has come between two partners, they may find it hard to resume their lives as if nothing had happened. The continued lack of interest may also become a challenge to intimacy.

One of the simplest ways to improve your sexual relationship with your partner and to reignite it after having had sexual problems related to thyroid dysfunction is to engage in more casual conversation with your partner. This will enhance affection. Also initiate more physical contact without actually thinking about sex.

You need to practice regular sessions of stimulation and caressing—at first without actually engaging in intercourse. Some of these techniques are described in books such as *The Gift of Sex: A Guide to Sexual Fulfillment.*[15] Have your partner rediscover your erogenous zones. You need to train your brain to respond to the stimulation that elicits arousal and excitement.

If sexual problems and symptoms of depression persist after correction of your hypothyroidism, consider changing your thyroxine treatment to a combination of T4 and T3 (see Chapter 20). This has helped many women with persistent depression and lack of sexual interest. If you are also taking an antidepressant, ask your doctor whether this medication could be the source of the sexual difficulties.

Sexual dysfunction caused by an antidepressant often alters your self-esteem, your mood, and your relationship with your sex partner. Sexual dysfunction occurs in 30–50 percent or more of people who take SSRIs for depression.[16] What causes the sexual dysfunction is the low dopamine associated with high serotonin, inhibition of nitric oxide, and sometimes high prolactin level. If you have sexual dysfunction caused by an antidepressant, discuss with your doctor the possibility of switching to another antidepressant, such as nefazodone or bupropion. These two antidepressants do not cause loss of libido; in fact, bupropion can enhance your desire to engage in sex. Adding bupropion to another antidepressant may be the antidote for the adverse sexual effects related to the first antidepressant.[17]

Menopause makes women more likely to suffer from hypoactive sexual desire syndrome. The lack of estrogens impairs their sexual thought process. Treatment with estrogen/progestin can increase sexual desire in premenopausal or postmenopausal women by giving them a better sense of well-being. Testosterone treatment in small amounts, as a gel or sublingual troche, may have a more clear-cut effect. It improves sexual desire, arousal, and sexual satisfaction. It helps with depression, headaches, and loss of energy.[18] However, testosterone treatment can promote hair growth in some women. And testosterone may not help with your hypoactive sexual desire syndrome if you continue to suffer from depression or relationship problems. Whether the use of testosterone for long periods of time causes any adverse effects has not been extensively studied. So if you take testosterone, make sure the dose is small and your testosterone levels remain in a normal range. You may also benefit from taking DHEA, which can improve your mood and sexuality.

If you have vaginal dryness due to lack of estrogens, you may want to consider one of the estrogenic intravaginal preparations in the form of cream, pessaries, tablets (such as Vagifem), and estradiol-releasing vaginal rings. Creams, rings, and tablets provide better results with vaginal dryness compared to nonhormonal gels.[19] I discourage you from using a cream made of conjugated equine estrogens. It can promote uterine bleeding, breast tenderness, and pelvic pain. The vaginal ring, however, not only is easy to use but will give you excellent results without causing discomfort.

Some couples who have experienced distancing and continue to suffer from lingering sexual problems after a thyroid hormone imbalance has been corrected may find it helpful to consult a psychotherapist or sex therapist. To obtain a list of sex therapists, contact:

American Association of Sexuality Educators,
Counselors, and Therapists (AASECT)
1444 I Street, Suite 700
Washington, DC 20005
Phone: 202-449-1099
Website: www.aasect.org

The sexual effects of thyroid imbalance described in this chapter are very common. In many couples, they are the main cause of relationship problems. In other couples, they are catalysts for relationship problems that are triggered by changes in the behavior and personality of the thyroid patient. This is one of the many facets of the big question, "Is it my brain, or is it my thyroid?" Thyroid patients and their partners must resolve this issue themselves or seek help from a sex therapist if the problem continues after the thyroid imbalance is corrected.

Important Points to Remember

- Optimal thyroid hormone levels are crucial for having normal libido and normal physical responses that lead to sexual fulfillment.
- An overactive thyroid can cause painful intercourse and a loss of interest in sex, or it can result in raging libido and careless behavior.
- An underactive thyroid often results in blunted sexual appetite, lack of lubrication, and painful sex.
- Sexual problems can continue after correction of a thyroid imbalance. You and your partner need to learn about these effects, discuss them openly, and seek help from a sex therapist if psychological problems and distancing persist.

12

"YOU'VE CHANGED"

When the Thyroid and Relationships Collide

Women and men are fundamentally different in how they communicate and interpret each other's language, behavior, and emotions.[1] Many couples come to recognize their real differences, accept them, and eventually learn to deal with them.

The intrusion of a thyroid imbalance into a couple's relationship very often exacerbates these differences. Subtle changes in how the afflicted person speaks and acts alter the dynamics of the relationship. Thyroid patients, particularly those suffering from an overactive thyroid, often become moody, anxious, angry, and irritable.[2] And many begin to have a distorted perception of their partner's behavior. Unfortunately, their partners may not understand what causes these changes. Inability to cope with changing demands and difficulty in communicating can lead to chaos, with misunderstandings, false expectations, and arguments over trivial matters. For many people, the relationship becomes a burden.

People with a thyroid condition are having terrible trouble understanding themselves and their new, confusing feelings, so they are unlikely to understand their partners. Indeed, thyroid patients are so overwhelmed by their new emotional problems that they cannot cope properly with the stress of the relationship, which becomes a cycle of reactions and counterreactions. Both partners then share the mental stress provoked by the thyroid condition.

Typically, when one of the partners is suffering from thyroid disease, the relationship undergoes two distinct phases, each characterized by its own distinct dynamics and thyroid-related effects. The first phase begins with the intrusion of the thyroid condition and ends when the diagnosis is made. In this phase, relationships frequently deteriorate and may even end because of the lack of understanding of what precipitated or caused the relationship problems. The second phase follows diagnosis.

In phase one, the intrusion is, in most instances, insidious. More often than not, the personality of the afflicted person changes drastically. Although people with thyroid conditions are capable of hiding their suffering to some extent, the disease quickly alters their behavior and language so significantly that other people easily recognize the change. As long as the cause of the change remains undetermined (that is, the thyroid condition has not yet been diagnosed), the couple will be unable to pinpoint the origin of their problems. The relationship suffers proportionately to the length of this period, which could last months or even years.

The paradox in this phase is that people with thyroid ailments do recognize that unusual things are happening within their bodies and minds, but they are unable to understand them, qualify them, or even describe them accurately. At the same time, their distorted perception of themselves and the world around them causes them to regard their partners' behavior as inappropriate. The thyroid sufferers truly believe that their partners are the ones who have changed and are responsible for their own emotional upheaval. In turn, spouses and other loved ones often react by blaming the patient. Hence, thyroid patients may experience guilt feelings resulting from disagreements that worsen their existing anxiety, stress, anger, and depression.

Distancing is inevitable because the patient becomes unable to deal with the stress of arguing. Although both hypothyroidism and hyperthyroidism can lead to similar behavioral changes, certain changes may be more characteristic of one condition than the other. Let's take a look at some of the changes that can ignite fighting, arguing, and distancing.

Ten Ways That Thyroid Conditions May Change Your Personality and Relationships

Many years of working with and observing people with thyroid conditions have allowed me to identify the following ten types of thyroid-related changes that cause trouble for many couples.

Thyroid patients often become impatient and irritable and may display excessive, unreasonable anger. A thyroid imbalance may make you excessively critical and lead you to pick fights with those around you and snap at them. Often anxiety and worries underlie the criticism and anger that people with thyroid imbalances direct toward others. Ironically, though, people with thyroid conditions do not handle criticism well themselves. Take Janice, for example. She had been happily married for four years when she began experiencing tiredness, anxiety, and weight gain. She then suffered for two years before being diagnosed with hypothyroidism at the age of twenty-seven. Janice tended to blame her husband's attitudes for their disturbed relationship. She said:

For instance, if I did not want to spend money on a certain thing and he wanted to, I would be unreasonably angry, and I would say things that were inappropriate. I told him he was selfish and that he wasn't working toward a common goal. I perceived any decision he made or anything he said or did as inappropriate. It is a miracle we are still together after what we went through in the past two years.

The situation Janice faced is all too real for people with thyroid ailments. They feel compelled to lash out at the very people to whom they need to turn in times of anxiety. In essence, their behavior is controlled by their affliction.

Another hypothyroid woman told me, "There was a lot of yelling and bickering at home. I was frequently very angry. I was disrespectful to my husband and would snap at him when he asked questions because I was upset about the bills or our financial situation. No matter what he did, I would not have been satisfied." Clearly this report goes to the heart of the matter in depicting the incredible conflict within the patient. For the person experiencing the disease, there is no right answer, and anxiety generates discord.

Similarly, Camille, a thirty-two-year-old housewife who suffered from an overactive thyroid due to Graves' disease, told of a family life filled with constant fighting, screaming, and arguing. She said, "Before I was diagnosed, I wasn't getting along well with my parents, which was annoying to me. I had a short temper with them. At home, I have been very cross and sarcastic with my kids. If one of my children left a shoe lying in the middle of the room, I got really annoyed and picked up the shoe and threw it across the room. I couldn't believe I did that. It was not the way I would normally react." This illustrates patients' common tendency to experience a sense of disbelief regarding their unexplained behavior. They know their behavior deviates from what is "normal" for them, but they have no clue as to why.

Another example reveals the common thread of discord that thyroid patients experience in their relationships. Darlene started noticing symptoms of hyperthyroidism three months after her wedding. She and her husband started fighting over trivial matters and ended up seeking help from a counselor. She confessed:

There are certain things that I should have compromised on. If I had been in a calmer mood, I would have been able to handle that. I did not have patience with my husband. Before the symptoms of hyperthyroidism, I tended to be less emotional. My husband is Jewish, and I'm Catholic. He didn't want to go home for Christmas. We had a big argument about that. He ended up going home by himself. If I had been more patient, we could have sat down and worked things out.

Darlene worked in a store's customer service department. She experienced the same impatience at work as she had at home and began having problems with her colleagues. She explained the situation like this: "I was lacking patience with the customers all the time. Many times I started crying over trivial matters. I had a big argument with my supervisor. She was irritating me! People say that I would talk really fast. I knew something was wrong, but I had no idea what. I didn't know about hyperthyroidism, where things move quicker."

Darlene's experience is typical of how people with an overactive thyroid are unable to explain their behavioral changes adequately. They feel as if everyone else is to blame, and their behavior is fueled by emotions laced with anger. The fast pace at which hyperthyroid people's brains work may make them regard everybody else as slow and lead them to rationalize the irritability and anger.

People with thyroid conditions may make unrealistic demands of partners, spouses, or family members. They frequently ask others to do things for them, and they also tell others how to do things. A hyperthyroid woman who had serious marital problems as a result of her Graves' disease told me, "I would tell my husband he was never home and that I needed him home. He is a student, and he is not at school full time, and I would get upset because he was not home to help with chores. But in fact, he was doing the best he could, and still I was not satisfied." This example shows how patients are incapable of viewing their relationships rationally. They cannot see situations clearly and may even provoke their partners with their unrealistic expectations.

Thyroid patients, particularly those with hypothyroidism, want peace and quiet. They feel the need to withdraw from activity and noise. They have a low tolerance for sound. In essence, they wish to insulate themselves in a surrealistic world of tranquillity. One hypothyroid patient told me, "I would want peace and quiet at home. If I didn't get it, I would start shouting at my children and at my husband. Anything that made a lot of noise or movement irritated me. The TV was a nuisance to me. I couldn't watch it. The children's making a lot of noise was a frustration."

Patients may become withdrawn from friends, and they do not want to talk or go out with people. They may lose all interest in doing things with their partners. A good example is Angel, a twenty-five-year-old woman who was suffering from an underactive thyroid. She said:

> All I wanted to do was sleep. I couldn't seem to get enough rest. Nothing made me happy. Ted wanted to take me out to eat, and I didn't want to go. He wanted to go to a movie, and I'd say no. If he rented a movie, I'd just fall asleep. I didn't want to be intimate. I didn't want to cook or clean. Then he would get frustrated, and I'd get really emotional and mad. He didn't understand that I'm more tired than he is.

He would try to talk to me, and it was so hard for me to tell him, "Ted, would you just shut up?" He just wanted to tell me about his day and to hear about my day. Questions, questions, questions, talk, talk, talk—and I was so irritable. At first, I think I wanted him to just shut up, then I didn't really want him to shut up.

I just want to feel better and to have more energy. One year ago, I could not have been happier. I felt good, looked good, and we were going out all the time.

Hypothyroid patients want to be left alone. They just want to sleep and withdraw from those around them. In some cases, they realize the people around them are doing the best they can, but they still want to maintain their isolation.

People with thyroid conditions may require more attention from their partners and often feel that they are not getting enough attention. They feel that whatever a partner might do to comfort them is not enough. Ironically, those with thyroid imbalances have mixed feelings about their loved ones. They want their loved ones to be there for them—but only on their terms. In other words, if loved ones do not follow the "rules" laid out for them by the person with the imbalance, he or she will not hesitate to turn on them. Many thyroid patients told me something like this: "I preferred him just to be there, hold my hand, and listen to me, but not to say anything. When he would say things, it would make me irritable and angry."

Mona, suffering from postpartum hypothyroidism, fought with her husband more than she ever had before. She felt she did not get the attention she needed. "The only thoughts I had during this time were that my husband was not helping me with the things that I needed. I had reached a point where I would have hit him in the face in public. I wanted to feel I was cherished. I was feeling very unattractive, like you do after you have a baby. I was extremely overwhelmed and overtired."

People with thyroid ailments may show a lack of commitment to doing things at home or for the family. They may not want to be asked to do things or may become angry if asked. A common source of disagreement is hypothyroid people's declining interest in doing things around the house. Because they are exhausted, they have difficulty handling even minor chores. Just going to the store can be an insurmountable task.

One patient summed this up as follows:

I felt that as long as he didn't ask anything of me, like cooking dinner when I didn't want to, I was comfortable. I wished he would have understood my emotions and feelings and symptoms, but he didn't at first. He kept pushing me. I guess he thought I was being lazy. I felt something was really wrong. I didn't want him to ask me to get out of bed, but he would. He felt it was all in my mind. He wasn't being empathic or sympathetic, so I would get angry with that.

Thyroid patients may exhibit unexplained hatred toward partners, spouses, relatives, and friends or contradictory, rapidly changing feelings. This problem is aptly demonstrated by the case of Jackie, who developed postpartum hypothyroidism. She described the situation like this:

> I had a very good relationship with my parents before. When my baby was two months old, I experienced a lot of irritation and anger toward my mother, who used to be my best friend. My mother became angry that I had become so withdrawn from her and so disrespectful. I was very hurtful to her, but I was sick and couldn't deal with her. I didn't feel connected to her at all. I didn't want her to come to my house. I didn't want her to help me in any way.

Jackie's case is typical in that she realized her relationships had changed, but she felt helpless to do anything about it. She knew things were not the way they used to be, but she was unable to see things in proper perspective. To her, feelings of hatred were unavoidable and unchangeable.

Similarly, Sylvia, who was very much in love with her husband and had had what she called a serene, peaceful relationship with him, told me, "My emotions toward my husband were shifting back and forth. Sometimes I liked to be with him and sometimes not." These shifting feelings are quite common among patients afflicted with thyroid imbalance. When coupled with the types of changes in sexual interest described in Chapter 11, they become a serious source of distancing and conflict.

Thyroid sufferers may become overly anxious about how their emotional changes and health are affecting their ability to do their jobs and earn a living. When work-related anxiety is brought home, it often leads to arguing, angry outbursts, and increased irritability. Poor job performance or even job loss due to hypothyroidism or hyperthyroidism's adverse effects on thinking and reasoning further lowers self-esteem. Issues pertaining to financial security and financial responsibilities often arise, burdening the relationship even further. In other cases, people with a thyroid condition become trapped in their work. Many patients, in trying to hold on to their jobs, devote most of their attention and remaining energy to the effort to maintain their job performance. This tremendous burden on the brain will often be expressed in outbursts at home as patients' frustrations and inability to fulfill emotional and physical responsibilities in their private lives affect partners or families.

Amanda, a teacher with a hypothyroid condition, described this conflict to me. "I became irritable with students," she said. "I had to exercise a great deal of self-control so that I wouldn't fly off the handle. This would tire me out so much that, when I got home, I was useless to my husband. I felt guilty, like I wasn't really all there to do the things we wanted to do. We would go dancing, and I couldn't remember to move my foot out for each step. It was very noticeable." When patients focus on doing the best they can at work, their home life inevitably suffers, because they have no energy left for family duties and obligations.

In the same fashion, a hyperthyroid person can become obsessed with work, which may alienate his or her partner. This was true for Kenneth, a thirty-two-year-old salesman who took on another part-time job when he hit the manic period of hyperthyroidism. His wife, frustrated by his behavior, said:

> For the two years that he was doing the part-time job, we grew apart. He was all work. I couldn't even catch him. Then he slept during the weekend. During that time, he had very little to do with us because he had to work. I felt that it was "Kenneth's life," and then it was me and the kids' life.
>
> People would say, "How do you put up with him?" "He is crazy." "How does he work like that?" "You don't have a life." You start examining your life then and asking yourself what you really have. I felt like he didn't love me or care about me. I saw the same distance between him and the kids and his parents. I kept telling him we were growing apart. I told him, "You're going to wake up one day and we are going to be miles apart." Whatever I told him, it didn't register.

Extreme anger and irritability may lead to violence. Whitney, a thirty-one-year-old woman, was living by herself and had been dating a man for a couple of years when she became hyperthyroid. She used to love this man, and they were making wedding plans when things gradually began to change. In her words:

> I had a fairly normal life. As my symptoms progressed, it seemed I was in conflict with everyone. I was disagreeing with everything. People would hurt my feelings easily. The man I was dating at that time refused to understand what I was going through. He was dismissing me and saying it was stress or that I was acting like a baby. He made me feel very small about my problems. He said I was lazy. I was so fatigued from my thyroid condition, but I did not know it. I am not a lazy person!
>
> I remember the intense anger I felt. One day I sat and fantasized about driving my car through his garage. It seemed like a wonderful thing to do. I didn't act upon that. I wouldn't even think of that today. I became more combative. We had lots of arguments that always ended up with me crying and walking out; my emotions would overtake me.
>
> My emotions caused me to have a continuous internal battle. I had no tolerance or patience. When it is your nature to be generous, giving, kind, tolerant, and basically easygoing, and then you're the complete opposite, it is hard to cope. I became mean and nasty, and I didn't know why I was unhappy. I had tantrums and violent spells. I actually could have killed someone.

Violent actions and thoughts plague many thyroid patients. In this way, the patients may become harmful to themselves and others and could end up facing legal problems as well as the problems associated with the disease itself. The thyroid patient's anger may sometimes be expressed as verbal or even physical violence, as was the case with Ryan, a middle-aged engineer.

Jeannine, Ryan's wife, said, "It was not so easy to talk to him. It was like he was on drugs. He was verbally abusive all the time. He was like a volcano: any little thing causes it to erupt."

Ryan related an episode that illustrates how trivial, unimportant matters can trigger bouts of anger and violence:

One day, Jeannine's sister stayed with us. She didn't like me, and she irritated me quite a bit. I sat down and listened to what my wife had to say, and then when I decided to say something, her sister locked herself in the bathroom because she didn't want to hear what I had to say. It totally infuriated me. I went to the bathroom door and started to knock on it. I told her to let me in the door. When she said no, I said, "Let me in the damn door!" When she said no again, the next thing I knew, my arm had just gone through the door. I don't even remember hitting the door, but my arm was through the door, and she was standing up in the shower screaming. I didn't hit her, but I felt like hitting her. She came back in the den, and I told her what I had to say, and I said, "Now if you want to go in the bathroom, you can."

Jeannine was a passive and submissive person. She remained in the marriage despite the lack of communication, anger, and distance between her and Ryan.

Hyperthyroidism may make someone act in ways that others may perceive as inconsistent and irrational. Paul and his father were partners in running a gas station. When Paul became hyperthyroid, the business began to do poorly because of his irrational behavior and aggressiveness with customers. As a result, Paul and his father eventually stopped talking to each other.

Friends would ask Paul's wife, "Why is he acting so nervous, and why does he have to speed to go somewhere when he is not in a hurry?" She said, "We would fly out of the driveway like it was an emergency. He acts as if he is crazy. Everything has to be fast."

According to Paul, "My personality really changed drastically. I got to where I really couldn't relax at all, and even at home, I couldn't stand to sit on the couch. I had to be doing something, or I would go into a mood swing where I would get agitated with any little thing." Paul's case is typical with regard to alienation and extreme personality change.

The Partner's Four Most Common Reactions

Not knowing that there is a physical or chemical reason for the personality change, the partner of the person with a thyroid imbalance often becomes confused. The reactions to this new situation vary from person to person. The spouse has been used to living with one person and now must live with a new person who has different perceptions, feelings, and emotions. The differences in perception and language between men and women become a real issue for most spouses because, for some time, they have coped with and adjusted to certain differences—and now those differences have changed. Lack of understanding can generate inappropriate reactions that may contribute to more arguing.

Here are some common reactions of partners:

Partners may pull away from the person with the thyroid imbalance. The distancing, which is the spouse's typical response, initially reflects avoidance of problems. The patient perceives this pulling away as a lack of caring, understanding, and empathy—as a statement that the partner is indifferent. Because of the lower self-esteem generated by thyroid imbalance, the patient tends to feel more anger and may attribute some of his or her problems to the distancing behavior.

This can be seen in the case of Sondra, who was suffering from hypothyroidism and was as confused as her husband about what had happened to their relationship. "We used to get along so well," she said. "I became irritable. I felt he was not really empathic with me for some reason. He does not talk to me very much anymore." Sondra focuses on the distance as a cause more than an effect of her behavior. The lines become blurred for patients when they try to fathom exactly what caused the relationship changes.

Partners may refuse to accept the personality changes associated with thyroid conditions and react with anger and criticism. This typically causes the fighting to escalate. The spouse may go overboard with criticism, which exacerbates the patient's feelings of low self-esteem. The patient may be blamed for deliberately creating arguments. "He took away my motivation and my self-esteem," one hyperthyroid woman said. "He makes me feel awkward about being sick. He asked me if I was doing it for attention. He doesn't have a clue that it is embarrassing. I never felt like he understood what I was going through. We would fight over stupid stuff, like what kind of shampoo to buy." After this couple had seen a counselor for several months with no improvement in their relationship, her overactive thyroid was diagnosed. When the husband learned that his wife's changing emotions were due to her thyroid condition, they stopped going to the counselor, and he became understanding, flexible, and compassionate.

Partners may be unable to cope and become depressed and anxious

themselves. When the wife has a thyroid condition, the husband may become anxious, realize the severity of their problems, and make an effort to understand or talk things over. He may even suggest counseling. During her hyperthyroidism, Ashley experienced a lot of anxiety and mood swings. Her husband, who is somewhat dependent, became anxious, which generated depression. Ashley said, "Initially, I was the one who had a lot of anxiety and anger, but quickly he also became nervous, had bouts of anger, and became depressed."

A few partners may recognize that their loved one has definitely changed and will make an effort to find a medical reason for the changes. Lynette, who had been married for fifteen years, had been very close to her husband since they were children and was supportive of him when he was in law school. They had learned to live with each other and were very close. Initially, when Lynette started having symptoms of hypothyroidism—such as outbursts of anger, irritability, and weight gain—he was quite supportive. He did not know that the problem was physical, however. Although Lynette became angrier and more irritable, they were so close that her husband quickly learned to adapt to the situation, and he concluded that Lynette's behavior stemmed from her weight problem. In a reassuring tone, he repeatedly told her that what was bothering her the most was really the weight. "You have to exercise and try to stay on a diet," he kept telling her. She followed his advice and worked out at the gym, but her condition remained unchanged. After her physicians dismissed Lynette as not having a medical problem, her husband continued to be supportive and started searching self-help books, which led him to suspect that she had a thyroid condition.

A thyroid patient experiencing a change in personality may not necessarily recognize that he or she is the source of the problem, although the person usually does recognize that problems exist. At this stage, however, most people who are close to someone with a thyroid imbalance do not make an effort to understand. Other partners, seeing that the relationship is deteriorating rapidly, often suggest that the couple see a psychologist. Under these circumstances, counseling may or may not be helpful because the source of the problem—the thyroid condition—is not recognized, and the irrational behavior, uncontrollable anger, and irritability continue, which perpetuate the arguing. Often, despite counseling, the couple grows further apart, and this may lead to a divorce, particularly if the thyroid condition has not been diagnosed and its role in the couple's problems recognized early enough.

At times, even basic communication may become a problem. Gene, the husband of a hyperthyroid woman, said, "What she is thinking comes out of her mouth several times. Either she might tell me something three times before I get angry, or she may think she told me something and she never uttered the words, and then she becomes infuriated."

When couples have preexisting problems, those problems may be exacerbated by the intrusion of the thyroid imbalance, and arguing can mount to unbelievable levels. Without counseling, the relationship will inevitably founder.

Relationships After Diagnosis

Once the condition has been diagnosed, the couple is frequently relieved because they have found an explanation for their problems. The treatment of the thyroid imbalance generally leads to a gradual resolution of the emotional stress, guilt feelings, and mental effects. Still, this often means that these factors may linger for several months or even years, depending on the complexity of the thyroid condition and its treatment.

After being diagnosed with hypothyroidism, Jamie was started on thyroid hormone treatment. She has not fully recovered and feels quite guilty about not being able to keep up with her husband or provide him with the attention he needs. She said:

> I am depressed because I feel like I can't give my husband what I want to give him. I still am not able to be there for him and to do things with him. I want to be intimate like I felt in our first year of marriage. I enjoyed having sex with him, going out, and doing things with friends. Then, after I changed, I didn't want to be intimate with him. That same touch would make me bristle. It was like I had an aversion to him. I felt like telling him, "Just leave me alone." Then I started feeling guilty.

After a few months, though, Jamie's personality returned to normal. Her husband, Andy, knew she had a thyroid imbalance, and Jamie's doctor had explained that it would take a few weeks until the thyroid was regulated. Andy said, "I became used to the change from her being happy to being a person who would snap. She never hollered at me, but she came back quickly with 'Leave me alone!' I knew this was not her." In this type of situation, both partners feel guilty, but the patient experiences the greater guilt because he or she feels responsible for having brought the disease into the relationship.

Monica, a thirty-three-year-old accountant, experienced a similar situation. She had suffered from Graves' disease for more than a year. The intrusion of the thyroid condition into her relationship with her partner, Jack, led to arguing, fighting, and distancing. Monica recognized that her behavior was the cause of some of the problems and felt guilty because she realized that she was not easy to live with.

"I have to say I'm probably hot-blooded also," she said. "I am this way about everything—kids, money, work. I'm sure it is hard for Jack. I can imagine that he had a hard time trying to decide what I was going to feel like today or maybe what I would feel like in thirty minutes. I probably was very hard to please."

To cite another example, one day a patient who had been suffering from Graves' disease for three years walked into my office. For the first time, her thyroid seemed to be well regulated, so I was surprised when she told me that she was getting a divorce. She said she had not felt this good for such a long time. Her mood swings, irritability, and anxiety had resolved. She had started working out and had been feeling good about herself. I told her that usually people get divorced before diagnosis, when their thyroid condition is affecting them the most. She said:

> I had been having marital problems for so long! It was an unhealthy relationship for a long time, and in fact, I feel that the stress of the marriage could have caused my Graves' disease. I felt like I had lost so much. I didn't have a job, money, or any control over my life or my health. Even though he was bad for me, I didn't have the courage or the strength to divorce him when I was ill. But now I have regained my self-esteem, and I see more clearly. I am more self-confident. I had to wait to feel this way to have the courage to divorce him.

What Partners Need to Know

Many people with thyroid disease have indicated the importance of receiving support and understanding from their partner or spouse after they are diagnosed and started on treatment. One hypothyroid woman said, "When I did see the doctor and was diagnosed, then my husband started being sympathetic and supportive. He let me sleep, and he would keep my son away from me, but it wasn't until after I was diagnosed. This was so helpful. That helped me recover quicker. Our arguing just stopped."

The partner's support and understanding are crucial for recovery because patients are still not the same as they used to be. They are still unable to control the anxiety, mood swings, anger, and irritability adequately.

Spouses of thyroid patients should also be involved in the management of the thyroid condition. A well-informed spouse will have a significant beneficial impact on the patient's recovery from the emotional effects and suffering due to the thyroid condition. Sometimes the spouse's support may even be as instrumental as the treatment provided by the physician.

Peter, a supportive husband, told me about his wife, who was still being treated for her thyroid condition. "When I see her slipping away," he said, "I know now what that is about, and it is not because she needs another pill. The process of recovery is slow and gradual. I think that thyroid patients need a lot of rest, and I encourage her to get it. Now I don't get upset when all she wants to do is sleep."

Many husbands, not understanding the impact of a thyroid imbalance, may refuse to put up with their spouses. Some may blame women for using hormones as an excuse for bad behavior. It is just as important for male partners to learn how hormones affect mood as it is for women with thyroid imbalances to become informed about their own condition. The imbalance in the brain takes time to normalize. Partners, unaware of these effects, quite often believe that the thyroid sufferer's reactions are psychological.

Some men embrace this challenge. When Loretta got remarried, her husband knew about her thyroid condition. He was an intelligent man and began to educate himself by reading about thyroid disease and its effects. He very quickly realized that he needed to be one of the primary supports for Loretta's recovery and to help her with her suffering. He was very much in love with her and became interested in her condition to the point that he knew perhaps even more about thyroid disease than Loretta did. He came to every office visit and was the one asking questions about therapy, testing, and the effects of thyroid imbalance on the body.

Other spouses, though, prefer to remain ignorant about the disease and its symptoms. When a partner chooses this method of coping with the situation, the patient is left feeling ignored and even guiltier. This will only exacerbate the situation and make the patient's suffering linger indefinitely.

The examples provided in this chapter illustrate how the intrusion of a thyroid condition can easily disturb the harmony of family life. Understanding the emotional aspects of a thyroid imbalance will not only help both patients and family members maintain their relationships; it will also help reduce the stress that can affect the course of the thyroid condition.

Important Points to Remember

- Thyroid disease can induce a dramatic personality change and can make the patient unrecognizable.
- Different kinds of relationship problems can occur as a result of a thyroid imbalance.
- Quite often, thyroid patients are misunderstood by their partners. It is important that the partner of a thyroid patient learn about the effects of thyroid disease and be as supportive as possible.

13

OVERLAPPING SYMPTOMS

Adrenal Fatigue, Fibromyalgia, Hypoglycemia, and Chronic Fatigue Syndrome

"I am tired. I am exhausted. I cannot function the way I used to!" I hear these complaints from patients all the time. Many of them come to me because for some time they have been unable to function as before. The tiredness and feeling of exhaustion have robbed them of any sense of joy in everyday life and have interfered with their lives at all levels. Obviously when someone suffering from fatigue sees a specialist in thyroid disease, the tired person often has a notion that a thyroid imbalance may be a contributing factor. Frequently I see in the patient's expression that I am his or her last hope.

Typically, these patients have already seen quite a few doctors for the same complaint and often bring with them copies of records and tests that had been requested by other physicians. The tests and the causes considered inevitably vary from physician to physician. The interpretation of fatigue tends to differ depending on the training, experience, and interest that a physician may have in a particular field of medicine. Most physicians, when faced with the symptom of severe fatigue, are primarily concerned with identifying a major physical condition causing the fatigue.

But when it comes right down to it, major medical conditions are found in only a small percentage of people struggling with fatigue. Each year, doctors record nearly 500 million patient visits to their offices for fatigue.

People say that they're tired so often that it is frequently ignored: feeling tired has become part of the normal way of living. If a person is suffering from several other symptoms, he or she might initially mention only the tiredness and exhaustion because of a perception that all the other symptoms are either part of the tiredness or caused by it. Many people figure, "This is stress. Everything will be fine." Many doctors, too, will often dismiss complaints of tiredness with the recommendation that the patient get more exercise, eat a better diet, or lose weight. Frequently this allows the symptoms of significant unexplained suffering to continue.

Being tired is indeed a common complaint, and only if you insist that you are more than just fatigued are your symptoms likely to be taken seriously by friends, relatives, or physicians. Studies of fatigue have suggested that there is a continuum ranging from "healthy normal" fatigue to severe and debilitating fatigue. Surveys of European and American communities have shown that fatigue is a common symptom and occurs in 6.9 to 33 percent of men and 10.9 to 42 percent of women.[1] One study conducted in a primary care setting showed that fatigue of a month's duration or more was reported as a major problem among 19 percent of men and 28 percent of women.[2]

Undoubtedly, regardless of the root cause of the fatigue, suffering from fatigue and the associated impaired quality of life has to do to a great extent with disturbances of one or more of the three major foundations of overall wellness: the brain, the immune system, and the endocrine system. Because the three systems interact with each other, many patients see their symptoms escalate and worsen, leading to extreme forms of fatigue and confusion as to what may be causing the suffering.

The Tripod of Wellness

Our well-being is under the scrutiny of three major systems: the brain, the endocrine system, and the immune system. I call this the tripod of wellness. These three systems, constantly interacting, allow us to appropriately react to and fight anything in the environment that threatens and interferes with our mental and physical health. The interactions among these three systems are so tight that in some cases a disturbance of one system ultimately will alter the functioning of the other two.

Once a dysfunction of the endocrine system such as a thyroid imbalance occurs, the other two components of the tripod of wellness (the brain and the immune system) are almost inevitably affected. A person with a thyroid imbalance may become depressed and overwhelmed with stress. The depression causes the immune system to weaken, resulting in infection and more fatigue.

A disturbed immune system causing an autoimmune attack can by itself promote depression. During the autoimmune process, the immune system produces chemicals such as cytokines, which in turn can affect brain neurotransmitters that regulate mood and behavior. Celiac disease is an example of an autoimmune disorder in which the immune system affects mood. Patients suffering from celiac disease have a much higher incidence of depression and panic attack, due primarily to the effects of the immune system on brain chemicals involved in mood and emotions.[3]

Quite rarely, the immune effects on the brain are so severe that a patient may end up suffering from a neurological condition called Hashimoto's encephalopathy.[4] Patients with Hashimoto's encephalopathy suffer from lethargy, involuntary muscle movements, muscle weakness, seizures, impaired cognition, abnormal behavior, and depression. This condition is treated with high doses of glucocorticoids to slow down the effects of the immune system. The treatment often results in a dramatic improvement of the symptoms within a few weeks.

This cascade of one system affecting another and thereby worsening the fatigue has a wide range of implications. The first is that it reduces the likelihood that a doctor will consider an endocrine problem as the source of the suffering, because now other systems of the body are involved as well. The second implication is that if a person has more than one condition causing fatigue, symptoms of both conditions may escalate, making it highly likely that one of the conditions will be overlooked. Finally, the escalation of symptoms can become extreme in some patients, who may end up suffering from chronic depression, fibromyalgia, and chronic fatigue syndrome.

Many patients who were diagnosed with fibromyalgia or chronic fatigue syndrome (CFS) and later found to be hypothyroid ask me whether having the two conditions was just a coincidence or whether the thyroid disorder triggered their fibromyalgia or chronic fatigue syndrome. The answer is not always straightforward. Did the stress or depression generated by a thyroid imbalance weaken the immune system, making the patient vulnerable to fibromyalgia or chronic fatigue syndrome? Or did the overwhelming stress and depression caused by the fatigue and the physical symptoms of fibromyalgia or chronic fatigue syndrome affect the immune system, resulting in a thyroid disorder? Or did the immune system affect brain transmitters and promote fatigue and depression? The relationship among stress, depression, and disorders such as fibromyalgia and chronic fatigue syndrome is complex but reflects interactions among the brain, endocrine system, and immune system.

An infection with a virus such as a retrovirus seems to play a major role in the occurrence of CFS. People exposed to high levels of stress may not recover from a viral illness as swiftly as people with lower stress levels (or better mechanisms for coping with stress). Now we understand that it is the psychological vulnerability of some people that makes their immune system weaker, and this causes the viral infection to linger for a long time.[5] For most people suffering from chronic fatigue syndrome, it is virtually impossible to determine which problem initiated the cascade of events—stress, depression, viral infection, disturbance of the immune system, or disturbance of the endocrine system.[6]

A series of studies has also established that the endocrine system is often disturbed in patients suffering from CFS. Many, for instance, are found to have low cortisol levels, an indication of slowing of the adrenal glands. But again, it is not clear whether such disturbances are the cause of the disorder or are the consequence of the depression and the stress associated with the disorder.

Adrenal-Related Fatigue

As an endocrinologist, I feel privileged to specialize in a major system of the body that regulates the largest and most significant components of human physiology. The endocrine system affects most facets of our well-being from minute to minute.

Although thyroid hormone imbalance is undoubtedly the leading cause of fatigue related to endocrine gland problems, deficiencies of the pituitary gland and the adrenals could be hidden causes of fatigue. Countless patients who have suffered fatigue as the result of a dysfunction of the endocrine system have wandered from physician to physician searching for help, when all it would have taken to uncover the source of their suffering was a blood test. In one way or another, most hormones regulate bodily energy levels. Literally, any deficiency of a hormone produced by the endocrine system can promote fatigue. Hormones are the chemicals that are dispersed to your organs and oversee the basic functions of the cells in your body. A typical example of a malfunctioning endocrine gland that may result in tiredness and exhaustion is adrenal insufficiency, or Addison's disease. In adrenal insufficiency, the root of the fatigue is an impaired production of cortisol. In nearly 70 percent of cases, this condition is due to an autoimmune attack on the adrenal glands. The attack and the destructive process that takes place in the adrenal glands are reminiscent of Hashimoto's thyroiditis. In fact, patients suffering from autoimmune disorders, including Hashimoto's thyroiditis or Graves' disease, are more prone to becoming afflicted by Addison's disease and vice versa.

Physicians often diagnose Addison's disease only when the disease and the cortisol deficiency have progressed to critical levels. Frequently patients suffer from fatigue for a long period of time before the diagnosis is made. An example of this is Betty, a forty-two-year-old woman who had lost nearly twenty pounds over two years. Her fatigue and exhaustion became debilitating. Her muscle weakness and loss of appetite were so severe that she had seen ten physicians. Some diagnosed her with depression, others with chronic fatigue syndrome or food allergies. Her misery turned out to be due to a deficiency of the adrenal glands, which also made her depressed. I gave her hydrocortisone treatment, and her fatigue and other symptoms resolved over the next month.

It is increasingly recognized that many people suffer from low-grade adrenal insufficiency related to immune system attacks on the adrenal glands. To make the diagnosis of adrenal insufficiency, your doctor will typically do a blood test to check your ACTH level. ACTH is the pituitary hormone that makes your adrenal glands produce cortisol in the right amount. Your doctor will also perform an adrenal challenge test, which consists of testing your cortisol level, then injecting ACTH into a vein and testing cortisol levels again thirty minutes and sixty minutes after the injection. In addition to fatigue, adrenal insufficiency can lower your blood pressure and cause other symptoms such as nausea, fainting, low blood pressure, muscle aches, and weight loss.

Cortisol also plays a role in response to stress. For example, if you fall ill or have surgery, your body's normal response is to produce high amounts of this crucial hormone to help you recover. This is one of the main reasons why testing your adrenals should be routine if you are suffering from an autoimmune thyroid disease. Clearly, having an autoimmune thyroid disease puts you at a much higher risk for having adrenal insufficiency. Overlooking this diagnosis can have serious consequences for your health.

Adrenal insufficiency may also be caused by damage to the pituitary gland from an immune system attack, resulting in a deficiency of ACTH.

Many people talk about "adrenal fatigue" in reference to a depletion of cortisol production that occurs when chronic stress shuts down the adrenal system. When you experience a tremendous amount of stress or have been a victim of post-traumatic stress syndrome, your adrenal glands secrete large amounts of cortisol in response, as I explained in Chapter 4. Too much cortisol can alter immune system functions, cause cells to function improperly, and promote thyroid hormone inefficiency. And when the stress becomes chronic, the need to continually produce such high levels of cortisol can exhaust the adrenal system; eventually the cortisol response slows down, which contributes to fatigue. The fact of the matter, though, is that the symptoms we often call "adrenal fatigue" are caused by a high level of free radical buildup in the cells of your body and are related to a significant cellular thyroid hormone imbalance—in essence, it is a form of cellular hypothyroidism. In these situations, your T3 levels are low because of the impaired conversion of T4 to T3, and your reverse T3 is elevated (see Chapter 2).

I do not recommend taking hydrocortisone treatment for "adrenal fatigue," since your adrenal glands are not damaged, as they are in Addison's disease or other forms of true adrenal insufficiency. Once an adrenal challenge test, such as the ACTH stimulation test described above, has ruled out true adrenal insufficiency, the best way to overcome the effects of too much cortisol and chronic stress is to engage in mind-body practices such as yoga or tai chi. You also need to get rid of the free radical buildup and make the conversion of T4 to T3 in your cells as efficient as possible. In order to do that, take a comprehensive mix of potent antioxidants, like those found in ThyroLife Optima, which I typically recommend to people suffering from adrenal fatigue (see Chapter 22).

Growth Hormone–Related Fatigue

Another often overlooked cause of persistent fatigue is pituitary fatigue. A study published by Australian researchers showed that growth hormone deficiency and cortisol deficiency due to pituitary dysfunction are quite common among patients suffering from fatigue.[7]

The pituitary gland, the master gland that controls most endocrine glands—including the thyroid, the adrenal glands, and the sexual glands—receives messages from both the brain and the glands that it regulates. The pituitary gland, although tiny and hidden in a small socket of the bone at the base of the skull (called the sella turcica), has tremendous effects on various aspects of bodily functioning. People in whom this gland is destroyed—by a tumor, for instance, or by an abrupt reduction in blood supply (as might occur during severe hemorrhage)—begin to suffer from hypopituitarism, a deficiency in the hormones produced by the pituitary gland. Among the wide array of effects that may result from hypopituitarism are an underactive thyroid, an underactive adrenal gland, a deficiency in sex hormones, and a deficiency in growth hormone. The end result is the occurrence of a wide range of symptoms including fatigue, depression, and low blood pressure. Among other effects, hypopituitarism can make you prone to cardiovascular disease, and this has to do with low growth hormone and inadequate levels of other hormones.[8] Patients with hypopituitarism may also experience symptoms of hypoglycemia, joint pains and aches, muscle aches, and dizziness.

If you have an autoimmune thyroid disease or another autoimmune condition, you become vulnerable to an autoimmune attack on your pituitary gland, which in turn can cause pituitary dysfunction. When this happens, your immune system produces high levels of pituitary-attacking antibodies. These antibodies are directed at the prolactin-secreting cells or other cells, including those that produce growth hormone. In one study, antipituitary antibodies were found in 22.2 percent of patients with various autoimmune conditions.[9]

Another research study has shown that approximately one of five patients with Graves' disease or Hashimoto's thyroiditis has pituitary-attacking antibodies.[10] Having pituitary antibodies in your system can make you suffer from severe growth hormone deficiency and even cortisol deficiency,[11] both important causes of fatigue and physical and mental exhaustion. If you have ongoing fatigue, you need to have your pituitary tested, particularly if you also have an autoimmune disorder. Also, if your thyroid imbalance has been corrected with treatment and you continue to suffer from lingering fatigue and depression, your residual symptoms could be due to an autoimmune attack on your pituitary.

In recent years, extensive research has shown that head trauma can cause some damage to the pituitary gland and cause deficiency in growth hormone, thyroid hormone, and even sex hormones.[12] Hypopituitarism can occur even decades after head trauma, often related to road accidents.[13] Patients with head trauma (traumatic brain injury) become very fatigued and have a significant deterioration in attention, concentration, learning abilities, memory, problem solving, and even language. Many of these symptoms are related to growth hormone deficiency, which is the most common pituitary abnormality among people with traumatic brain injury.[14]

Pituitary hormone deficiencies can also occur as a result of an "empty sella," a herniation of the subarachnoid space within the sella turcica.[15] It can be caused by excess pressure in the brain or by a pituitary tumor. Head trauma, radiation, and surgery can also produce an empty sella. Nearly one of five patients with empty sella suffers one or more pituitary hormone deficiencies.

Although growth hormone promotes growth in children (a deficiency in infancy or childhood will result in dwarfism), growth hormone deficiency in adults was, until recently, thought not to affect health. However, expanding research has shown that a deficiency in growth hormone in adults often results in fatigue, reduced capacity for exercise, muscle weakness, impaired cognition, and decreased muscle mass.[16] One study showed that 61 percent of patients with adult-onset growth hormone deficiency suffer from atypical depression.[17] This is simply because growth hormone, like thyroid hormone, regulates chemical transmitters in the brain. Growth hormone deficiency can promote significant mental distress, lead to social isolation and anxiety, and cause fibromyalgia. Growth hormone deficiency could account for as many as one-third of all cases of fibromyalgia.[18] Growth hormone deficiency can make you gain weight and have an abnormal body composition. In addition to losing muscle, you will gain fat around the abdomen. This in turn promotes inefficiency of insulin and high levels of inflammation in your fat tissue. Growth hormone deficiency increases your risk of cardiovascular disease and lowers cardiac performance.

Treatment with daily injections of growth hormone will improve your energy, sleep, emotions, and cognition. It will make your muscles stronger, will make you lose fat, and will improve levels of cholesterol and triglycerides. It will also improve your bone density. After two months of treatment, your depression will lift. Growth hormone treatment helps thyroid hormone to work efficiently and promotes good skin health. However, it can cause carpal tunnel syndrome, peripheral swelling, joint pains and swelling, gynecomastia, and high blood sugar. If you are receiving growth hormone treatment, avoid taking oral estrogens. Oral estrogens may lessen the body composition benefits of the treatment.

Three months of low-dose growth hormone therapy is generally enough to predict if you will benefit from the treatment. If you do, you may need to continue the treatment for a long time. According to research, growth hormone treatment over a ten-year period seems to be safe.

Thyroid Imbalance and Fibromyalgia

If you have struggled with fatigue and musculoskeletal pains and aches in several areas of your body for at least three months, you could be suffering from fibromyalgia. In this condition, the pains and aches often wax and wane, and you may become sensitive to pressure applied on painful spots, or even clothing. The diagnosis of fibromyalgia is typically made when your doctor triggers pain in at least eleven musculoskeletal areas of your body by finger examination.[19] You may also suffer from headaches and morning stiffness. The fatigue associated with fibromyalgia might improve throughout the day but typically recurs in the late afternoon and evening. Sleep disturbances are common—your sleep becomes light, restless, interrupted, and nonrefreshing. As a result of the pain, aches, sleep problems, and fatigue, you feel disabled and debilitated. A minimal physical effort makes you more tired, and this affects your life at work and at home. You may experience other symptoms, such as irritable bowel syndrome, urinary frequency due to cystitis (an inflammation of the bladder), emotional distress, anxiety, and irritability. You also may become easily distressed by daily hassles. You become frustrated because people surrounding you, including your relatives, see you as healthy, but you do not feel healthy.

Fibromyalgia affects 5 percent of the population. More than 80 percent of those who suffer from fibromyalgia are women, and the onset of the condition is usually between the ages of twenty and fifty. Symptoms may be worse during the menstrual period.

Once dismissed as not being a real medical condition, fibromyalgia is now viewed as a disorder of pain processing in the brain, in which the brain's pain centers become exquisitely sensitive to any painful stimulus in your body. It's as if the brain is exacerbating the sensation of pain. Current research suggests that there may be a strong genetic component in the development of fibromyalgia, though environmental factors also seem to play an important role. For instance, a physical injury, a major emotional stress, and even infectious diseases such as hepatitis C, Epstein-Barr virus, parvovirus, and Lyme disease can trigger fibromyalgia. Even exposure to heavy metals, vitamin D deficiency, iron deficiency, and growth hormone deficiency can be contributing factors. It is, however, not yet clear how these factors actually cause the brain's abnormal response to pain.

I strongly believe that immune system reactivity plays a major role in fibromyalgia. There is clearly a high level of association between autoimmune conditions such as autoimmune thyroid disease and fibromyalgia. Just as stress can trigger an autoimmune thyroid condition, it can also trigger fibromyalgia. In addition, like autoimmune thyroid disease, fibromyalgia is associated with a severe state of inflammation, and treatments that target reducing inflammation lead to symptom improvement of the condition.

Research has suggested that free radicals and nitric oxide in muscles play an important role in the condition.[20] For this reason fibromyalgia patients need to take antioxidants, omega-3 and omega-6 fatty acids, and vitamins.[21] While a precise mechanism that can explain all cases of fibromyalgia has not been identified so far, the thyroid system clearly plays a major role in promoting its occurrence.

In fibromyalgia there is a constant low-level activation of the coagulation system.[22] The coagulation abnormality does not produce a blood clot, but generates a soluble fibrin monomer (SFM), which coats the inside of small blood vessels and thereby limits oxygen and nutrient flows into the cells. The decreased oxygen supply to the cells leads to fatigue, muscle pain, brain fog, and sleep disturbances. Your genes could make you produce too much SFM. Environmental factors, including trauma, exposure to heavy metals, and toxins coming from viruses, yeast, and bacteria, can also promote excessive production of SFM. The SFM coating of the small vessels favors the growth of yeast, bacteria, and mycoplasmids, which can hide in the coating and escape destruction by the immune system. The clotting abnormality and the hidden infection make thyroid hormone work less efficiently.[23] For this reason, some doctors advocate treatment with the active form of thyroid hormone, T3, to overcome this resistance and to treat the symptoms of fibromyalgia. People suffering from fibromyalgia can improve or even be cured when they are treated with high amounts of T3 in conjunction with taking nutritional supplements, eating a wholesome diet, and exercising.[24] In one report, 75 percent of patients improved when they followed this treatment program, and nearly 40 percent were cured.[25] The doses used, however, almost inevitably make the patients hyperthyroid. In my opinion, you may get similar benefits if you take lower doses of T3.

Immune attack on the thyroid is common in patients with fibromyalgia. One of three patients with fibromyalgia has an autoimmune thyroid disease.[26] Patients suffering from fibromyalgia are four times more likely to have an autoimmune thyroid disease than people without fibromyalgia. Patients with fibromyalgia in conjunction with an autoimmune thyroid disease often have had depression or another mental ailment.[27]

If, on top of fibromyalgia, you become affected by an autoimmune thyroid condition, your fatigue and depression will become worse. This is clearly an example of how the immune system's production of inflammation chemicals can exacerbate fatigue and depression in patients with other conditions.

Doctors refer to fibromyalgia caused by hypothyroidism as "hypothyroid fibromyalgia," as opposed to "euthyroid fibromyalgia" (meaning fibromyalgia not caused by a dysfunctioning gland). Nearly 12 percent of all cases of fibromyalgia are caused by an underactive thyroid.[28] If you have been diagnosed with fibromyalgia, you need to be tested for underactive thyroid. Doctors typically diagnose fibromyalgia months or even years after a person has been diagnosed with hypothyroidism. Often the patient has complained of fatigue, aches, and pains before therapy, but these symptoms were initially attributed to hypothyroidism. After the thyroid has been adequately regulated, however, the patient continues to complain of these and a few other symptoms that, taken together, are consistent with fibromyalgia.

Elaine, age forty-two, was suffering from numerous symptoms quite typical of fibromyalgia with a significant component of depression. When she was diagnosed with hypothyroidism after three years of going from doctor to doctor seeking an answer, she was happy and relieved, thinking that all of her problems were due to her thyroid. Although correction of her thyroid imbalance did result in some improvement, it did not completely resolve her suffering.

During Elaine's first visit to me, before she was started on thyroid medication, her husband said:

> Every 60 or 120 days, she will sit down and write a list of how she's feeling in anticipation of seeing a new doctor. These symptoms range from being dizzy to one cheek going numb, to an uncontrolled spasm in the muscle, weak knees, depression, dry eyes, pains and aches in her joints, stiffness, sleep problems, aches in muscles, and legs and toes tingling. It is rare that these lists get to the doctor's hands because it's easy to type the list, but there is a fear in handing it to the doctor. He or she looks at this long list of symptoms that Elaine says she is experiencing all the time and concludes, "This is one physically and mentally sick puppy and it's beyond me," or "This can't be happening."

My findings indicated that Elaine was suffering from two separate conditions, fibromyalgia and hypothyroidism. The underactive thyroid might have promoted the fibromyalgia and was exacerbating its symptoms. As noted earlier, after treatment of her thyroid imbalance, many of Elaine's symptoms improved, but many related to the fibromyalgia persisted.

Doctors' frequent dismissal of patients like Elaine and their lack of support, education, and recognition of the syndrome often lead patients to consult physician after physician, and sometimes to opt out of the medical establishment altogether. They may seek help from unreliable healers, subjecting themselves to quackery, and even accept dangerous treatments that have not been proven effective.

Fibromyalgia can also be triggered following treatment of an overactive thyroid. Poor correction of an overactive thyroid or repeated rapid swings of thyroid levels during treatment (causing abrupt shifts from hyperthyroidism to severe hypothyroidism) can provoke onset of fibromyalgia (see Chapter 17).

Activation of the adrenal system, excess cortisol, and excessive production of substance P and release of inflammatory chemicals may be at the root of the problem in some patients with fibromyalgia. Many people suffering with fibromyalgia can be helped with the serotonin-3 receptor antagonist tropisetron. In addition, the flavonoid quercetin, which slows down inflammation and lowers the activation of mast cells, helps with the symptoms.[29] Melatonin, 1 to 3 mg at bedtime, can improve your sleep and the pain and aches. Sleep disturbances can also be reduced by taking a growth hormone secretagogue (GHS).[30] If you are premenopausal, your symptoms tend to worsen during menstrual periods. Women tend to have more severe pain after menopause. Twenty-five percent of postmenopausal women with fibromyalgia indicate that their symptoms started at the time of menopause.[31]

Before accepting the diagnosis of fibromyalgia, discuss other disorders with your doctor. Some of the symptoms of fibromyalgia are also symptoms of connective tissue disorders, such as rheumatoid arthritis, Sjögren's syndrome, polymyalgia rheumatica, polymyositis, and lupus. These conditions can cause generalized pain syndrome, as can parathyroid disease and osteoarthritis. Also, many patients with fibromyalgia suffer simultaneously from a connective tissue disorder such as Raynaud's phenomenon or Sjögren's syndrome.

Fibromyalgia, whether caused by or co-occurring with an underactive thyroid, is not necessarily a crippling disease. There are ways to control the symptoms. Strength training significantly improves muscle strength and joint function in women with fibromyalgia.

Small doses of tricyclic antidepressants such as amitriptyline improve sleep and pain from fibromyalgia, but these do not work in everyone. Newer agents such as the dual serotonin-norepinephrine reuptake inhibitor duloxetine and the antiseizure drug pregabalin are quite effective and often work better than the tricyclic antidepressants.[32] Research has shown that pregabalin at a dose of 450 mg per day improves symptoms of fibromyalgia, including sleep and fatigue.[33] It is a well-tolerated treatment and improves the quality of life. Deep-water running seems to be a safe exercise that has a positive impact on the pain. In addition, it helps tremendously with the emotional aspects of the condition.

A muscle relaxant taken in the evening may be helpful in reducing aches and pains and sleep problems in fibromyalgia patients. Achieving aerobic fitness and avoiding a sedentary lifestyle will gradually improve the symptoms. Excessive exercise, on the other hand, can exacerbate the symptoms. Massage has helped many patients. Antioxidant supplementation helps with pain and aches. I have found that avoiding caffeine in the afternoon and evening improves the quality of sleep. Also, patients should avoid too much noise at night. A low-salt vegan diet rich in lactobacteria and emphasizing uncooked foods has been shown to improve the symptoms of fibromyalgia.[34]

Hypnotherapy seems to be more effective than physical therapy in persistent fibromyalgia. Counseling and biofeedback have helped many patients as well. Cognitive behavioral therapy and spiritual healing techniques such as prayer can also be of tremendous benefit.

Research has also shown that tai chi, which combines physical exercise and mind-body therapy, improves the symptoms of fibromyalgia.[35] Meditation therapy and living mindfully also help. Meditation will improve anxiety, pain, and depression, enhance mood and self-esteem, and reduce the perception of stress.[36]

Acupuncture treatment seems to be quite effective in patients with fibromyalgia. A study published by researchers at the Southern California University of Health Sciences showed that acupuncture is effective in improving pain and depression in patients with fibromyalgia.[37]

One trial demonstrated that the subcutaneous administration of growth hormone daily was found to be effective in improving the symptoms of fibromyalgia, particularly the aches and pains, fatigue, and reduced capacity for exercise in patients with low IGF1 levels.[38] Another treatment modality for fibromyalgia is hyperbaric oxygen therapy. This treatment greatly helps the symptoms of fibromyalgia patients.

Available Treatments for Fibromyalgia

- Tricyclic antidepressants
- T3 medications (T4/T3 therapy for hypothyroid fibromyalgia)
- Serotonin and norepinephrine dual reuptake inhibitors
- Antiepileptic drugs (pregabalin, gabapentin)

- Selective serotonin reuptake inhibitors (though results have been inconclusive)
- Sedative-hypnotic compounds (zopiclone and zolpidem can improve sleep and reduce fatigue, but not usually pain; sodium oxybate has been shown to improve all symptoms)
- Pramiprexole (a drug used in Parkinson's disease to help reduce limb movement)
- Tizanidine
- Tramadol
- Cognitive behavioral therapy
- Exercise
- Muscle relaxants
- Hypnotherapy
- Antioxidants
- Acupuncture
- Relaxation techniques (tai chi, meditation)
- Massage
- Swimming

Thyroid Imbalance and Chronic Fatigue Syndrome

The Centers for Disease Control define chronic fatigue syndrome as a new onset of persistent or relapsing debilitating fatigue or easy fatigability that does not resolve with bed rest and is made worse by exercise. Also called immune dysfunction syndrome, chronic fatigue syndrome is caused by common viral infections in people who have additional risk factors such as a genetic predisposition and immune system dysfunction. Chronic fatigue syndrome is associated with high levels of inflammation chemicals. Like fibromyalgia, CFS seem to be strongly related to immune system reactivity and could easily correlate with thyroid autoimmunity. In general, the diagnosis is considered if the fatigue has lasted at least six months.[39] Other symptoms that may occur in chronic fatigue syndrome are chills, sore throat, painful regions, generalized muscle weakness, muscle pain, prolonged fatigue after exercise, headaches, joint pains, neuropsychological symptoms, and sleep disturbances.

Epidemiologic studies conducted in several countries have shown that the frequency of chronic fatigue syndrome in the general population is 0.3 to 1 percent.[40] The neuropsychological symptoms of both depression and chronic fatigue syndrome are quite similar. However, certain physical effects (low-grade fever, night sweats, swollen lymph nodes, and pharyngitis) will point to CFS rather than depression. The psychological impairment can lead to social pressure and isolation. Patients may be described as "crazy" or "lazy."

Patients with chronic fatigue syndrome view themselves negatively, and the way they perceive and describe their illness may perpetuate their symptoms. For this reason, social support is of tremendous importance. Research has shown that lack of social support perpetuates the fatigue and the functional impairment.

Involvement of the central nervous system and deficiency of the hypothalamic-pituitary-adrenal system contribute to the disorder. Low DHEA-sulfate and inflammation may be contributing to the disrupted functioning of the immune system. Inflammation and high levels of oxidative stress, and perhaps lack of antioxidant defense, account for the occurrence of chronic fatigue syndrome. Supplementation with antioxidants and probiotics improves the functioning of the immune system and reduces the symptoms of chronic fatigue syndrome.[41]

Research has shown that zinc levels are quite low in patients with CFS, and the lower the zinc levels, the more severe the symptoms. Low zinc promotes more inflammation and more disturbances in the T lymphocytes.[42] Taking zinc supplements should be part of the treatment program. Deficiencies in other vitamins and micronutrients, including deficiency in B vitamins, vitamin C, magnesium, sodium, L-tryptophan, L-carnitine, coenzyme Q10, and essential fatty acids, are also blamed for the occurrence of CFS.[43] For this reason patients with chronic fatigue syndrome are often prescribed a high-potency vitamin and mineral supplement.

Some studies have shown that mild cortisol deficiency related to a hypothalamic-pituitary defect may contribute to CFS. If testing shows cortisol deficiency, treatment with hydrocortisone can help relieve symptoms.[44]

Although there is no cure for CFS, several other treatments have been shown to help some patients, including graded exercise therapy and cognitive behavior therapy. Potentially helpful medications include antidepressants, injections of high doses of immunoglobulin, intramuscular injections of magnesium sulfate, and consumption of high doses of essential fatty acids. Because serotonin levels are abnormal in patients with CFS, the serotonin precursor 5-hydroxytryptophan can be helpful in some people. Homeopathic medicine can also diminish your symptoms of fatigue.

Because the symptoms of hypothyroidism and CFS are quite similar, some patients with underactive thyroid may be misdiagnosed as having CFS. In such patients, the right treatment is achieving and maintaining a perfect thyroid balance with thyroid hormone therapy. Also, if you suffer from both CFS and a thyroid imbalance, you will not get full benefit from the currently available treatments for CFS unless your thyroid imbalance has been properly corrected and monitored.

Hypoglycemia: The Mysteries of Blood Sugar

Another cause of fatigue and mood changes that can lead to confusion and misdiagnosis is hypoglycemia. Hypoglycemia (a below-normal blood sugar level) can cause fatigue, headaches, and rapid heartbeat. Other common symptoms of hypoglycemia are an inability to concentrate, confusion, irritability, bizarre behavior, trembling, anxiety, sweating, and hunger. The symptoms occur because the brain is not receiving enough sugar, and ordinarily will resolve rather quickly when you eat carbohydrates.

Many of the symptoms of hypoglycemia result from the activation of the autonomic nervous system, the same system that causes some of the physical symptoms of an anxiety disorder. Hypoglycemia, widely publicized in popular magazines and books, has been often cited as a common cause of tiredness, poor work and study performance, and sexual dysfunction. As a result, many people suffering symptoms due to depression or anxiety disorder are erroneously diagnosed as hypoglycemic.

The standard test for hypoglycemia is an oral glucose tolerance test, which consists of measuring blood sugar before and several times after the ingestion of glucose. In healthy people not suffering from hypoglycemia, the blood sugar rises after glucose ingestion and then gradually decreases to low levels two to three hours after the ingestion of sugars. After the drop in blood sugar, the levels will typically return to normal. It has been estimated that 20 percent of normal healthy people have a reactive low blood sugar two to three hours after food intake but do not experience symptoms.[45] Doctors will make the diagnosis of true reactive hypoglycemia only if you have experienced symptoms when the blood sugar is low during the glucose test.

I have seen quite a few people who were labeled hypoglycemic for a long time, yet the source of their symptoms turned out to be depression or an underactive thyroid. Even though the explosive epidemic of mislabeling seemingly everyone as hypoglycemic that occurred in the 1970s and 1980s[46] is slowly receding, this problem has continued to affect a substantial number of people. If you were diagnosed as hypoglycemic based only on symptoms, or if your glucose test was not interpreted correctly, you may become debilitated by the diagnosis itself. Many supposed hypoglycemics refuse to eat in restaurants, don't drive a car, or become "dietary cripples" who are afraid of certain food choices.

If true hypoglycemia is not the reason for the symptoms of fatigue and anxiety after a meal, why, then, do some people experience fatigue, sleeplessness, difficulty concentrating, and even rapid heartbeat and sweatiness after eating? If you absorb sugar faster than average, insulin levels in response to the sugar surge are, in general, higher. This often happens when you have too much thyroid in your system. The high increase in insulin levels in your bloodstream typically causes the blood sugar to drop quickly after the abrupt rise. Even if you do not experience clear-cut low blood sugar, the rapid decline of blood sugar could trigger an exaggerated response of the adrenaline-activated nervous system, which results in symptoms. In essence, a person can experience symptoms of hypoglycemia without actually having hypoglycemia.

The timing of symptoms is important in differentiating true hypoglycemia from what I call "rapid blood sugar drop syndrome." With true reactive hypoglycemia, symptoms typically begin three hours after meals. They also coincide with a low blood sugar reading. In contrast, symptoms related to "rapid blood sugar drop syndrome" generally occur earlier, one hour after eating.

The type of foods consumed determines the magnitude of the rise in blood sugar. Researchers have developed a scale, called the glycemic index, that scores foods according to the degree of rise in blood sugar that occurs after they are eaten. The higher the glycemic index, the higher the insulin response and the more rapid the subsequent fall in blood sugar. Simple sugars have a higher glycemic index than complex carbohydrates. What determines the glycemic index is not only the type of carbohydrates (simple versus complex) but also the amount of fat, protein, and fiber, as well as the method of food processing and cooking. Thus, to avoid a rapid drop in blood sugar, select foods that have the lowest glycemic index. (Consult the ThyroLife Diet in Chapter 21 for a more thorough discussion of the effects of different foods on blood sugar.)

Equally disturbing are vague suggestions that connect hypoglycemia to hypothyroidism[47] and imply that hypoglycemia is a common occurrence in hypothyroidism. These have led some people to conclude that a person suffering from symptoms of hypoglycemia could be treated with thyroid hormone. Thyroid specialists often see patients who were diagnosed as hypoglycemic because of symptoms of fatigue, headaches, and sleep disturbances, and who were then inappropriately placed on thyroid hormone treatment for these symptoms, even though these patients have a normal thyroid gland.

Making the Diagnosis

To determine the likelihood that you are suffering from chronic fatigue syndrome, fibromyalgia, hypothyroidism, or a combination of these conditions, complete the following questionnaires and score yourself for each of the symptoms you are experiencing.

QUESTIONNAIRE A:
SYMPTOMS COMMON TO FIBROMYALGIA,
CHRONIC FATIGUE SYNDROME, AND HYPOTHYROIDISM

Indicate whether you have been experiencing each of the following symptoms. When you answer no, proceed to the next symptom; when you answer yes, score the severity of your symptom (1 = mild, 2 = moderate, 3 = severe) before proceeding to the next one.

Fatigue	Yes	No	___
Lack of endurance	Yes	No	___
Dizziness	Yes	No	___
Joint stiffness	Yes	No	___
Depression	Yes	No	___
Anxiety	Yes	No	___
Difficulty concentrating	Yes	No	___
Muscle weakness	Yes	No	___
Headaches	Yes	No	___
Worsening PMS	Yes	No	___
Mood swings	Yes	No	___
Irritability	Yes	No	___
Word mix-ups	Yes	No	___
Joint pains and aches	Yes	No	___
Swollen fingers	Yes	No	___
Brain fog	Yes	No	___
Panic attacks	Yes	No	___
Memory blanks	Yes	No	___
TOTAL SCORE			___

Add up your total score. If it is higher than 15, you may be suffering from fibromyalgia, chronic fatigue syndrome, or an underactive thyroid and should proceed to questionnaires B, C, D, and E.

QUESTIONNAIRE B:
CHRONIC FATIGUE SYNDROME/FIBROMYALGIA

Have you suffered, for six months, from fatigue occurring
even at rest and not relieved by rest that has affected
your ability to participate in your usual work, social,
or personal activities? (If you answer yes, give
yourself 10 points.)   Yes   No   ___

Do you feel exhausted, dizzy, and about to faint
after a hot shower? (If you answer yes,
give yourself 5 points.)   Yes   No   ___

Do you feel drained and exhausted for more than
twenty-four hours after exercising? (If you answer
yes, give yourself 5 points.)   Yes   No   ___

Did your symptoms begin abruptly? (If you answer
yes, give yourself 5 points.)   Yes   No   ___

Have you experienced since the onset of the fatigue,
but not before, any of the following symptoms
in a persistent or recurrent fashion? If so, score
the severity of each symptom as follows: 1 = mild,
2 = moderate, 3 = severe.

Changing joint pains	Yes	No	___
Bad days, good days	Yes	No	___
Trouble sleeping in the middle of the night	Yes	No	___
Increased thirst	Yes	No	___
Dry eyes, dry mouth	Yes	No	___
Visual blurring	Yes	No	___
Rapid heartbeat	Yes	No	___
Loss of appetite	Yes	No	___
Nausea	Yes	No	___
Severe malaise	Yes	No	___

TOTAL SCORE   ___

If your score is 25 or higher, you may be suffering from either fibromyalgia or chronic fatigue syndrome and should proceed to questionnaire C.

QUESTIONNAIRE C: FIBROMYALGIA

Have you had for at least the past three months pain or
   achiness in many parts of your body, affecting both
   sides of the body (right and left), above and below the
   waist and in the midbody (that is, any part of the
   spine)? (If you answer yes, give yourself 5 points.)   Yes   No   ___
Has your doctor been able to trigger pain in at
   least eleven places by pressing on the eighteen
   spots on your body called trigger points? (If you
   answer yes, give yourself 10 points.)   Yes   No   ___
Have you experienced any of the following
   symptoms? If so, score the severity of each
   symptom as follows: 1 = mild, 2 = moderate,
   3 = severe.
Muscle spasms   Yes   No   ___
Numbness and tingling   Yes   No   ___
Sensitivity of your eyes to light   Yes   No   ___
Bruising   Yes   No   ___
Irritable bladder   Yes   No   ___
Irritable bowel   Yes   No   ___
Eye pains   Yes   No   ___

TOTAL SCORE   ___

If your score is 25 or higher, you may be suffering from fibromyalgia.
Regardless of the score, proceed to questionnaires D and E.

QUESTIONNAIRE D: CHRONIC FATIGUE SYNDROME

Do you experience recurrent or persistent fevers?
   (If you answer yes, give yourself 10 points.)   Yes   No   ___
Have you had tender lymph nodes lasting for several
   weeks? (If you answer yes, give yourself 10 points.)   Yes   No   ___
Have you experienced any of the following symptoms?
   If so, score the severity of each symptom as follows:
   1 = mild, 2 = moderate, 3 = severe.

Night sweats   Yes   No   ___
Sore throat   Yes   No   ___
Increased thirst   Yes   No   ___
Frequent infections   Yes   No   ___

TOTAL SCORE   ___

If your score is 25 points or higher in questionnaire D, you may be suffering from chronic fatigue syndrome. Now, regardless of your scores in questionnaires B, C, or D, proceed to questionnaire E.

QUESTIONNAIRE E: HYPOTHYROIDISM

Have you experienced any of the following symptoms for at least one month? When you answer no, proceed to the next symptom; when you answer yes, score the severity of your symptom (1 = mild, 2 = moderate, 3 = severe) before proceeding to the next one.

Hair loss   Yes   No   ___
Dry skin   Yes   No   ___
Constipation   Yes   No   ___
Slow pulse   Yes   No   ___
Increased appetite   Yes   No   ___
Weight gain   Yes   No   ___
Sleep apnea (heavy snoring and brief, intermittent
   cessation of breathing during sleep)   Yes   No   ___
Yellow palms   Yes   No   ___
Muscle cramps   Yes   No   ___
Increased sleep   Yes   No   ___

TOTAL SCORE   ___

If you score higher than 10 in questionnaire E, you may be hypothyroid. If you also scored 25 or more in questionnaire C or D, you may have both hypothyroidism and chronic fatigue syndrome or fibromyalgia.

Important Points to Remember

- If you are suffering from fatigue, do not assume that your other symptoms are caused by the fatigue. To help your doctor uncover the source(s) of your fatigue, describe *all* your symptoms as precisely as possible.
- Remember, a person may have more than one disorder causing fatigue. Thyroid imbalance can coexist with other conditions that typically cause fatigue, including adrenal insufficiency, adrenal fatigue, growth hormone deficiency, fibromyalgia, and chronic fatigue syndrome.
- Keep the tripod of wellness (the endocrine system, the immune system, and the brain) in mind while you are trying to find out what is causing your fatigue.
- If you have fibromyalgia, a thyroid condition could be the root cause.
- Do not easily accept the diagnosis of hypoglycemia unless your symptoms coincide with low blood sugar levels.
- To avoid being misdiagnosed, use symptom questionaires that help you determine which one of the three overlapping syndromes (fibromyalgia, chronic fatigue syndrome, and thyroid imbalance) is causing your symptom(s).

PART III

WOMEN'S
THYROID PROBLEMS

Your Symptoms Are Not All in Your Head

14

PREMENSTRUAL SYNDROME
AND MENOPAUSE

Tuning the Cycles

From puberty to menopause, women's bodies and brains are influenced by continuous cycles of hormones. These hormones are crucial not only for reproduction but also for the nature of a woman's feminine identity. Sex hormones—including estrogen, progesterone, testosterone, and DHEA—also play an important role in thinking and memory, and they interact with chemicals in the brain that regulate mood, emotions, and sex drive.

The well-defined pattern of women's monthly cycles is tightly regulated by messages from the hypothalamus and pituitary gland. Even though the thyroid system and the sex hormone system are two independent systems governed by the same "master gland," the pituitary, there are important relationships between the two.

First, thyroid hormone affects the levels of sex hormones and the way they work in your body. A thyroid hormone imbalance frequently causes either heavy, prolonged menstrual periods (especially in hypothyroidism) or brief, scanty menstrual periods, or even cessation of periods (in hyperthyroidism and also in severe hypothyroidism).[1] Thyroid hormone is also critical for conception and for a successful, healthy pregnancy.

Second, sex hormones seem to play a role in the occurrence of thyroid disease. In females, autoimmune thyroid disorders become more common at puberty. As a woman enters her reproductive years, the frequency of both Hashimoto's thyroiditis and Graves' disease increases sharply. At menopause, the frequency of Hashimoto's thyroiditis and low-grade hypothyroidism also increases, with 13 to 15 percent of postmenopausal women having some thyroid hormone deficit.[2] One study showed that Hashimoto's thyroiditis occurred more frequently in women who had a longer reproductive span (that is, more years between puberty and menopause).[3]

Other facts clearly indicate that sex hormones have a major effect on the activity of the thyroid gland and may even affect the triggering of an autoimmune reaction in the thyroid. For instance, many women with dormant Graves' disease may have a flare-up in the first trimester of pregnancy or after delivery. The important hormonal changes that occur after delivery also seem to account for the high frequency of postpartum thyroid disease. The triggering or worsening of thyroid conditions throughout these periods of hormonal shifts is probably related to effects of sex hormones on the immune system.

Sex hormones also have a significant effect on how a thyroid imbalance is manifested physically and mentally. The chemistry of both brain and body is influenced in normal and abnormal conditions by the thyroid and sex hormones. A thyroid hormone imbalance will exacerbate the symptoms of hormonal shifts, so a woman who usually has few or no symptoms related to hormonal changes will begin to experience more symptoms when a thyroid imbalance occurs.

These complex ways in which thyroid problems cause escalation of symptoms are most apparent during three important periods of the hormonal cycle: the luteal phase of the menstrual cycle (after ovulation, when an egg is released—the time when most women experience premenstrual syndrome, or PMS), the postpartum period, and menopause. This chapter focuses on the relationship between the thyroid, luteal phase syndrome (PMS), and menopause. (Postpartum depression is discussed in Chapter 15.)

PMS: Chemical Imbalance or Hormonal Shifts?

During the last part of the menstrual cycle (that is, five to seven days prior to the menstrual period), many women suffer mood swings, irritability, anger, loss of energy, difficulty concentrating, appetite changes (particularly food cravings), anxiety, depression, loss of interest in ordinary activities, exhaustion, and sleep pattern changes, including insomnia. This mix of symptoms, casually called premenstrual syndrome, is reminiscent of a depressive type of cyclic mood disorder. During the course of the reproductive years, this cyclic change in emotions and mood often begins in an insidious fashion. Gradually, women who experience PMS learn to cope with the episodic and recurrent suffering.

Because the symptoms of PMS are similar to those of cyclic depression, it's often thought that a subtle chemical imbalance is responsible for the mood effects. PMS tends to become more noticeable to the woman during the last few days of the menstrual cycle. This is when estrogen levels, after increasing following ovulation, tend to decline. At the same time, the levels of progesterone, which had been produced in great quantities in the second part of the menstrual cycle, tend to decrease as well. These hormonal shifts have been thought to be the basis for premenstrual syndrome. Hormonal shifts also explain the physical discomfort—including bloating, aches and pains, breast tenderness, headaches, migraines, and gastrointestinal symptoms—that you may experience during PMS.

Premenstrual syndrome is one of the least understood syndromes in medicine. Endocrinologists, reproductive endocrinologists, psychiatrists, and gynecologists have all attempted to understand the basis for the syndrome, yet none has been able to declare authoritatively what causes PMS. For the most part, the various specialists have addressed only the facets of the syndrome that apply to their field. Endocrinologists have found multiple abnormalities that could account for the fluid and salt retention that occurs during the premenstrual period. Reproductive endocrinologists and gynecologists have explained the changes in hormone levels occurring in the last part of the menstrual cycle. Psychiatrists have focused on the emotional aspects of premenstrual syndrome and have provided some criteria for making a correct diagnosis.[4]

Researchers from the various fields have proposed that the cause of premenstrual syndrome could be an increased sensitivity in some women to the hormonal shifts of the menstrual cycle. Research has shown that the functioning of the serotoninergic system in the brain changes throughout the menstrual cycle, and this has to do with the changes in hormone levels. Estrogen enhances the activity of serotonin in certain regions of the brain and regulates mood, emotion, and cognition.[5] Estrogens also regulate interactions between the brain and the endocrine system. Some women are more sensitive to the serotonin changes caused by hormones, making them more likely to suffer from PMS. In essence, some women may have an underlying subtle chemical imbalance that predisposes them to suffer PMS. Thyroid hormone, cortisol, and sex hormones (that is, estrogen, progesterone, and androgens) regulate to some extent the amount of chemicals in the brain and their effects on the body and mind.

As estrogen levels decline in the premenstrual period, serotonin activity declines as well, which explains the changes in mood and behavior. The rise in progesterone that occurs after ovulation also contributes to the decline in serotonin activity and affects the neurotransmitter GABA, which is equally involved in regulating mood, emotions, and eating behavior. In fact, progesterone causes the same negative effects on mood as benzodiazepines, barbiturates, and alcohol.[6]

Recent research has shown that the hormone leptin, which regulates appetite and metabolism, contributes to the occurrence of PMS. Leptin regulates reproduction and emotions as well. Patients suffering from PMS have higher leptin levels during the second part of the menstrual cycle.[7] They tend to eat more fat, more simple sugars, and less protein before their menstrual periods, and to eat more often, making it hard for them to follow a weight management program.

The importance of neurotransmitter changes and their interactions with hormones can be highlighted by the fact that being overweight makes a woman more predisposed to have PMS. Recent research has shown that PMS is three times more common in obese women than in nonobese ones.[8] Tobacco smokers, too, are more prone to suffering from PMS than nonsmokers. If you suffer from PMS, you also will be more likely to consume heavy amounts of alcohol.[9]

Nearly 50 percent of all women experience some discomfort during the premenstrual period,[10] but the majority of them have mild changes that they perceive as normal and similar to what other women experience. When asked whether they have symptoms of premenstrual syndrome, such women will typically respond, "Oh, yeah, I have those." But in some cases the symptoms are far more severe.

A menopausal woman who suffered from PMS for years told me once:

I am so happy to not have periods any longer because my PMS was severe. I would describe it as viciousness, vicious irritability around PMS! It was like, "Mark your calendar, don't come near me." I didn't want to go out in public during those times because I was afraid I'd have an altercation—I'd say something to somebody because they looked at me wrong.

Yet this woman kept her suffering a secret. She never sought medical help.

As with many mental conditions, psychiatrists have proposed rigid criteria for determining whether a woman has PMS. According to psychiatrists, you are considered to be a PMS sufferer only if you have several severe symptoms and only if you receive the diagnosis of "late luteal phase dysphoric disorder." Just 3–8 percent of women meet these criteria. However, according to the much less rigid criteria used by the American College of Obstetricians and Gynecologists, you will be considered to be a PMS sufferer if you have only one mood-related symptom and one physical symptom. As you can see, you may be suffering from PMS, but you may not receive the proper diagnosis if you are evaluated by a doctor who uses the psychiatric criteria. Research has suggested that 13–18 percent of women have premenstrual symptoms severe enough to cause distress and suffering.[11] Yet many of these women are dismissed as being normal. You need to record your symptoms and the way you feel in daily diaries and use the less rigid criteria for diagnosis to get the help you need.

Premenstrual symptoms tend to worsen as you get older. They worsen even more during the time a woman is about to become menopausal, so the symptoms of PMS and perimenopause may become intermingled.[12] At this stage of their reproductive lives, women are often surprised to hear that PMS symptoms could be causing their discomfort. The symptoms may become continuous as their ovulation becomes irregular and their menstrual periods become heavier and irregular.

There is in fact a tight link between suffering from PMS and the likelihood of experiencing menopausal symptoms including hot flashes, poor sleep, decreased libido, and even menopausal depression. Research has shown that one of four women suffering from perimenopausal depression had previously suffered from PMS, but less than one of ten depression-free menopausal women had experienced PMS.[13] This tells you that if you have suffered from PMS, whether the root of the problem is a thyroid imbalance or not, you become more vulnerable to perimenopausal depression.

Women who suffer from chronic, undiagnosed mood or anxiety disorders in addition to having PMS can find it particularly difficult to get diagnosed properly. If you already suffer from depression or an anxiety disorder, you will be more likely to suffer from PMS. Clear-cut exacerbation of depressive symptoms occurs in 80 percent of patients suffering from depression.[14] In these women, the emotional suffering related to their mood disorder worsens in this vulnerable period of the menstrual cycle. For several days before the menstrual period, they experience a mixture of discomfort and suffering related to both the PMS and the mood disorder, with the symptoms sometimes becoming severe and disabling. This intensification of symptoms represents a strong argument in favor of a subtle chemical imbalance in the brain being at the root of PMS.

Thyroid Hormone Imbalance: The Link to PMS

Endocrinologists have studied various facets of the body's hormonal systems in order to explain some of the symptoms occurring in premenstrual syndrome. They have found some abnormalities in many hormonal systems, including the thyroid system. Since thyroid hormone affects levels of brain chemicals known to affect emotions and mood, several researchers have attempted to determine whether PMS could be caused by a thyroid imbalance.

Dr. Peter Schmidt and his coworkers from the National Institutes of Health showed in a study of a large number of women fulfilling the clinical criteria of premenstrual syndrome[15] that 10.5 percent of women with PMS had a thyroid imbalance, frequently low-grade hypothyroidism. Utilizing TRH stimulation testing, the most sensitive test available for detecting a very minor thyroid hormone deficit, they also found that 30 percent of women with PMS who have normal basal TSH levels had a minor thyroid imbalance. The frequency of low-grade hypothyroidism determined by TSH measurement in large samples of women of reproductive age has generally been 3.6 to 7.5 percent, so the rate found in this study was higher than expected.

An open trial conducted by Dr. Nora Brayshaw showed that a high dose of thyroid hormone caused relief of symptoms in women with PMS. Most of the women studied had low-grade hypothyroidism.[16]

These results suggest that thyroid imbalance, including low-grade hypothyroidism, may play a role in the occurrence or exacerbation of PMS in some but not all women. It is possible that a deficit of thyroid hormone in the brain is the basis of premenstrual syndrome in some women. The similarities between the symptoms of hypothyroidism and those of premenstrual syndrome make this hypothesis plausible. Some of the common symptoms include weight gain, poor regulation of temperature, lethargy, irritability, mood swings, and anxiety. The effectiveness of thyroid hormone treatment in some women who suffer from PMS but have normal thyroid glands is reminiscent of the effectiveness noted in women suffering from depression.

Martha, a thirty-two-year-old manager, had never had symptoms of PMS until two years before her gynecologist made the diagnosis of hypothyroidism. She said:

Initially, I was happy most of the time. Then, two years ago, I started getting tired and depressed and having headaches before my period. Little by little, I became very emotional and couldn't get out of bed. I would get up, shower, get dressed, and just sit there.

For several months, my periods would last two weeks, so it was like basically the whole month on PMS. I would be irritable the whole time. When I was diagnosed with hypothyroidism and started thyroid hormone treatment, my symptoms started decreasing. My headaches started decreasing, and then my symptoms went away.

Martha's case is not unique. Women may visit their doctor because of PMS symptoms and turn out to have a thyroid disorder.

Many women diagnosed with Graves' disease who have had some experience with PMS state that Graves' disease can be described as PMS multiplied many times. The symptoms of hyperthyroidism and PMS may be so similar that you may attribute symptoms of hyperthyroidism to worsening PMS. Some women with mild overactive thyroid will notice thyroid-related symptoms only in the premenstrual period.

While it is clear that thyroid imbalance can promote the occurrence of premenstrual syndrome, immune system reactivity and inflammation chemicals related to autoimmunity are likely to play a role in the high incidence of PMS in thyroid patients. The hormonal swings that occur in the later part of the menstrual cycle preceding the menstrual period could make the immune system become more reactive, leading to increased release of cytokines, substances that affect mood and emotions as well as exacerbate inflammation, fluid retention, and bloating. In essence, if you have Hashimoto's thyroiditis and low-grade hypothyroidism, you are at higher risk for having more severe PMS, since the effects of the immune system dysfunction are adding to the effects of the thyroid imbalance.

How Thyroid Dysfunction Can Exacerbate PMS

For women suffering from mild premenstrual syndrome, the occurrence of a thyroid imbalance (either hypothyroidism or hyperthyroidism) may aggravate PMS symptoms.

Billie was thirty-two when her gynecologist diagnosed a goiter. Thyroid testing showed hypothyroidism. Billie had started having PMS at the age of twenty but coped with the symptoms quite well. Over the preceding three-year period, though, her symptoms had gradually worsened. She saw numerous physicians, who recommended different treatments without results. The worsening of PMS resolved when her hypothyroidism was corrected.

Before treatment, Billie described her symptoms as follows:

> I have been suffering from these symptoms for some time. I wanted to break up with my boyfriend, or I didn't like him or something. Then I started noticing that, even when he was gone, I still had that. My symptoms became much worse in the past three years. It was like clockwork. Same feelings, same anxiety. A physician diagnosed PMS and prescribed Prozac. Prozac helped a little, but then I had side effects. I stopped taking it.
>
> I had gotten it down pretty much. Twenty days out of the month I am okay. I know any day I'm waiting for it to come. All of a sudden, it feels like something comes in my body and takes over.
>
> My mind all of a sudden changes. My appetite goes crazy. I never can get satisfied. The imbalance almost drives me crazy. My emotions become overwhelming.
>
> It comes and goes in waves. I would cry and not know why. One minute I would be on top of the world and be doing things with my family, and then five minutes later something would make me mad and I would be yelling at my friends or husband. I'm not the same person. It's like dual personalities.
>
> I went to a PMS specialist. He handed me a brochure and said, "This is what PMS is, and I'm sorry I have nothing to tell you. Take these birth control pills and see if that helps." They made me tired and made me gain weight. Another doctor read my history and told me that I might be suffering from a bipolar disorder. One doctor told me I had cyclothymia.

Billie's PMS became much more severe at the onset of her hypothyroidism. With thyroid hormone treatment, her mind felt clearer all the time and her symptoms improved. She said:

> I stayed on more of an even keel. My appetite was more regular. My energy level was more consistent. I didn't do a lot of things at one time. I was more method-

ical. I usually try to get a lot of things going at the same time—baking, cooking, doing laundry. I don't tire out as I did. I'm calmer. My responses are more thought out. I didn't have any other improvement like this with any other medication.

Thyroid hormone excess or deficiency gives a different shape to premenstrual syndrome. It not only amplifies preexisting PMS symptoms but also adds new symptoms to the mix. The additional suffering differs depending on the type and severity of the thyroid imbalance.

Whereas hypothyroidism combined with PMS means more sudden depressed moods, crying spells, feelings of despair and loss of control, sleepiness, guilt feelings, and anger, the combination of hyperthyroidism and PMS results in more anxiety symptoms, restlessness, and altered sleep patterns. Hyperthyroid women experiencing panic attacks may find that those attacks increase in both frequency and severity during the last part of the menstrual cycle. In general, the mood swings, irritability, and anger become mixed with a higher degree of anxiety and agitation during the premenstrual period.

How to Cure Your PMS

If you have a thyroid imbalance and have suffered from PMS, obviously the first step in improving or curing your PMS is to properly address the thyroid imbalance and have it adequately corrected. If you have an underactive thyroid, you are more likely to benefit from a combination of T4 and T3. The active form of thyroid hormone, T3, enhances serotonin activity in the brain and helps alleviate the mood-related symptoms. However, even with proper thyroid treatment, you may continue to suffer from residual PMS symptoms. To cure these symptoms, you may need to take a contraceptive pill containing a low dose of estrogen to prevent the hormonal swings related to ovulation. This has become the most widely accepted treatment for PMS. Oral contraceptives containing only progestin do not improve PMS symptoms and may even make things worse. Newer formulations such as Yasmin, containing low-dose estrogen in conjunction with the progestin drospirenone, help the most.[17] This kind of oral contraceptive also reduces the water retention so common in PMS.

Selective serotonin reuptake inhibitor (SSRI) antidepressants are quite effective in treating both the mood symptoms of PMS and physical symptoms such as bloating and headaches. Research has shown that more than 60 percent of patients suffering from PMS respond to these medications.[18] Sertraline, fluoxetine, and extended-release paroxetine have been approved by the U.S. FDA for PMS. One study showed that citalopram is effective in patients who failed to respond to other SSRIs. These drugs can be effective when taken intermittently in the second phase of the menstrual cycle. However, some women do better when they take the SSRI continuously.[19] Tricyclic antidepressants can be used as an alternative, but I do not recommend antianxiety medications such as buspirone or alprazolam, as they are seldom effective.

Changing your diet can help with PMS, too. Soy foods, which are rich in isoflavones, can improve serotonin activity in your brain and can reduce PMS symptoms.[20] Increase your calcium and vitamin D intake. According to recent research published in the *Archives of Internal Medicine,* low calcium intake and vitamin D deficiency contribute to the occurrence of PMS.[21] Women suffering from PMS generally have a much lower calcium intake than women not suffering from PMS. Calcium supplementation has been shown to help PMS symptoms. You also need to take adequate amounts of chromium, copper, and manganese, as blood levels of these minerals have been found to be low in patients suffering from PMS.[22] Nitric oxide is released in high amounts as a result of hormone swings[23] in PMS sufferers and could be contributing to the occurrence of PMS symptoms.

If you suffer from irritable bowel syndrome, you are more likely to experience depression, anger, and cognitive impairment premenstrually.[24] You then need more aggressive treatment, including practicing relaxation and following a strict diet. You also need to stop smoking and engage in a weight management program. Losing weight will improve your PMS symptoms tremendously. Supplementation of 50 to 100 mg of vitamin B_6 in conjunction with 200 mg of magnesium is also quite helpful.[25] These supplements improve the anxiety symptoms related to PMS. I have found that taking a comprehensive mix of antioxidants and ingredients that lower systemic inflammation, such as selenium, glutathione, alpha-lipoic acid, quercetin, and curcumin, helps PMS symptoms tremendously. (For details on useful antioxidants, see Chapter 22.)

Research has demonstrated that chiropractic therapy can be highly effective in reducing PMS symptoms.[26] Acupuncture, which works on the serotoninergic and opioid neurotransmitter systems, has been shown to significantly improve symptoms in 77.8 percent of patients, compared to 5.9 percent of women treated with placebo.[27] Other medications can be of some benefit, too. Spironolactone, a potassium-sparing diuretic, helps some patients, but the benefits are less than those obtained with an SSRI. In some severe cases, growth hormone treatment has been shown to significantly improve PMS. Cognitive behavior relaxation therapy, aerobic exercise, and L-tryptophan may also be of use.

The Thyroid and Perimenopause

Endocrinologists have noticed that the occurrence of hypothyroidism can be a more significant stress in the perimenopausal period (the roughly five to ten years leading up to the onset of menopause) than when it occurs at other times. Also, the symptoms of hypothyroidism may intensify as a result of hormonal shifts that precede menopause. As estrogen levels decline prior to menopause, lower serotoninergic activity in the brain caused by lower estrogen will make you more sensitive to the effect of low thyroid on mood and emotions. A long-standing, untreated thyroid condition during the perimenopausal period can cause more depression, irritability, and anger and may trigger personal problems and more menopausal symptoms.

Symptoms of menopause and hypothyroidism are astonishingly similar, leading many patients suffering from mild hypothyroidism to be dismissed as perimenopausal. If a woman is in the perimenopausal or postmenopausal period, the first thing that tends to come to a gynecologist's mind is that symptoms of mood swings or fatigue are due to a hormonal imbalance. A woman may even suggest this possibility to the physician. Should these symptoms persist despite adequate hormone replacement therapy, only an astute and thorough gynecologist might eventually test the thyroid as a possible reason for the symptoms.

The Thyroid's Effects on Menopause

For most women, menopause is a physiological reality. It is not only a marker for the end of the reproductive years but also a critical period during which hormonal and sociocultural influences reshape how a woman perceives herself. Wide fluctuations of hormone levels affect your neurotransmitters and may make you more susceptible to depression and anxiety. Vasomotor instability may make you experience hot flashes and night sweats. Your sleep may become disturbed, and your sexuality may change. You are at a higher risk for bone loss, impaired cognition, and cardiovascular disease. Your metabolism slows down, and you may begin to gain weight.

Through this transition, you will also have a higher risk of developing a thyroid imbalance. Because of the hormonal changes and for other poorly understood reasons, women become more vulnerable to immune attacks on the thyroid when they become menopausal. The frequency of low-grade hypothyroidism increases sharply at menopause, with at least one in eight women becoming afflicted with hypothyroidism.[28]

A thyroid imbalance often makes symptoms of menopause worse, as its effects may prevent women from being able to cope with the broad range of physical and emotional stresses that occur with this transition. Thyroid disease during menopause may have a significant effect on how a woman perceives her menopausal symptoms and even on the nature of those symptoms. Even low-grade hypothyroidism can ignite hot flashes, sleep problems, depression, and worsening anxiety.

Nora, a forty-nine-year-old woman, described to me the mix of symptoms that she experienced when she became menopausal a year earlier:

My periods started being further and further apart, and coinciding with an increase in symptoms of fatigue. Not fatigue like, "Oh, I just can't do anything today," but sleepiness and tiredness that just had to be addressed. I would sometimes wake up in the morning, have my cup of coffee, do whatever, and not have the energy to get dressed. I would lie back down for another hour. Maybe around noon I would finally feel refreshed. It really took a long time to get recuperated, I guess. I would go to the mall for two hours and come home and crash!

My hot flashes have been a subject matter for jokes. I think I had hot flashes for about six months. They were increasing in intensity, and I realized it wasn't a joke. I would want to cry when I felt them coming on, because I knew that for up to the next 20 minutes or so, I would not be able to think about anything but cooling off. I was carrying the fan around, people were laughing at me, and I would laugh back. This was on top of the lethargy and the three-hour naps, sometimes two times a day! If it hadn't been for the menopause, things hadn't been accentuated enough for me to take action and have my thyroid evaluated.

I was never depressed, as far as I knew. But then when the menopause hit, I felt like I was becoming seriously depressed. That bothered me, and it concerned me, and I wondered if it would ever change.

For Nora, hormone replacement therapy helped only a little. Through the transition her thyroid gland became underactive and caused her to have an escalation of symptoms. Only after addressing and treating both components did she feel normal again. She said, "I just felt more well-rounded, more balanced, more optimistic." Her fatigue, depression, and hot flashes all went away.

Today, many women live one-third of their lives or more after menopause. Despite the recognition of the need for comprehensive care for women and of the importance of preventive medicine and education to ensure women's good health, healthcare delivery systems have not emphasized the importance of early detection and adequate treatment of thyroid imbalances. Education about thyroid disease should be a part of a woman's health program.

Thyroid Patients in the Hormonal Transition

If you have suffered from a thyroid imbalance during the reproductive years, you are more likely to experience menopausal symptoms such as headaches, depression, and constipation when you reach the transition and afterward.[29] Even if your thyroid levels have been stable with treatment prior to menopause, the activity of the immune system can change during the transition, destabilizing your thyroid levels and making your menopausal symptoms worse.

The physical and emotional symptoms of menopause have been widely assumed to be due to a decline in estrogen levels. For most women, however, hormonal changes probably do not account for all the changes in well-being or the physical symptoms of menopause. If they did, all women would experience menopausal symptoms when they reach the transition. In fact, only 50 to 60 percent of women suffer from hot flashes. Not all women become depressed or emotionally unstable. What does seem to have a great effect on the occurrence of menopausal symptoms is the amount of stress experienced prior to menopause. Studies done in Japan and the United States have shown that the expression of the symptoms of menopause and the frequency of these symptoms differ significantly between Japanese and American women.[30] For instance, approximately 38 percent of American women experienced a lack of energy, compared to only 6 percent of Japanese women. Some 30 percent of American women experienced irritability, whereas this symptom was reported by only 12 percent of Japanese women. Many other symptoms of menopause, such as depression and trouble sleeping, were on average three times more common in American women than in Japanese women. American women also complained of more hot flashes and night sweats than their Japanese counterparts. The differences are so striking that they can be explained only by sociocultural factors.

One study found that stress from bereavement, divorce, or friends moving away is closely associated with the psychological and physical symptoms of menopause.[31] Other factors, such as low educational and socioeconomic status, are also associated with more symptoms of depression than are generally found among middle-class women. Women with lower monthly incomes were shown to have a higher incidence of nervous complaints at menopause.[32]

People with a tendency toward mood swings can feel helpless to anticipate and cope with major life changes. Consequently, if your thyroid condition has made you more prone to becoming depressed, you may feel unable to control the changes that occur during menopause. You are also likely to perceive those changes in a more negative way. The depression worsens, and the stress is perceived as overwhelming. Women who are more affected by menopausal symptoms are likely to be those who are under high levels of stress and/or who have particularly negative beliefs about menopause. Christiane Northrup, a doctor and women's health specialist, pointed out that "expectations of problems in menopause lead to problems."[33]

Immune system reactivity, which is naturally enhanced during the hormonal transition, can provoke or exacerbate some menopausal symptoms, including fatigue, low mood, anxiety, and even hot flashes. The triple impact of hormonal changes, thyroid hormone imbalance, and a rising tide of inflammation chemicals released by a reactive immune system can mean that some women struggle with severe menopausal symptoms. For such women, I treat their thyroid imbalance, address their hormonal imbalance via carefully and individually tailored hormone replacement therapy, and use measures to make the immune system less reactive. To learn more about the measures I recommend to reduce immune system reactivity, consult Chapter 3.

Get the Help You Need Through the Transition

As explained earlier, if you have suffered from a thyroid imbalance and you are perimenopausal or postmenopausal, you are more likely to have escalation of symptoms related to both lack of estrogen and thyroid-related symptoms. Even if your thyroid levels become normal with treatment, you will be more likely to experience hot flashes, night sweats, sleep disturbances, low mood, and irritability. You probably sense that estrogens could improve many of the symptoms but wonder whether hormone replacement therapy (HRT) is the right choice for you. Research has shown that HRT may increase your risk for breast cancer and may be associated with cardiovascular disease. This research, however, has been criticized and its conclusions questioned. You need to be well informed concerning benefits and potential adverse effects prior to making the decision about taking estrogen therapy.

The Women's Health Initiative (WHI) study, published in July 2002, reported that there was a decreased risk of colorectal cancer and osteoporotic hip fractures in women receiving estrogen in combination with progesterone (0.625 mg conjugated equine estrogens and 2.5 mgs medroxyprogesterone). However, there was an increased risk of breast cancer, coronary heart disease, stroke, and blood clots in the veins. According to this study and other research, heart attacks and other vascular problems tend to occur within the first year of treatment.[34]

The fact of the matter is that the potential health problems seen in some of the women receiving conjugated equine estrogens/medroxyprogesterone combination treatment may not occur in women receiving other dosages of hormones or other forms or types of hormone replacement. For instance, it is possible that transdermal forms of hormone treatment and other ways of taking estrogens are quite safe and do not promote the same side effects reported in the WHI study. It is also possible that the use of low-dose hormone treatment helps without causing major health issues. Despite this, a significant amount of fear has been generated in the public and the medical community, making it difficult for physicians to provide women with the best advice concerning the use of hormones.

A serious problem with the WHI study is that the women studied ranged from fifty to seventy-nine years of age, and many of them were predisposed to having coronary artery disease and cerebrovascular disease to start with. The women who experienced cardiovascular problems were older women who were already at high risk for having these health issues. It is also possible that the culprit in the occurrence of adverse health effects is progesterone. When taken continuously, it may eliminate the benefits of estrogen on the heart and the brain. In fact, women treated with estrogen only in the WHI study have not suffered from a higher occurrence of cardiovascular disease. In contrast to the WHI study, extensive research has shown that estrogens protect against cardiovascular disease. Prior to menopause, women are less likely to have heart attacks than men simply because estrogens have a cardio-protective effect.[35]

If you start estrogen treatment early, you may lower your cardiovascular risk.[36] After menopause, women are more likely to have higher cholesterol levels, high blood pressure, and hardening of the arteries as a result of low estrogens. Estrogens, alone or in combination with progesterone, lower your bad cholesterol (LDL) and increase your good cholesterol (HDL).[37] Because the risk of experiencing cardiovascular problems after starting HRT proba-bly applies only to women who have a high risk to start with, before begin-ning hormonal treatment you need to assess your risk factors, have a good cardiac evaluation, and begin lifestyle changes involving diet, weight loss, regular exercise, smoking cessation, and adequate control of high blood pres-sure, diabetes, and cholesterol problems.[38]

As noted, the dose and type of hormone and the delivery system may also have an effect on your risk of cardiovascular problems. At present we have little information concerning any real risk of using the transdermal patch or gel delivery system for HRT. You should use the lowest dose of estrogen that relieves your symptoms, as low-dose estrogen replacement may turn out to be safe and can provide you with what you need to prevent bone loss and cure your symptoms. Also, if you need progesterone treatment, you should take the lowest dose and, if needed, take it in a cyclic way. You may also use hor-mone treatment for only a limited period of time.

If you are being treated with thyroid hormone for an underactive thy-roid, transdermal estrogen is also preferred because it does not affect the dose of thyroid hormone you need. In contrast, oral estrogen will make your requirement for thyroid hormone higher. Approximately 5 percent of all postmenopausal women receive estrogens in conjunction with thyroid hor-mone.

The overinflated and distorted negative information provided by the media after the release of the results of the Women's Health Initiative made nearly two out of three women receiving HRT stop the therapy. However, half of those women restarted the treatment months later.[39] Instead of stopping HRT because of fear of heart disease and then ending up restarting the treatment, it may be wiser to switch to a lower dose.

Another issue related to HRT is the risk of developing breast cancer. Your risk of breast cancer starts going up significantly after five years of treatment, but it may not go up at all if you are not taking progesterone. If a risk exists, it could be related to the dose and the duration of use.[40] Five years after stopping hormonal replacement therapy, the risk of breast cancer will be the same as for women who never used HRT.[41] You may wonder whether having a thyroid condition increases your risk of breast cancer. Research conducted in the Netherlands showed that there was no direct relationship between breast cancer and blood markers for autoimmune thyroid disease; however, postmenopausal women who suffer from hypothyroidism seem to be at a slightly increased risk for breast cancer.[42] Even if a link exists between autoimmune thyroid disease and breast cancer, it is very minimal, and should not affect your decision concerning hormonal therapy.

You need to have a mammogram before you start HRT. If you do not have risk factors for breast cancer, you should repeat the mammogram every two years. When there is increased breast density as a result of estrogen treatment, ultrasound will be useful simply because mammography becomes less reliable as a screening method for breast cancer.

If you have had a hysterectomy and want to take estrogen, it should be taken alone, without progesterone. If you have an intact uterus, however, taking estrogen alone can increase your risk of uterine cancer. The reason is that estrogen causes a thickening and proliferation of the internal lining of the uterus (endometrium), which over time can cause a predisposition to cancer. It is prevented by taking progesterone, preferably in a cyclic fashion, which causes shedding of the buildup.

The drawback of progesterone treatment is its interference with your brain chemistry.[43] Progesterone lowers serotonin in the brain, resulting in more symptoms of depression. Women taking estrogens and progesterone may have more symptoms of depression than women taking estrogens alone. Also, the higher the dose of progesterone, the greater the likelihood that a woman will experience depressed mood. On the other hand, progesterone may help relieve hot flashes. There are different progesterone medications. The effect on mood and anxiety symptoms differ from one preparation to the next.[44] The type of progesterone that you should take will depend on your symptoms, and on how you react to the medication.

If you have mild depressive symptoms, often HRT is enough to treat the depression. Estradiol (as a patch or in gel form) and vaginal progesterone are the best combination because vaginal progesterone is less likely to enhance depressive symptoms or to counteract the benefits of estrogens on depressive mood.

The hormone regimen I recommend to my thyroid patients depends on the severity of their hot flashes, whether low mood is a problem, and whether they become emotional, anxious, and fatigued when they take progesterone. A particular hormone regimen may work for one patient but not for another. However, I tend to recommend a low-dose regimen with a cyclic progesterone treatment for women who need it. Generally speaking, the estrogen replacement that I prescribe most often is pure estradiol in gel form, such as Divigel, Elestrin, and Estrogel, applied daily. These preparations tend to provide the most even blood levels of the hormones.

Taking hormones in a low dose in a cyclic fashion does reduce hot flashes, night sweats, and other menopausal symptoms. It also improves the elasticity of the skin, reduces wrinkling, and makes the skin less dry. Research has shown that estrogen replacement slows skin aging.[45]

HRT improves disruption of sleep in menopausal women. A combination of low-dose estrogen and 100–200 mgs of progesterone at night seems to provide a greater benefit to women who have sleep disturbances than the more conventional combination of equine estrogens and medroxyprogesterone.

A new medication called Angeliq, which combines low-dose estrogen (estradiol 1 mg) and drospirenone (2 mgs), a new progestin that is less likely to cause blood clots, seems to be a promising new form of HRT with fewer adverse effects.[46] The new progestin contained in this medication also causes less water retention than other synthetic forms of progesterone.

One reason why menopausal women note a decrease in lean body mass and an increase in fat is the drop in hormone levels. Estrogen treatment in early menopause can help minimize these body changes. Some women think estrogen treatment will make them gain weight, but research has not confirmed that estrogen/progesterone treatment causes weight gain. In fact, if you take estrogens in addition to low-dose testosterone, you will increase your lean body mass and reduce fat in all parts of your body.[47] Your sexuality and quality of life will also improve more than if you take estrogens only.

As you age, dehydroepiandrosterone (DHEA) levels become lower. Low DHEA promotes aging of the body and many age-related disorders that come with it. One study showed that taking 25 mgs a day of DHEA will reduce age-related decline of the endocrine system and improve physiological functions.[48] Animal research has also shown that DHEA reduces fat accumulation in certain parts of the body and enhances insulin efficiency. The benefits are similar to the benefits of estrogens. However, I discourage you from taking DHEA in pill form, as when it's taken orally it goes straight to the liver, and the long-term safety of taking DHEA this way is not known. Rather, I recommend that you take DHEA in smaller doses and in a sublingual compounded form. This will give you more stable levels of DHEA and greater benefits without any risk.

"Natural" or bioidentical hormone therapy refers to hormone treatment with individually compounded recipes of some steroids in various dosage forms. These include DHEA (dehydroepiandrosterone), pregnenolone, testosterone, progesterone, estrone, estradiol, and estriol. Bioidentical hormones have become increasingly popular and are thought to be more effective than the pharmaceutical forms of HRT. Although very little research has compared the two, the use of bioidentical hormones can provide you with a greater flexibility with respect to the dose and type you need. It also gives you the same hormones that your body normally produces and in the amounts that your body needs.

If you suffer from disturbing hot flashes and your choice is not to take hormones or hormone treatment has not been effective, you may want to use an SSRI or SNRI (serotonin-norepinephrine reuptake inhibitor). Research has shown that these antidepressants have a beneficial effect on hot flashes.[49] Another option is to increase your intake of phytoestrogens. Phytoestrogens are polyphenol compounds of plant origin that have a similar molecular structure to 17 beta-estradiol. Soy isoflavone extracts can help relieve hot flashes, but they are not as effective as estrogens or antidepressants.[50] I encourage you to take omega-3 fatty acids for your menopausal symptoms, whether you have elected to receive HRT or not.

After the release of the Women's Health Initiative results, numerous dietary supplements have been proposed for women in menopause. Research has shown that extract of black cohosh (*Cimicifuga racemosa L.*) improves menopause-related symptoms; however, it can cause liver damage.[51] Your doctor may recommend dong quai (*Angelica sinensis*), ginseng, garlic, *Rhodiola rosea*, or evening primrose oil. However, there has been little research done on these herbs, and it is possible that some of them will increase your risk of breast cancer. The semipurified isoflavone red clover leaf extract provides little benefit. Another alternative is Femal, which is an herbal compound made from pollen extracts. It may improve your hot flashes and other symptoms of menopause.[52]

Tibolone is another option to treat hot flashes and vaginal dryness. Tibolone regulates estrogen effects. It also improves your libido and your energy. Tibolone, however, does not affect breast tissue. Selective estrogen receptor modulators (SERMs), such as raloxifene, will also help with menopausal issues. The over-the-counter supplement 5-hydroxytryptophan can also help your hot flashes and other menopausal symptoms.[53]

For menopausal women and women about to become menopausal, relaxation techniques, adequate correction of the thyroid imbalance, and lifestyle modification are crucial to prevent or treat the lingering effects of thyroid imbalance (see Chapter 18). Sex hormones, thyroid hormones, and stress influence mind and body. How these effects manifest in terms of mood or physical discomfort varies from woman to woman, and how a physician diagnoses his or her patient's suffering depends on the physician and what appears to be the source of the most prominent symptoms. One physician may blame hormones, another may cite stress, and a third may implicate depression or anxiety. Regardless of the type and severity of symptoms, I recommend that you embrace my thyroid mind-body program detailed in Chapter 22.

Important Points to Remember

- If you are a new PMS sufferer, an underactive or overactive thyroid may be the cause of your symptoms.
- If you have suffered from PMS but your symptoms have recently worsened and your menstrual periods have changed, have your doctor consider a thyroid condition.
- PMS is essentially a brain chemistry disorder, and changes in hormones that regulate your brain chemistry appear to be important contributing factors. Keep in mind that thyroid hormone is a major player in brain chemistry.
- If you have experienced a severe thyroid imbalance in your reproductive years, you are likely to experience unpleasant times at menopause. Adequate thyroid treatment and embracing my mind-body program may be the solution.
- Menopause is a vulnerable time for women. The frequency of Hashimoto's thyroiditis and hypothyroidism increases sharply during this period.
- The symptoms of menopause and thyroid imbalance are quite similar. If you begin to experience depression, fatigue, and mood swings, do not necessarily attribute your symptoms to menopause. Have your doctor test your thyroid.
- Thyroid imbalance worsens symptoms of menopause and vice versa. Unless all the effects of menopause and thyroid imbalance are addressed, your symptoms may continue and escalate over time.

15

THYROID BALANCE FOR
HEALTHY PREGNANCY

Even before the era of sophisticated, precise thyroid testing, doctors were aware of the effects of thyroid imbalance on reproduction. At the turn of the twentieth century, physicians administered thyroid hormone to women to improve their fertility and treat menopause. Today's doctors recognize that adequate thyroid hormone levels are essential to help regulate the production of sex hormones (that is, estrogen and progesterone) and the hormonal cycle responsible for ovulation. Both an excess of thyroid hormone and, more commonly, a deficiency of the hormone alter the harmonious functioning of the reproductive system and sometimes prevent ovulation. Even if ovulation and conception occur, a thyroid imbalance can lead to a deficit in progesterone, which can render the uterus unsuitable for implantation of an embryo. This, in turn, prevents a normal pregnancy.

A number of important advances have occurred in the past several years in the field of infertility medicine. Less publicized have been the findings that link thyroid hormone imbalance with impaired reproduction, infertility, and miscarriage.

Both an underactive thyroid and an overactive thyroid can cause infertility problems and affect the outcome of a pregnancy. Nevertheless, because hypothyroidism is much more common than hyperthyroidism, thyroid-related infertility and miscarriage problems are more frequently caused by an underactive thyroid. For this reason, this chapter focuses on hypothyroidism as a cause of these difficulties.

Infertility is a common condition. Doctors estimate that one of every six couples of childbearing age has a problem with fertility.[1] With modern infertility protocols, which are frequently expensive and time-consuming, approximately two-thirds of all couples can be treated and successfully conceive.

Infertility can be considered a type of chronic illness. The afflicted person lives with a constant but shaky hope that "it" will go away or be cured. An inability to conceive can generate a profound feeling of failure, which can lead to a state that psychologist Erik Erikson described as "stagnation and personal impoverishment."[2] Many infertile couples become obsessed with their childlessness and feel inferior when they see other people with babies. The countless doctor appointments, the expenses, the effects on employment, and the monthly hopes and expectations may eventually overburden the couple and cause them to feel they have no control over their lives, leading to depression and marital problems.

Quite frequently, women being treated for a thyroid imbalance enter infertility programs with no idea that their thyroid condition could be preventing conception and a normal pregnancy. Even more alarming, a significant number of reproductive endocrinologists and gynecologists who treat infertile couples are unaware that a minimal thyroid imbalance can cause infertility. Nor do many of these doctors realize the importance of detecting subtle thyroid abnormalities.

Although we don't know how frequently minimal hypothyroidism contributes to infertility, recent research has clearly demonstrated that it is an important contributing factor. One study showed that approximately 25 percent of women referred to one infertility clinic had low-grade hypothyroidism.[3]

When a couple seeks help for infertility, a female-related issue is identified 45 percent of the time. The most common identifiable female-related issues are ovarian dysfunction, tubal disease, and endometriosis. One study showed that even when the woman has an identifiable cause of infertility, she is more likely to have an autoimmune thyroid condition and thyroid dysfunction as well than a woman not having an infertility issue—antithyroid antibodies were elevated in 18 percent of infertile women, compared to 8 percent for healthy women.[4] The female issue that is more frequently associated with autoimmune thyroid disease and thyroid imbalance is endometriosis. As you can see, the thyroid can be an additional contributing reason for infertility, even if there are other issues that could explain your infertility problem.

If you're experiencing problems with fertility, discuss with your gynecologist the possibility of a thyroid imbalance before you spend two years engaging in an infertility protocol. Ask to have your thyroid tested. Often an imbalance will show up only if you have a TRH (thyrotropin-releasing hormone) stimulation test.[5] Among patients found to have low-grade hypothyroidism, the infertility may be reversed with thyroid hormone treatment.

Because thyroid testing is not routinely done when patients enter fertility clinics, many women with minimal hypothyroidism struggle for a long time attempting to conceive. Maria, age thirty-three, had gone through infertility protocols for almost two years. She was outraged when she learned that she had had symptoms of hypothyroidism for some time but that her gynecologist had not checked her thyroid at the outset of her treatment. She told me, "I had a hard time getting my weight off, and there were some other telltale thyroid signs that I think a doctor who was knowledgeable in this area should have been able to see." Maria became pregnant two months after beginning thyroid hormone treatment.

I have cared for several women with minimal hypothyroidism whose infertility problems were reversed within two to three months after they began thyroid hormone treatment. Prior to the thyroid problem's being identified, all of them had suffered significant emotional and financial burdens as well as altered relationships with their spouses. Many of these women actually wondered whether their marriages could survive. Although infertility usually affects both partners, the person suffering from infertility usually has greater feelings of guilt, inadequacy, failure, and low self-esteem. Infertility issues are more common in women than men. Also, given our culture's tendency to blame women, infertile women often take on even more guilt and suffering than men, and their feelings of inadequacy may be magnified.

The Burden of Stress and Anxiety

Quite frequently, when a woman is infertile, her husband makes her feel it is her responsibility to become pregnant. One patient described her situation as follows:

> My husband told me it was my "job" to get pregnant. I remember the therapist telling me, "I think part of the reason you feel so bad every month when you're not pregnant is because your husband has told you that it is your job, so you're failing at your job."
>
> My husband thought of it as my sole goal. My measure of self-worth became whether the pregnancy test came back positive or negative. So every time the test came back negative, I felt like a complete and total failure. This made me even more depressed. Because I had to suffer in silence, it made it harder to deal with all these emotions. I was filled with sadness.

Generally speaking, infertile couples feel so bad, sad, or ashamed of their problem that they do not tell other people about it. Cut off from friendly support, the infertile person or couple often feels isolated and struggles even more with the emotional upheaval brought on by this problem. It is very important for women to reach out for support during this time. RESOLVE, a national support group for women with infertility issues, has chapters that meet regularly in all major cities around the country. RESOLVE members help each other with medical information and emotional support.

The effects of infertility on a woman suffering from a thyroid dysfunction become exaggerated when she is unaware of the thyroid imbalance. The multiple effects of the thyroid imbalance on the woman's emotions may render the suffering quite unbearable and exacerbate the conflicts between spouses. Typically, if she were not hypothyroid, the woman could hide her sadness from friends or relatives, because it would be related to her infertility. When she is hypothyroid, even minimally, the effects of thyroid imbalance may make her depression worse and leave her unable to cope with the stress of infertility. Take steps to prevent this escalation. If you are becoming increasingly depressed over your infertility problem, get a thyroid-stimulating hormone (TSH) test.

The anxiety that occurs during the months when a woman is taking fertility drugs typically intensifies any anxiety caused by thyroid problems. She worries about whether she will become pregnant this month and how this will change her life. Due to the incredible anxiety she faces, the disappointment of a negative pregnancy test result may be magnified. As a consequence, some women experience worsening PMS and increased anger, mood swings, irritability, and arguing with their husbands.

A hypothyroid woman who is obligated to have intercourse even on days when she may have an aversion to sex often feels even more guilty and inadequate. Roselyn, a thirty-three-year-old secretary, has been married for five years. She tried to conceive for three years and went through infertility protocols with no success. The cause of the infertility was, however, a low-grade hypothyroidism that was uncovered only when they had almost given up the idea of having a baby. Roselyn said:

I could not believe how much stress I felt from trying to get pregnant. Month after month, we spent thousands and thousands of dollars. I had to make the two-hour round-trip to my doctor's office ten to twelve days a month. There was no apparent reason that the fertility protocols I tried were not working for me. It was totally unbelievable. What made it even worse for me was that I didn't feel like I got a lot of support from other people. When I would tell someone we were trying, they would just say, "Oh, all you have to do is relax. My best friend and her husband went on a second honeymoon, and she got pregnant!" I knew that in my case relaxation had nothing to do with whether I got pregnant. Finally, I just stopped talking about it even to my closest friends.

My infertility affected every aspect of my life. My husband is extremely introverted, and he doesn't discuss things with people besides me. So that made it much harder. My PMS has gotten worse, and I often find myself crying and sad. I was experiencing a lot of anxiety and couldn't sleep at night.

When the time of the month came when we had to have sex, I almost dreaded it. I was starting to resent even being touched by my husband. Important aspects of sexuality, like intimacy and spontaneity, are lost when you're going through infertility because the doctors tell you when to have sex, how to do it, who is supposed to do what, where to do it, and for how long. That's not the way it is supposed to be. For me, it just led to a lot more stress.

I couldn't understand what was happening. Nothing made any sense! The fighting and arguing between my husband and me kept escalating over the months. We started going to a therapist, sometimes five or even seven days a week.

I got hysterical. I ranted and raved. The monthly disappointment of not getting pregnant was just unbelievable. I would wait and wait and think, well I'm going to be pregnant. No, yes, maybe . . . and then, sure enough, I wasn't pregnant. It was totally devastating.

Everything I did had to be planned around when I needed to be at the doctor and when I needed to do this and that. There were many times that I really felt like just giving up. I think my husband got to that point, too.

I kept asking myself, "Is this even worth it?" Without even taking into consideration my time and other inconveniences, I bet we spent over $50,000. That was money out of our pockets.

Because of the repeated failures, Roselyn became quite depressed. As she described it, "I finally quit my job and stayed home. I didn't cook; I didn't do anything. I just sat around the house all day."

Many women like Roselyn become obsessed with their condition and undertake their own determined search for the cause of their infertility. Roselyn eventually became inspired to go to the library and do her own research. She says:

I looked at every infertility book. One book mentioned the thyroid. In this case, my doctor resisted, telling me it would cost $150 to run that test. I said to myself, "I'm already spending $500 every time I come in here, so what's another $150?" He agreed to run the test, and to his surprise, it showed I was hypothyroid. At the time, I was angry that this test had not been performed $50,000 and a year earlier.

When I began taking thyroid hormone, there was an improvement in how I was feeling—the cold, the dryness, the hair. I was a little aggravated that it took a couple of months. I thought you could just start me on thyroid hormone on Monday and I could be pregnant on Tuesday. It didn't work that way. Even so, it was the first step in getting me out of what was the worst situation I have ever been in in my entire life.

I also wonder whether anyone would ever have figured out that I had a thyroid problem had I not pursued the fertility research. I even had fertility-related surgeries before I was diagnosed as hypothyroid. Now I think all that was unnecessary.

To avoid the needless suffering that Roselyn went through, ask your reproductive endocrinologist if thyroid testing is part of the infertility workup. If not, have your doctor request the test.

When Inadequate Hormone Treatment Leads to Infertility

If you have already been diagnosed with an underactive thyroid and are being treated for it, your infertility may be caused by an under- or overcorrected thyroid imbalance. If you are taking thyroid hormone to treat hypothyroidism, make sure that your treatment is adequate before trying to become pregnant. Insufficient dosage can also cause infertility.

One evening I was giving a talk on the health effects of mild hypothyroidism to a patient support group made up of laypeople. As I was pointing to a slide illustrating that minimal thyroid hormone deficiency could be responsible for both infertility and miscarriages, I noticed the face of a young lady sitting in the back. She noticeably brightened up, and her expression changed from frustration to what appeared to be relief and hope. Following the lecture, she asked me a few questions about how a small deficit in thyroid hormone could affect ovulation and then indicated that she had a thyroid condition and would make an appointment to come and see me. She stated that she had been frustrated and that her stress levels had become high as a result of being unable to conceive. One week later, Felicia was in my office. She told me:

> I was diagnosed hypothyroid at the age of nineteen. I was then placed on thyroid hormone by my physician. My thyroid has been at the same level for probably the last eight years. I had been going to an internist who once a year had been running TSH tests, and it had been staying pretty stable. He would maybe adjust the dosage once in a while, but it was never anything drastic. I got married four years ago, and we were ready to have children. Initially, we had the attitude that if it happens, it happens. We weren't really on a schedule at any point. It was maybe a year and a half after we were married that we started to concentrate on it, and nothing happened. I had been seeing a gynecologist who happened to be an infertility specialist.
>
> I have been going through cycles of drugs to induce a pregnancy, and we have not been successful. I was wondering if my thyroid had anything to do with it.

I asked Felicia whether she had other symptoms. "I did notice that I started to get bad night sweats, and I was suffering from hair loss and very dry and scaly skin. I mean, you could run a brush across it and it would flake off, especially on my legs," she said.

Her marital relationship was affected significantly. Her husband constantly blamed her and made her feel as if something was wrong with her. She explained:

> It made me feel less of a woman. I began to envy women who don't have to go through all the battles of medications and timing and ovulation testing.

The worst part was the distance that grew between me and my husband. Sex became a chore after a while because you are concentrating on it so much that it isn't spontaneous and fun anymore. Then you come to the end of the month and you're still not pregnant, and you have to face at least another whole month of this routine that is now old and tiring.

In reviewing the records that Felicia had brought, I noticed that her TSH levels in the past two years, while she had been taking 0.15 mg of synthetic L-thyroxine, were 6.0 and 4.5 (normal TSH is 0.4 to 4.5 mIU/L). The fact that her levels were high suggested to me that she was not taking enough thyroid hormone. If that were the case, I thought the resulting mild thyroid hormone deficiency might account for her infertility. I increased her L-thyroxine dose and asked her to wait a few months before resuming the fertility drugs.

Two months later, Felicia got pregnant immediately, without fertility drugs. "We thought there is no way that it could have worked like that because of all these other obstacles that we had encountered in the past. It is amazing that we tried with medications for two years and we were not successful, and with a small increase in the dosage, I became pregnant right away."

When she returned to my office six weeks pregnant, Felicia was both happy and angry. She said, "What upsets me the most is that my internist knew I was struggling with infertility. I do feel like we wasted a lot of time and money because no one considered that the thyroid was a problem."

Any woman who has an infertility problem should have her thyroid checked. This simple test may help prevent much of the struggle, mental stress, and financial burden associated with infertility. Even a minute thyroid imbalance can result in correctable infertility. By the same token, any woman who is currently being treated for a thyroid imbalance or has previously been treated for such a condition should be thoroughly tested before attempting to conceive.

When a Miscarriage Intervenes

As difficult as infertility is, its hardships can pale compared to the trauma of a miscarriage. Many women, especially those who have had repeated miscarriages, experience tremendous stress and may also suffer from low self-esteem, depression, and marital conflicts.

Although recurrent miscarriages can be due to genetic problems or to a wide range of medical conditions, a high rate of recurrent miscarriages has also been demonstrated among women with thyroid disease. The relationship between pregnancy and thyroid problems has been known for some time. Three to four decades ago, gynecologists treated women who had multiple miscarriages with thyroid hormone, which was noted to prevent further pregnancy loss in a significant number of women. Research has shown that minimal thyroid imbalance can cause recurrent miscarriages and an inability to carry a normal pregnancy.[6] Even Hashimoto's thyroiditis not severe enough to make the thyroid gland underactive may be associated with miscarriages.[7]

Emily was happily married and, at the age of thirty-five, had her first child. Two years later, she decided to have a second child and stopped taking birth control pills for five months. Soon afterward, she says,

> I started gaining weight like a bear preparing for winter. The only difference was that I was barely eating and I was exercising daily. The weight problem started taking over my life. I was severely tired and depressed all the time, and all I wanted to do was sleep. When I decided to seek help, I went to a weight-loss clinic.
>
> The physician informed me that I had a goiter and suggested that I see my personal physician before beginning the weight-loss program. When my doctor informed me that I was pregnant, I thought the weight gain and the excessive lethargy were due to the pregnancy. The pregnancy made me excited, and I even ignored the thyroid problem.

Emily was already thinking about a name for the baby, but at the end of the first trimester, she had a miscarriage. She did not understand how this could have happened and felt that she had failed her husband and family.

While Emily was telling me her story, I was somewhat amazed that her physician had found a goiter but did not test her thyroid function. In retrospect, it was clear that she had many symptoms of hypothyroidism. The miscarriage was probably related to hypothyroidism because, two months later, tests were performed and showed that her thyroid was indeed underactive.

Emily's thyroid imbalance was diagnosed early on, and she had only one miscarriage. Months later, her thyroid hormone levels returned to normal with treatment, and she had no difficulty carrying a pregnancy to term. Any woman who has had several miscarriages should be tested for a thyroid problem. Even mild thyroid imbalance never suspected by physicians can cause a pregnancy to fail.

Beyond Infertility and Miscarriage:
How Thyroid Imbalance Can Affect Your Pregnancy

In addition to potentially impairing your ability to conceive and promoting miscarriages, thyroid hormone imbalance can cause a wide range of adverse consequences for your health and your baby's health.

Throughout pregnancy, thyroid hormone is essential for fetal growth and development. In the early stages of pregnancy, the mother's thyroid begins to produce more thyroid hormone to provide for both herself and the fetus, causing the gland to swell by about 20 percent in size. The baby is dependent on free T3 and free T4 from the mother's bloodstream until sometime during the second trimester, when the baby's thyroid becomes somewhat self-sufficient. Toward the end of pregnancy the baby's thyroid becomes crucial for its continued growth and development.

During the period in which the growing fetus receives all of its thyroid hormone from the mother, too much or too little in the mother's bloodstream can impact how the baby grows. Both hypothyroidism and hyperthyroidism during pregnancy have been associated with smaller babies and low birth weight. Hypothyroidism in the mother, even if it's low-grade, can result in neuropsychological deficits in the baby,[8] including decreased intelligence and poor motor skills,[9] and may even lead to fetal death. Research has shown that one out of four women with a TSH level higher than 4 mIU/L will miscarry between 7 and 20 weeks of gestation. It is possible that fetal death related to thyroid disease is linked both to thyroid hormone deficiency and to autoimmunity. And thyroid levels that are lower than normal toward the end of pregnancy give the baby a greater risk of respiratory distress.

Thyroid disease is the most common endocrine disorder in pregnant women. Hyperthyroidism is diagnosed in 0.4 percent of pregnant women and is usually related to Graves' disease. It is estimated that overt hypothyroidism is experienced by roughly 2 to 4 percent of all pregnant women,[10] and that subclinical, low-grade hypothyroidism is present in many more. Whether the hypothyroidism is overt or low-grade, the root cause of the thyroid condition is often Hashimoto's thyroiditis.

Toward the later stages of pregnancy, even slightly low thyroid hormone levels place you at high risk for the dangerous complications of preeclampsia and even eclampsia,[11] especially if the low thyroid levels occur toward the end of pregnancy. In preeclampsia, blood pressure rises, and there is the potential for damage to other organs, especially the kidneys. Symptoms of preeclampsia include swelling of the hands and face, sudden weight gain over a short period of time, headaches, belly pain below the ribs, irritability, and even vision changes. Preeclampsia can be mild, but it can easily progress to severe preeclampsia or even eclampsia, in which potentially life-threatening high blood pressure and seizures may occur.

Consequences of Thyroid Imbalance During Pregnancy

- Increased risk of neuropsychological impairment in newborns
- Increased risk of preterm birth
- Low birth weight

- Increased likelihood of admission to neonatal intensive care unit
- Increased newborn morbidity and mortality
- Pregnancy-induced high blood pressure
- Preeclampsia and eclampsia
- Abruptio (separation of placenta from the uterus)
- Anemia
- Postpartum hemorrhage
- Abnormal fetal head position at delivery (correlates with the severity of thyroid imbalance)

Because thyroid imbalance is common in pregnant women and can cause serious consequences for you and your baby, I recommend that all women with no history of thyroid disease be tested for thyroid imbalance and auto-immunity before conceiving, in order to minimize infertility and miscarriage issues. I also recommend that they get retested at six weeks and then every two to three months throughout pregnancy to detect a thyroid imbalance early and prevent its deleterious effects. If you have a history of thyroid disease or thyroid surgery, a family history of thyroid disease, a goiter, or any autoimmune condition, you need to be even more diligent about being tested before and during pregnancy.

If you have already been diagnosed with hypothyroidism and are taking a thyroid medication prior to becoming pregnant, it is essential to be tested before conception and throughout the pregnancy as well. Note that 50 percent of women treated with thyroid medication require a higher dose as the pregnancy progresses. For this reason, I recommend that you have your thyroid tests performed every six to eight weeks throughout pregnancy and the dose of medication adjusted according to the test results. Routine monitoring of your thyroid tests will make it easy to keep your thyroid hormone levels as well balanced as possible throughout the entire pregnancy.

Authorities in the thyroid field have debated about what optimal TSH levels should be for pregnant women being treated with thyroid medications. Even though there seems to be a consensus that TSH should be maintained at levels below 2 or 2.5, my opinion is that for pregnant women, TSH levels should be kept between 0.6 and 1.5 mIU/L. I have advocated this range for several years, and this has provided the best pregnancy outcome for my patients.

If you test positive for antithyroid antibody just before conception or in the first trimester of pregnancy, you will be at a much higher risk for becoming hypothyroid during pregnancy, even if your thyroid tests are in a satisfactory range. For many women who have normal thyroid tests during early pregnancy, thyroid imbalance shows up during the second or third trimester. When you are pregnant, do not rely on symptoms to alert you to a thyroid imbalance. Many normal pregnancy symptoms are similar to symptoms of thyroid disease. Remember, however, that the most noticeable symptoms of hypothyroidism during pregnancy include weight gain (more than expected for a pregnant woman), fatigue, hair loss, muscle cramps, and insomnia.

The most noticeable symptoms of hyperthyroidism when pregnant include a much faster heart rate than expected during pregnancy, very warm skin, heat intolerance, and excessive sweating. Excess thyroid hormone in your system can also make you experience significant vomiting, preeclampsia, eclampsia, congestive heart failure, or a thyroid crisis such as thyroid storm (see page 94).

In Chapter 2 I explained the importance of several micronutrients in maintaining optimal thyroid health. Pregnant women, whether they have a thyroid disease or not, need to pay even more attention to these essential nutrients to ensure thyroid function stability and perfect thyroid hormone balance that are so important for both you and your baby. If you are a thyroid patient being treated with thyroid medication for low thyroid, these micronutrients are even more critical. If you lack one or more of them, your thyroid levels can deteriorate and become imbalanced, even if you are taking the prescribed dose of thyroid medication. Of all the micronutrients that contribute to your thyroid health, pregnant women need to pay particular attention to iron and iodine.

Many pregnant women are iron deficient or even anemic. Iron deficiency has been shown to affect the thyroid, which in turn can cause neuropsychological problems in the fetus. Low iron levels in expecting mothers may lead to higher TSH and lower thyroid hormone levels.[12] It is therefore very important to have iron levels tested throughout pregnancy. If you have any form of iron deficiency, I recommend that you take iron supplementation at lunch and/or dinner. It is extremely important to make sure that you take any iron supplement at least four to five hours from the time you take your thyroid medication, in order to prevent any interference with the gastrointestinal absorption of the thyroid medication.

By now you know that iodine is one of the most crucial micronutrients required for the gland to manufacture thyroid hormone. In pregnancy, when the demand for thyroid hormone has drastically increased, your thyroid gland will require much more iodine than before. Also remember that as your pregnancy progresses, your baby's thyroid gland is developing and, at some point, will need iodine to be able to function on its own. Because iodine deficiency during pregnancy is not uncommon and has such potentially serious consequences, such as low IQ and neuropsychological deficits in the future baby,[13] I recommend that you select a prenatal multivitamin that includes the right amount of iodine. You also need to make sure that the prenatal vitamin includes all the essential vitamins, minerals, and antioxidants necessary for optimal functioning of the thyroid gland, both yours and your fetus's. The recommended iodine intake during pregnancy is 250 mcg daily, so be sure the prenatal vitamin contains somewhere between 200 and 250 mcg per daily serving. All this being said, beware of excess iodine, as it can cause a deterioration or impairment of thyroid hormone production, which can affect the outcome of your pregnancy and the health of your future child.

Important Points to Remember

- Thyroid imbalance, and low-grade hypothyroidism in particular, may be the overlooked reason for your infertility problems.
- Before you spend two years pursuing an infertility protocol, discuss with your gynecologist the possibility of a thyroid imbalance, and ask to have your thyroid tested thoroughly.
- Infertility can make you depressed because you may feel as if you have failed at your "job" of becoming pregnant. Thyroid imbalance may worsen your depression, leaving you unable to cope with the stress of infertility. If you are becoming increasingly depressed over your infertility problem, consider the possibility of a thyroid imbalance.
- If you find yourself trapped in the dilemma of lacking sex drive and feeling obligated to have sex, consider the possibility of a thyroid imbalance as the culprit for both the low sex drive and the infertility.
- If you are taking thyroid hormone to treat hypothyroidism, make sure that your treatment is adequate before you try to become pregnant. Both insufficient and excessive dosages can cause infertility.
- Thyroid disease is an often-overlooked cause of recurrent miscarriages as well. Have your thyroid checked if you have repeatedly failed to carry pregnancies to term.

16

POSTPARTUM DEPRESSION

The Hormonal Link

Bringing a new baby into the world typically brings happiness, joy, and relief. It also brings increased worries, responsibilities, sleepless nights, and, quite often, tremendous stress. In the period immediately after birth, you may experience temporary tension, anxiety, mood swings, anger, difficulty sleeping, and crying spells. For most women, these emotional changes last for only a few days and then resolve. Some new mothers, however, continue to suffer mild to moderate mood disturbances for several weeks.[1] Others longer-lasting, bona fide postpartum depression.

Over the past two decades, thyroid researchers have shown that various forms of autoimmune thyroid disorders are quite common during the postpartum period.[2] Clearly in a large number of women suffering from postpartum depression, thyroid imbalance is either a trigger of the depression or a contributing factor.

The Hidden Suffering of Postpartum Depression

Postpartum mental disorders have been recognized since antiquity. Descriptions of patterns of mental disorders related to childbirth have been available since a report by the Frenchman Jean-Etienne-Dominique Esquirol in 1838.[3] Nonetheless, postpartum mental disturbances were seldom talked about until recently, and women afflicted with postpartum depression hid their suffering out of shame. Serious interest by the medical community in postpartum conditions and recognition of both the high frequency of such suffering and its effects on the woman, child, and family began in 1982, when an English physician organized a conference on postpartum psychiatric illness.[4] This led to the founding of an international organization to promote advances in knowledge and treatment of postpartum psychiatric illness. Scientific advances in the field of psychiatry, the formation of support groups, and increased public awareness through media coverage have since revealed much of the hidden suffering associated with postpartum depression.

Postpartum depression is quite common in our society. It has been estimated that one of four women experience the postpartum blues,[5] and nearly 20 percent suffer depression in the first three months of the postpartum period.[6] Most women are depressed for a few weeks and then get over it spontaneously, whereas in more severe cases the depression may last up to a year.

In many cases, both the women themselves and their gynecologists attribute the emotional troubles that occur in the postpartum period to just caring for a new baby. Quite often, women struggle through this depressive state without receiving treatment or support from their spouses or families. In fact, most husbands of women going through postpartum depression have trouble coping with the changes in their wives' mood and behavior, which tends to isolate the women further and exacerbate their depression. Therefore, more often than not postpartum depression is undiagnosed, and its symptoms are frequently attributed to the stress that the mother is going through.

If you are suffering from postpartum depression, you are less likely to provide the affection and the care that your infant needs. You are also less likely to continue to breast-feed your infant. Postpartum depression in the mother can make a child more vulnerable to having cognitive impairment and attention deficit hyperactivity disorder. Research has shown that other consequences of maternal postpartum depression for the child may include violent behavior and difficulty controlling anger.[7] The longer the mother's depression, the more likely the child's behavior will suffer negative effects. Another effect of postpartum depression on the infant is impaired growth and diarrhea.[8]

Unfortunately, postpartum depression continues to be dismissed and not taken seriously. Psychiatric help is sought only in extremely severe cases of depression, when a person becomes suicidal, and many women suffering from postpartum depression remain undiagnosed and are not treated properly.

Fluctuations in the levels of bodily hormones have been held accountable to some extent for the occurrence of postpartum psychiatric conditions. Postpartum symptoms are increasingly thought to be tied to the rapid fall of hormone levels (that is, estrogen and progesterone) from the high levels during pregnancy to the low levels of the postpregnancy state.[9]

If hormone shifts were the only trigger, then all women would suffer from postpartum depression, but this is not the case. First, your genes can make you susceptible to postpartum depression; research has suggested that in many instances postpartum depression is familial. Women with a history of depression prior to pregnancy and women who suffer from severe PMS are also more likely to suffer from depression in the postpartum period.[10] If you experience depression, anxiety, or just "the blues" during pregnancy, you are at higher risk for suffering from postpartum depression. Equally important, if you experience a great deal of stress during pregnancy or immediately after delivery, if you have marital relationship issues, if you are not receiving adequate familial or social support, if you are subjected to physical, sexual, or emotional abuse or a significant financial hardship, if your pregnancy was not desired to start with, or if you have had pregnancy-related health issues, you are more vulnerable to having postpartum depression.[11] Women who frequently go to the doctor during pregnancy and those who take frequent sick leaves are also more susceptible to postpartum depression. If you have depressive symptoms in the third trimester of pregnancy or in the early postpartum period, this could be a clue that you will suffer from postpartum depression. What also can make you more vulnerable to postpartum depression is fatigue from caring for the infant and lack of sleep. In fact, if you are very tired and feel exhausted by the end of the second week postpartum, you have a high risk of suffering from postpartum depression, according to research.[12] In addition, if you experienced mild symptoms of elation early on after delivery, this may be another clue that you will suffer from postpartum depression.[13] This may indicate as well that you have a mood disorder of the bipolar type.

Depression is not the only type of mental suffering that can occur in the postpartum period. Women in the postpartum period perceive stress in an exaggerated way and often experience anxiety. According to research, one of three women suffers from a generalized anxiety disorder in the postpartum period, and a third of women who deal with anxiety also have depressive symptoms.[14]

It is obvious that the high vulnerability to mental suffering that many women have in the postpartum period increases the likelihood of postpartum depression if they have a co-occurring postpartum thyroid disease.

How Common Is Postpartum Thyroid Imbalance?

More than a century ago, a committee of the Clinical Society of London noted the role of thyroid imbalance in causing postpartum mental distress.[15] This report pointed out that many patients with an underactive thyroid were severely ill after childbirth. It has since become clear that a thyroid imbalance can cause or exacerbate postpartum depression. In fact, women who suffer postpartum depression have a higher frequency of positive antithyroid antibody, a marker for autoimmune thyroid disease.[16] It has also become obvious that thyroid imbalance tends to occur quite frequently in the postpartum period.

Research has shown that 5 to 12 percent of all women have postpartum autoimmune thyroiditis.[17] One-half to two-thirds of these women experience hyperthyroidism, hypothyroidism, or both in the postpartum period.[18] One study done in Wisconsin on women evaluated at six and twelve weeks postpartum showed that 11.3 percent of them had thyroid disease and 6.7 percent had either hypothyroidism or hyperthyroidism.[19] White women seem more likely to have postpartum autoimmune thyroiditis than African American women (8.8 percent versus 2.5 percent). The high frequency of postpartum thyroid dysfunction has to do with the immune system becoming more active and disturbed in the postpartum period. For instance, research has shown that as many as 45 percent of patients who suffer from Graves' disease during the reproductive years are diagnosed in the postpartum period.[20] Women who have had children have a higher risk for suffering from Graves' disease down the road than women who have never been pregnant. The rebound autoimmunity that occurs in the postpartum period is explained in part by hormonal shifts. Stress and depression can also make the immune system more reactive.

Quite often, however, postpartum thyroid imbalance occurs in women who already have an autoimmune thyroid disease prior to delivery. Research has shown that more than half of women who have thyroid antibodies (an indication of Hashimoto's thyroiditis) during pregnancy experience thyroid dysfunction in the postpartum period.[21] If you have positive thyroid antibodies during pregnancy, your risk of suffering postpartum depression becomes much higher as well.[22] You also are at risk for having postpartum thyroiditis if you consume high amounts of iodine.[23]

The Many Faces of Postpartum Thyroid Imbalance

The onset of a thyroid imbalance may occur as early as one to two months after delivery, and the imbalance may show up in different patterns. The most typical pattern has three distinct phases: a transient or temporary hyperthyroidism lasting two to three months, followed by a period of hypothyroidism, and then spontaneous return of thyroid levels to normal. This pattern occurs in 25–30 percent of women with postpartum thyroiditis. In a significant number of women, the function of the thyroid gland returns to normal by seven to eight months into the postpartum period. In essence, many cases of thyroid imbalances occurring in the postpartum period are temporary. Some women, however, will have a persistent and even permanent imbalance.

The reason for this pattern is related to a rapid autoimmune attack on thyroid cells, similar to the condition of silent thyroiditis (see Chapter 6), which tends to occur in people with Hashimoto's thyroiditis. During the first phase, the destruction of thyroid cells results in the release of thyroid hormone into the bloodstream, causing hyperthyroidism. As the destruction subsides, thyroid hormone levels decrease. This frequently results in hypothyroidism because the cells that were healthy and previously making adequate amounts of thyroid hormone are no longer present to maintain normal thyroid levels. Once the patient becomes hypothyroid, thyroid cells begin to regenerate. It takes a few weeks before the thyroid completes its recovery and thyroid hormone levels return to normal.

Kathy, age twenty-six, had several symptoms of postpartum thyroid dysfunction. She was diagnosed only after her thyroid function was on its way back to normal. Her symptoms were indicative of hyperthyroidism, which lasted for two months, followed by three months of hypothyroidism. But she and her husband, an anesthesiologist in a teaching hospital, had attributed all of her symptoms to the stress associated with having a baby and moving to a different city. Kathy described her symptoms as follows:

> I felt hyperactive after I had my baby. I was running around so much after she was first born to the point that I had uterine bleeding again. I was breast-feeding, but I would run around and try to do all these things.
>
> By the time my daughter was four months old, I'd lost twenty-six pounds. I felt hot, shaky, and sweaty. I remember sitting in the closet and crying and being very upset. I had rapid heartbeats. We thought it was just stress.
>
> Two months later, I felt depressed and all of a sudden tired and exhausted. I regained the lost weight plus another fifteen pounds. My skin was dry. I was so sleepy that when my little girl napped, I would nap, too. I went to see my doctor, and he said my thyroid was big.

What Kathy described was a period of hyperactivity and hypomania caused by hyperthyroidism, followed by a period of depression caused by hypothyroidism.

In general, hyperthyroidism tends to occur earlier than the first two to three months after delivery, whereas hypothyroidism usually occurs at a later point, at around four months after delivery. Hypothyroidism occasionally occurs as late as eight months after delivery of a baby.

In some women, destruction of the thyroid cells and the resulting hyperthyroidism are not severe enough to precipitate a phase of hypothyroidism. In such women, hyperthyroidism is present for several weeks, followed by resumption of normal thyroid function. Many of these women are not diagnosed unless systematically tested.

Another common pattern is just a transient hypothyroidism lasting two to three months. This may be followed either by the recovery of normal thyroid function or by the persistence of hypothyroidism, which requires life-long thyroid hormone treatment. Women who progress into permanent hypothyroidism may have a more severely destructive Hashimoto's thyroiditis than women who recover from this imbalance. Even women who experience transient low-grade hypothyroidism are at a high risk of becoming permanently hypothyroid years down the road. Graves' disease also frequently occurs in the postpartum period. In some women, dormant Graves' disease may flare up in the immediate postpartum period and cause postpartum Graves' disease. The risk of having Graves' disease in the postpartum period is greater in women older than thirty-five.

If you have experienced postpartum thyroid dysfunction once, you are at a higher risk for experiencing the same thing after future pregnancies as well. Also, many women who develop postpartum thyroid dysfunction will have some type of thyroid abnormality later. For instance, one study showed that 23 percent of women who experienced postpartum thyroid dysfunction were found to be hypothyroid twenty-four to forty-eight months later.[24] The striking finding was that half the women who experienced just hypothyroidism, as opposed to hyperthyroidism followed by hypothyroidism, in the postpartum period continued to suffer from an underactive thyroid. The older a woman is when she has the postpartum thyroid dysfunction, the greater the risk of having permanent hypothyroidism later. Also, for reasons that are unclear, women who have had multiple pregnancies and previous miscarriages are at a higher risk for having permanent hypothyroidism.

Effects of Postpartum Thyroid Imbalance on Mind and Mood

In the postpartum period, a thyroid imbalance is likely to induce, aggravate, and even perpetuate mental suffering, simply because the woman is already in a vulnerable state. Dr. Clifford C. Hayslip and his coworkers from Walter Reed Army Medical Center[25] have shown that women who suffered from postpartum hypothyroidism were depressed and had impaired concentration and memory as well as other complaints more frequently than did women who did not have postpartum thyroid dysfunction. A hypothyroid woman is likely to become careless and to make more mistakes in the postpartum period. She also tends to complain of fatigue, weight gain, cold intolerance, and nervousness. Hyperthyroidism causes fatigue, pains and aches, impaired memory, and irritability, and can promote depression in the postpartum period. Nearly half the women with postpartum hypothyroidism have nightmares, compared to 5.5 percent of women with normal thyroid function.

The rarest psychiatric condition that can occur in the period following birth is postpartum psychosis, characterized by hallucinations, delirium, and agitation. After the psychosis passes or is medically resolved, depression may follow. Although most cases of postpartum psychosis are not caused by a thyroid imbalance, such an imbalance has been implicated in rare cases.[26]

Because the effects of thyroid imbalance on mood and emotions in the postpartum period are little publicized, many new mothers are at risk for suffering significantly at just the time in their lives when they—and their families—would expect to feel the most joy. Typically, the depression due to postpartum thyroid disease is indistinguishable from that of postpartum depression, although in many instances the onset of depression due to postpartum thyroid disease occurs later. And many women who have postpartum depression unrelated to thyroid disease experience a worsening of their depression as a result of postpartum thyroid imbalance. Thyroid dysfunction in the postpartum period can intensify a woman's perception of stress and increase the difficulties of coping with the demands related to having a new infant. She may feel a lot of guilt about her inability to provide the care that her infant requires. Certainly, stress, an unconscious fear of mothering, marital conflicts, and real or perceived lack of support from husband and family exacerbate postpartum depression.

Grace, a twenty-nine-year-old nurse, described her suffering from major depression due to postpartum hypothyroidism after the birth of her daughter. She was feeling alone because her husband was out of town quite often and her mother had just been admitted to the hospital for cancer treatment. She said:

> For about four weeks, I would get up in the mornings and somehow function in a normal manner. Six weeks after I had my baby, I had a complete nervous breakdown. I would still be in my nightgown and have no recollection of the day at all. One night I went to the store and bought formula and a bottle, and I wrote down all the instructions on how to make the formula, and I sat down and could not move. I wanted to cease to exist for a period of time. I wanted to raise my child, but with everything that was happening, or that I perceived was happening, I couldn't deal with it at that time. I couldn't seem to articulate it, or nobody was listening to the type of help I needed. I needed to rest. They had me diagnosed with major postpartum depression. A few days later, they told me I had severe hypothyroidism.

Grace was treated with thyroid hormone and an antidepressant, which made the depression go away. The depression never came back, even months after stopping the antidepressant. This underscores again the importance of testing for a thyroid condition whenever a postpartum mother is depressed.

When a postpartum thyroid imbalance occurs in a patient with a history of depression, frequently the imbalance triggers a recurrence of the depression. One patient of mine had had trouble with recurrent depression for years and took medication intermittently, but her worst episode of depression occurred after she had her second baby. Unfortunately, her psychiatrist considered postpartum hypothyroidism only after she made two suicide attempts.

As explained earlier, the root cause of most cases of postpartum thyroid imbalance has to do with a flare-up of immune system reactivity that occurs after a woman delivers her baby. The peak of immune system reactivity often coincides with thyroid hormone imbalance and depression. I detailed in Chapter 3 how nonspecific inflammation chemicals produced by the immune system when you have autoimmune thyroid disease can affect brain function and mood. In the postpartum period you are especially vulnerable to these inflammation chemicals and the concomitant thyroid hormone imbalance that the immune system has provoked. For these reasons, to overcome postpartum depression in the most efficient way, you need to address all the components that are contributing to your depression and lower quality of life, including measures to reduce immune system reactivity.

Curing Postpartum Depression

Correcting the thyroid imbalance is a prerequisite for addressing your depressive symptoms in the postpartum period. With thyroid treatment, your symptoms may improve or resolve completely. If you have an underactive thyroid, I recommend a combination of T4 and T3 (see Chapter 20). But often thyroid hormone treatment may not be enough, and you need to take an antidepressant for the depression to resolve completely. If you do not get adequate treatment for your depression, it could become a severe and persistent depression that will affect you and your child.

Sertraline is the most prescribed antidepressant because it is viewed as safe for the nursing infant. Bupropion SR is also quite effective and safe. By and large, however, no major adverse effects have occurred in infants exposed to other antidepressants through breast-feeding.[27] However, to minimize the infant's exposure to the medication, you should take the lowest dose that will help your symptoms, and I recommend that your child be monitored carefully for any effect.

You will also benefit from cognitive behavioral therapy in conjunction with an antidepressant. Using both will help you get more benefits than if you used only an antidepressant. Psychotherapy can help resolve any underlying issues that may affect your relationship with your child. Group interpersonal therapy is also quite beneficial.

I cannot emphasize enough the importance of taking a comprehensive mix of antioxidants, vitamins, and minerals that support optimal thyroid and immune system health. These will help you with your mood, energy, and overall well-being. Most importantly, they will help you lower the immune system reactivity that is the root cause of your postpartum thyroid disease and depression. You also need to follow, step by step, all the components of my mind-body program detailed in Chapter 22. Take 1,000 to 2,000 mg of omega-3 fatty acids, either from fish oil or as a supplement. Research has shown that increasing consumption of these fatty acids will help depression.[28]

It is likely that the drop of insulin levels after delivery contributes to the occurrence of postpartum depression. For this reason, you may be able to improve your symptoms by increasing your intake of carbohydrates.[29] This will stimulate the release of insulin from the pancreas.

When postpartum depression and postpartum thyroid dysfunction occur at the same time, one cannot with certainty implicate the thyroid disease as being the only reason for depression. Although research has shown a link between postpartum depression and postpartum thyroid imbalance, no one can be certain whether the depression would have occurred if the thyroid disease had not been present. Nevertheless, thyroid testing needs to be done in any woman suffering from postpartum depression. Treating the thyroid imbalance may make the depression go away. Most physicians do not take postpartum symptoms seriously because, culturally, it is expected that women will go through some mood changes and emotional instability in the postpartum period. Our society unfairly expects these new mothers to "tough it out" and push their way through the sometimes overwhelming emotional and physical effects of postpartum depression. Doctors, spouses, and families often tell new mothers to ignore their own symptoms and "think of the baby" and the joy they "should" feel. Despite the frequency of postpartum depression and postpartum thyroid dysfunction, physicians often ignore both problems and neglect thyroid testing of depressed women in the postpartum period. This tendency *must* change to prevent serious consequences for both mothers and infants.

Important Points to Remember

- In some women, a thyroid imbalance makes postpartum depression worse. Have your thyroid checked if you become overwhelmed by sadness, crying spells, distancing from your spouse, or an inability to care for your baby.
- Thyroid imbalance in the postpartum period often exhibits a pattern of transient hyperthyroidism followed by hypothyroidism, then recovery of normal thyroid function.
- Some women, however, experience only transient hyperthyroidism or transient hypothyroidism. Others develop a permanently overactive thyroid due to Graves' disease or a permanently underactive thyroid due to Hashimoto's thyroiditis.
- Once you have had thyroid trouble after delivering a baby, your risk of having thyroid problems after subsequent pregnancies is increased. Also, you become at risk for having permanent hypothyroidism down the road.
- The postpartum period is a vulnerable one for women, many of whom experience the onset of their thyroid imbalance after delivering a baby.

PART IV

OVERCOMING
THYROID DISEASE

The Journey to Wellness

17

TREATING THE IMBALANCE

Being diagnosed with a thyroid imbalance can be a relief for people who have long suffered from its symptoms, because they expect that all their problems will disappear very quickly with treatment. They cannot wait to get on with their lives, feel good again, and function normally. Their doctors will often assure them that their thyroid tests will become completely normal over the next few weeks and they will start feeling better. Typically, when patients begin the treatment, they will perceive a gradual improvement. For weeks or months, however, they may continue not to feel at their best. Many find it hard to admit to other people, either at work or at home, that they are still not feeling good.

In fact, some symptoms may resolve only after a period of thyroid stability. Often, after correction of a thyroid condition, emotional effects may persist as a result of what I call the "shake-up" of the brain by the thyroid imbalance. In order to shorten this period of recovery and avoid the persistence of symptoms, you need to work with your doctor to reach and maintain normal thyroid hormone levels as soon as possible. You also need to avoid wide fluctuations in your thyroid levels, which are likely to occur if your doctor has little expertise in treating thyroid disorders.

This chapter teaches you how to reach and maintain a proper balance. It also addresses many of the problems that commonly occur during the treatment of thyroid conditions. It highlights cases of undue suffering resulting from stereotypical treatment approaches and limited awareness of the effects of thyroid imbalance during treatment. It also shows you how to avoid these pitfalls and speed up your recovery.

Finding the Right Doctor

To regain your mental and physical wellness, your physician not only needs to be experienced in adjusting and fine-tuning medication, but also needs to have adequate knowledge and experience about autoimmunity and about the emotional effects of thyroid disease.

The emotional effects of thyroid imbalance may make you feel alone and helpless. The physician's attitude will have a significant effect on the way you will feel. You have the right to expect your doctor to explain the nature and effects of thyroid imbalance. Some doctors are not prepared to deal with the emotional and mental effects of thyroid imbalance during treatment, however, and will instead focus almost exclusively on normalizing your blood tests. This can be very frustrating to patients whose emotional and mental changes haven't been explained adequately. Some patients, who haven't been told about the effects of thyroid imbalance, may find themselves wondering whether they are not sick but "crazy." You should expect more from your doctor than just analyzing blood tests and adjusting thyroid medication. Your doctor should explain the dynamics of the disease and lay out what is likely to happen as a result of it.

While treating Cassandra's overactive thyroid with medication, the endocrinologist's primary concern was to adjust the dose of medication and try to achieve normal blood tests. Meanwhile, Cassandra was experiencing unexplained emotional problems. She described her encounters with her physician:

We would have a very brief discussion and do an exam. Sometimes she would chastise me for not working. I felt she couldn't understand how truly ill I was. I was reporting all the anxiety and depression, and she was very dismissive of that. I went every two weeks for a period of months.

I didn't think enough aggressive measures were being taken to subdue my symptoms. I was so angry with the endocrinologist. I was thinking maybe I wasn't being a good patient. But I was a very compliant patient. I wanted to feel better. It was like I was in a big black hole trying to climb out, and nobody could reach in to get me. I felt helpless. It was very depressing. I felt trapped. My self-esteem was terrible.

One day, the nurse announced I was in the exam room, and I heard the doctor say, "Again?" She often didn't communicate with me outside of the office. Her office staff would call, or I would get messages in the mail to adjust my dosage.

I expected her to have a greater understanding of what I was going through symptomatically and emotionally.

Cassandra had great willpower. She wanted to feel normal; she wanted to understand. She wanted to communicate with her physician. She attempted to describe her emotional, debilitating suffering, but her doctor seemed unconcerned. Unlike Cassandra, many people may not feel at ease talking about their suffering. Many have severe anxiety or panic attacks and do not express the symptoms to their physicians for fear of being taken for fools. Yet it is important to express these symptoms, both to ensure better understanding and to obtain optimal treatment. To avoid undue suffering generated by lack of communication between you and your doctor, choose a thyroid specialist who can deal with your emotions.

Treating the Underactive Thyroid

As I've explained, hypothyroidism due to a damaged thyroid gland causes high TSH levels. The higher the TSH, the more severe the hypothyroidism. Your doctor's treatment goal is to give you the amount of thyroid hormone needed to reduce TSH to normal levels. In general, the higher the TSH, the higher the thyroid hormone dose needs to be for you to reach and maintain normal thyroid balance.[1] Therefore, the TSH level obtained at diagnosis may allow your doctor to predict from the outset the dosage range needed to achieve close-to-normal thyroid levels. Thus, it is not uncommon for doctors to increase the dose gradually over the first few weeks of treatment without monitoring TSH until the estimated dose has been reached and stabilized for a few weeks.[2]

Although synthetic levothyroxine, currently the most widely used form of thyroid hormone to treat hypothyroidism, became available in the 1950s, its use became widespread only in the early 1970s, when researchers discovered that animal-derived thyroid extracts were causing unstable and inconsistent blood levels of thyroid hormones. Desiccated thyroid contains T4 and T3 in variable amounts, depending on the preparation process used by the manufacturer and the iodine content in the diet of the animals from which the thyroid glands were taken. Also around the same time, scientists discovered that when people take synthetic thyroxine (T4), some of it is converted to T3 in bodily organs, thus providing stable levels of both T4 and T3. The stability of thyroid hormone levels and TSH levels achieved by using synthetic levothyroxine is also due to the fact that T4 has a very long life in the body. When taken on a daily basis, the thyroxine pill allows for a steady and continuous production of T3 in bodily organs.

Pharmaceutical companies manufacture levothyroxine tablets in different strengths, ranging from 25 mcg (or .025 mgs) up to 300 mcg (0.3 mgs). The availability of these different strengths facilitates the fine adjustment of the dose of thyroid hormone so that blood levels can be maintained in the normal laboratory range as long as you continue taking the medication. The three most commonly used brands of levothyroxine are Synthroid, Levoxyl, and Unithroid. When you fill your prescription, make sure you are not given a generic preparation, since generics may not contain the exact amount of thyroid hormone prescribed.[3]

In June 2004, the Food and Drug Administration determined that many generic levothyroxine medications are equivalent to and as safe as brand-name preparations.[4] The methods and the criteria that the FDA used to reach this conclusion might have been appropriate for many medications, but certainly not for thyroid hormone replacement treatment. Despite a difference in potency of more than 10 percent between the various levothyroxine preparations, the FDA is still considering them as equivalent.[5] Yet such difference obviously can lead to significant difference in your blood tests. The FDA's decision means that now pharmacists can give you any levothyroxine preparation, including a generic, instead of the brand prescribed by your doctor. As you can imagine, the ruling made by the FDA has, to say the least, displeased endocrinologists throughout the country. Medical associations such as the American Association of Clinical Endocrinologists and the American Thyroid Association have been seriously concerned about the potential health-related adverse effects of substituting generic levothyroxine preparations for brand-name products. I urge you to be proactive and demand that your pharmacist give you the exact brand of medication that your doctor has prescribed. In fact, to avoid any instability in your blood levels generated by substitution, try to keep taking the same brand throughout your treatment. Also, if for financial or insurance reasons you have to take a generic product, make sure that your pharmacist gives you the same generic for refills; this will minimize significant changes in your thyroid levels during treatment. It is to be hoped that these issues will be resolved once the FDA takes steps to change the methods and criteria for evaluating the equivalence of thyroid medications.

The choice of the levothyroxine preparation used to treat your low thyroid condition also needs to take into account the kinds of inactive ingredients (additives) that are used to make the tablet. If you are suffering from an autoimmune thyroid disease, it is possible that your immune system is reactive to gluten, lactose, soy, cornstarch, potato starch, food coloring, or other additives. Such potential immune system irritants might promote immune-system-related lingering symptoms and can even affect the gastrointestinal absorption of the active thyroid hormone, causing instability and ineffectiveness of the treatment. For instance, some levothyroxine preparations such as Unithroid and Tirosint claim to be gluten-free. Of all the generic products, only levothyroxine made by Mylan Pharmaceuticals claims to be gluten-free. Many other brands and generic formulations cannot guarantee whether the tablets are gluten-free or not. For some patients, I had to use levothyroxine in a compounded dye-free form for optimal stability of thyroid levels and for the patient to feel at his or her best. In essence, your thyroid hormone treatment is not just a matter of adjusting doses; it also involves selecting the right thyroid medication, one that does not provoke immune system reactivity.

In Chapter 20 I will explain why many thyroid patients benefit from a combination of levothyroxine and T3 treatment for optimal wellness. Combining the two hormones the right way will make the two thyroid hormone levels (T4 and T3) well balanced, as if the thyroid gland were functioning in a perfect way. I do not, however, recommend that you take only a T3 medication for the treatment of your low thyroid condition. Many healthcare professionals continue to prescribe high doses of medications that contain both T4 and T3. The three most frequently prescribed medications that contain both T4 and T3 are Armour Thyroid, Westhroid, and Nature-Throid. Armour Thyroid (desiccated thyroid hormone) comes in several strengths ranging from ¼ grain to 5 grains. The gluten status of Armour Thyroid is not certain; however, it is soy free and does not contain potato starch or cornstarch, but does contain lactose. Westhroid is also available in dosages ranging from ¼ grain to 2 grains. It is gluten free, corn free and soy free, does not contain cornstarch but contains lactose. Nature-Throid is available in doses ranging from ¼ grain to 5 grains. It is gluten free and soy free, and it does not contain cornstarch, potato starch, or lactose.

Be aware that the higher the dose of these T4/T3 combination medications, the higher the amount of T3 you will get in your system after taking the medication. Surges of T3 can trigger cardiac arrhythmias and can be damaging to your muscles, brain, and immune system. Although I use these medications on a routine basis, I use them in low doses in conjunction with levothyroxine if necessary to avoid imbalanced T3 levels in my patients.

If your doctor doesn't do the dose adjustments properly, you are likely to continue to experience symptoms for a long time. For Tracy, whom I recently saw for a second opinion, it took a year and a half to reach normal thyroid levels after her initial diagnosis. She said, "My doctor was having so much trouble getting me regulated to a normal TSH level. Every four months, I'd be going back in and complaining I wasn't feeling well, and sure enough, the blood test would show that I was correct. The adjustments made by my doctor were never enough to make me normal again."

In people with severe hypothyroidism, the initial dose of thyroid hormone should be small and increased gradually to the dose required. Abrupt and rapid administration of high doses of thyroid hormone to severely hypothyroid patients may cause health problems, especially in older people. For example, while a person is hypothyroid, his or her heart works slowly and has adapted to the low metabolism. Rapid correction of hypothyroidism in someone with a preexisting heart condition, which may be unknown to the patient and physician, could quickly accelerate the heart function and induce a heart attack. It is clearly better and safer to start at a dose of 25 mcg a day and in-crease the dose weekly by 25 mcg until the estimated dose is reached. For patients under forty-five years of age who are otherwise healthy, the dosage may be stepped up faster. In older patients and those with heart disease or anxiety symptoms, the dosage should be stepped up every two weeks.

Severe mood disorders that can be quite alarming may also occur when doctors prescribe high doses of thyroid hormone at the beginning of treat-ment. Often such patients have a history of high anxiety or emotional prob-lems. These symptoms may occur four to seven days after they begin taking the high dose of thyroid hormone. If you experience mental effects, you need to have your doctor reduce the dose of thyroid hormone immediately. Doc-tors have had to hospitalize patients because of mania or other reactions to excessive thyroid hormone. Patients may become severely agitated, their thoughts may race, and they may exhibit inappropriate behavior. Some may even experience hallucinations and delusions.[6]

A high amount of thyroid hormone commonly worsens an existing anxi-ety disorder, which may be a source of confusion for you and your physician. Myra, age forty-nine, had had a great deal of stress in her life and had been suffering from a generalized anxiety disorder for quite a few years. She was intermittently prescribed Valium and other medications, which helped con-trol her anxiety, and she had learned through the years to manage her symp-toms. When she was diagnosed as hypothyroid, her doctor prescribed a high dose of thyroid hormone from the beginning instead of starting her at a low dose and stepping it up gradually. After a few days on the medication, Myra began to experience severe panic attacks and increased anxiety symptoms. She woke up in the middle of the night with a rapid heartbeat, a hot and sweaty feeling, and a choking sensation "as if somebody was pressing on my neck."

She took the thyroid pill for a couple of weeks, but her symptoms kept getting worse. She reached the point of experiencing ten to fifteen panic at-tacks a day. Finally, she concluded that this might be caused by the thyroid medication and stopped taking it on her own, which caused the anxiety symptoms and panic attacks to diminish. Later, even small doses triggered panic attacks. It became a vicious cycle in which Myra associated the thyroid hormone treatment with a worsening of her symptoms. After I counseled her about the nature and cause of her symptoms, she finally agreed to try the graduated dosage method. The dose was eventually increased, her thyroid levels became normal, and the exaggerated anxiety symptoms were resolved. In fact, Myra now suffers from less anxiety than she did before the doctors diagnosed her thyroid condition. Myra's anxiety disorder was probably caused in part by the underactive thyroid, but when too much thyroid hor-mone entered her system at once, the anxiety became worse.

Approximately six weeks after you reach the estimated dose that is expected to bring your thyroid levels close to normal, your doctor will typically order a TSH test so the dose can be adjusted. The size of the adjustment needed should be determined based on the result of the new TSH test. How fast this adjustment is made also depends on your age and on whether you suffer from a heart condition.

The dose of thyroid hormone may need to be adjusted once or twice before you reach a normal TSH level. Do not have your TSH tested more often than every six to eight weeks at the beginning. The criterion for successful therapy is to finally get TSH within a normal range and keep it there.

PROBLEMS DURING THE MAINTENANCE PHASE
OF TREATMENT OF HYPOTHYROIDISM

Once your thyroid test levels have stabilized, you need to make sure that your doctor does not prescribe too much or too little thyroid hormone. In one study, 14 percent of hypothyroid patients taking thyroid hormone were over-replaced, and 18 percent were underreplaced.[7]

People taking too much thyroid hormone will have a low TSH reading and may develop cardiac problems.[8] Postmenopausal women will have accelerated bone loss, which predisposes them to osteoporosis.[9] Even minimal thyroid hormone excess may make you irritable and cause you to suffer from undue nervousness, anxiety, or hypomanic behavior.[10]

Consider the case of Catherine, a thirty-four-year-old sales manager who was diagnosed with hypothyroidism by her internist. The dose of thyroid hormone she was receiving exceeded her needs. She began suffering from shakiness, insomnia, and palpitations; she also noted that her eyes seemed to be locked in a stare. She described symptoms of hypomania. "I couldn't sit still for any length of time," she said. "I became too energetic and obsessive-compulsive about cleaning my house and working long hours. I would get up in the middle of the night to clean up."

Catherine felt she was possessed and had lost control of her body. Deep inside, she noted that the person she had become was not her usual self. She experienced rage for no apparent reason and felt compelled to ride a bicycle in a remote area, pedaling as hard and fast as she could, until she felt the rage subside.

These changes had occurred so quickly that Catherine didn't understand what was happening to her. She thought she was losing her mind. Her heart was beating at such a fast pace that she was afraid to go to sleep for fear she would have a heart attack in her sleep. "I wanted so badly to be my old self— the me that I knew and loved. I was afraid of this new person, and I wanted to feel healthy again." Catherine did indeed feel healthy again once her dose of thyroid hormone was reduced to a more appropriate level.

Do not increase the dose on your own or insist that your physician increase the dose because you have not felt an improvement and believe that a higher dose would make you feel better. Increasing the dose may cause new problems. Do not decrease or stop the thyroid medication on your own or skip taking it once or twice a week either. Some patients phone their doctors and try to convince them to alter their prescription without testing and/or follow-up. This can lead to a cumulative deficit or excess in thyroid hormone, which can cause a great deal of suffering.

Sophia had been receiving 150 mcg of levothyroxine daily for three years. One day, she called her physician and mentioned that she had heart palpitations. These were in fact due to anxiety over another family member's health problems. Sophia's physician decreased the dose from 150 mcg to 75 mcg and told her to come to his office for repeat thyroid testing three months later. Because of her personal problems, Sophia did not take the time to have a follow-up test until a full year later. During that year, she had a wide range of symptoms that she attributed to stress but were actually related to low thyroid hormone levels.

When Sophia finally did return to her physician for follow-up, her tests showed hypothyroidism because she was taking only half the dose required to maintain normal thyroid levels. After the dose was readjusted, her symptoms gradually disappeared. In fact, she became better able to cope with her family problems.

Another unfortunate problem that still happens to some hypothyroid patients taking thyroid hormone occurs when general practitioners instruct them to stop taking their medication. Crystal, who was hypothyroid, was taken off thyroid hormone by her general practitioner when he saw that her thyroid test results were normal while she was taking thyroid hormone. What this physician probably overlooked is that the test results were normal because of the treatment. Three or four months after she stopped taking the medication, Crystal suffered from serious depression and had many symptoms of hypothyroidism. She went back to her doctor, and he said her symptoms were caused by stress. When I tested Crystal and found her hypothyroid, I placed her back on thyroid hormone treatment, and she has done well ever since.

The likelihood that you are under- or overmedicated is extremely high if your physician does not monitor TSH when you are taking thyroid hormone. Many physicians unfortunately continue to run T3 and T4 tests and often try to make treatment decisions based on these tests instead of TSH. T4 and T3 test results are also easily misinterpreted when the levels of the proteins carrying thyroid hormone in the blood are abnormal (see Chapter 7). In addition, several medications can alter thyroid hormone levels. For instance, Dilantin and aspirin may lower the total T4 reading, even though thyroid function is normal.

To achieve a good balance, you need to have your TSH maintained between 0.5 and 2.0 mIU/L while receiving thyroid hormone treatment. A TSH ranging between 2.0 and 4.5 may mean some thyroid hormone deficiency (see Chapter 7). Yet a recent survey comparing how thyroid specialists and primary care physicians administer thyroid medication to hypothyroid patients indicated that primary care physicians are in general satisfied when the TSH is maintained between 0.5 and 5.0 mIU/L.[11] Often all it takes to restore normal thyroid status is a small increase in the dose, which might have significant effects on the way you feel. If, despite having a normal TSH for at least three to four months, you continue to suffer from depression or symptoms of underactive thyroid such as lack of energy, cognitive changes, low mood, tiredness, dry skin, and pains and aches, you may experience an improvement by combining T4 and T3 in your treatment program (see Chapter 20). Your system may still be lacking some T3 even though your blood test results are normal.

OPTIMIZING YOUR USE OF THYROID HORMONE PILLS
Many foods, nutrients, and drugs can interfere with thyroid hormone absorption. For example, if you take iron at the same time as thyroid hormone, it will bind with some of the thyroid hormone and block its absorption. Fiber, coffee, as well as calcium supplements, if taken close to thyroid hormone intake, may interfere with absorption of the hormone.

Several medications, when taken together with thyroid hormone, can also decrease the availability of the hormone by interfering with its absorption in the gastrointestinal tract. Common medications that can affect thyroid hormone absorption are drugs used to lower cholesterol (cholestyramine, colestipol, and colesevelam), antacids containing aluminum (Maalox and sucralfate), proton pump inhibitors used to treat GERD (Prilosec, Losec, and Omesec), the weight-loss medication orlistat (Alli and Xenical), and raloxifene (Evista), used to prevent and treat osteoporosis.

To avoid this interference effect, take your thyroid hormone at least three to four hours before or after you take calcium, iron, or any of these medications. I recommend that you take your thyroid pill at the same time every day, at least forty minutes to one hour before breakfast on an empty stomach with one large cup of water. Take your nutritional supplements and drugs at lunch and suppertime.

Some medications increase the rate at which your body clears thyroid hormone. If you are taking a stable dose of thyroid hormone and were recently prescribed the drugs Dilantin (phenytoin), Tegretol (carbamazepine), or phenobarbital, you may need a change in your dosage. Do not forget to mention these new medications to the physician treating your hypothyroidism so your thyroid can be retested.

Generally speaking, it is quite safe for women with a thyroid imbalance to use oral contraceptives, even while taking appropriate thyroid medication. Oral contraceptives containing estrogen and estrogen replacement therapy cause a slight increase in the need for thyroid hormone replacement, because estrogens cause an increase in thyroid-hormone-binding proteins in your bloodstream.[12] If you have been receiving a stable dose of thyroid hormone and have begun taking an oral contraceptive or hormone replacement therapy, it is wise to have your physician order a TSH test three months after you start the estrogens. By that time, your blood levels should have stabilized so that the TSH test result will be reliable for the purpose of a dose adjustment. If you have taken tamoxifen, an antiestrogen used for the treatment of breast cancer, for more than one year, you may require more thyroid hormone.[13]

HOW OFTEN SHOULD YOU BE RETESTED?

Some doctors recommend that when a patient's thyroid function has returned to normal with a specific dose of thyroid hormone replacement, further thyroid tests should be done once a year. I simply do not agree with this approach, because your thyroid condition may not be stable. Not only could the function of the gland deteriorate significantly in the interim, but patients with Hashimoto's thyroiditis may have a concomitant Graves' disease that may be more active at some times than at others. If you have hypothyroidism due to Hashimoto's thyroiditis and are taking a stable dose of thyroid hormone, a flare-up of Graves' disease and production of the antibodies that stimulate the thyroid gland may make you require less thyroid hormone.[14] Rarely, it can even cause the rapid onset of hyperthyroidism and require stopping thyroid hormone treatment.[15] Several of my patients with underactive thyroids suffer from frequent fluctuations in the activity of the gland. You need to be aware that the residual activity of the gland affected by Hashimoto's thyroiditis does change and can fluctuate over time.[16] As a result, patients with an underactive thyroid may require frequent adjustments in the dose of thyroid hormone.

Retesting patients once a year will ignore possibly significant changes in their thyroid activity. Some patients may suffer from the effects of thyroid hormone excess or deficiency and not know it. Because changes in thyroid levels in patients receiving stable doses of thyroid hormone are common, a better recommendation is that thyroid tests be done regularly every six months and that the test results be closely scrutinized in conjunction with a careful assessment of symptoms.[17] Unfortunately, hypothyroid patients are in general not monitored adequately. One recent study showed that only 56 percent of hypothyroid patients treated with thyroid hormone were monitored at the minimum recommended frequency.[18] If you are hypothyroid as a result of the treatment of Graves' disease, you may need more frequent testing (every three to four months), at least initially.

Three years previously, doctors in her managed care health program had diagnosed Wanda with an underactive thyroid. The thyroid hormone she was taking made her symptoms subside. She was retested once and was told to continue the same dose of medication. A few months later, she began experiencing tremendous stress at home. She complained of many symptoms that her primary care physician never attributed to possible hypothyroidism. She had understood from her physician that her thyroid problem was taken care of as long as she took the medication.

Wanda said, "I was absolutely zonked out. I would walk in and lie down and go to sleep at six-thirty. I was very depressed. When I told my primary care physician I was having dizziness, he put me on motion sickness medicine, which I took only one time because it made me feel bad."

When Wanda was finally tested again two years later, she was quite hypothyroid. Adjustment of her thyroid medication resolved her tiredness and other symptoms. After that experience, Wanda decided to change her health insurance coverage and her doctor.

Many patients believe that having an underactive thyroid means that the gland has quit working and all they have to do is take the same pill for their entire lives. Therefore, they try to get refills for their medication over the phone, believing that there is no need to be examined or tested. This may result in unhappy surprises.

The Barnes and Wilson Treatment Methods

In the 1950s, it was recognized that symptoms such as fatigue, headaches, irritability, menstrual irregularities, muscle aches and pains, lethargy, and emotional instability in women could be interpreted in different ways by different doctors.[19] Based on these symptoms, an endocrinologist might diagnose hypothyroidism, whereas a psychiatrist might diagnose depression or melancholia.

The late Broda O. Barnes, in his book *Hypothyroidism: The Unsuspected Illness*,[20] advocated thyroid hormone treatment for people suffering from various symptoms of an underactive thyroid such as headaches, fatigue, infections, skin conditions, infertility, arthritis, and weight problems. Barnes suggested that the way to diagnose hypothyroidism and to monitor treatment is to take the patient's basal temperature. This approach was based on research he published in the early 1940s showing that hypothyroidism is associated with low basal temperature and that many people with low basal temperature and symptoms of hypothyroidism improved with thyroid hormone treatment.[21]

Some patients treated according to the Barnes method with natural thyroid hormone do indeed have hypothyroidism and do respond to the treatment. Thus, a number of physicians began to advocate thyroid hormone as a treatment for patients suffering from tiredness, depression, or other nonspecific complaints accompanied by a low basal temperature—without thyroid testing. They believe that low basal temperature is always an indication of low thyroid. A low temperature, however, could merely be an indication that the patient's metabolism is slower than normal. It could also be seen in patients with depression, post-traumatic stress syndrome, eating disorders such as anorexia nervosa, and renal failure. If the symptoms improve or resolve with thyroid hormone treatment, it could in many cases be due to the antidepressant effect of the medication rather than the correction of hypothyroidism. Ideally, the use of body temperature to diagnose and monitor treatment of hypothyroidism should be abandoned.

Other doctors also advocate the use of thyroid hormone to treat symptoms that follow a major stress, attributing them to low levels of T3 in our bodies. For instance, Dr. E. Denis Wilson, in his book *Wilson's Syndrome: The Miracle of Feeling Well,* described a particular syndrome as a cluster of debilitating symptoms brought on especially by a significant physical or emotional stress that can persist even after the stress has passed.[22] Wilson attributed this persistence to maladaptive slowing of metabolism, characterized by a body temperature that runs, on average, below normal and thyroid blood tests that are often in the normal range. Curiously, many of the symptoms he referred to—fatigue, depression, headaches, migraines, premenstrual syndrome (PMS), anxiety, panic attacks, irritability, hair loss, decreased motivation and ambition, inappropriate weight gain, decreased memory and concentration, insomnia, and intolerance to heat and cold—are symptoms of depression. He also included irritable bowel syndrome, delayed healing after surgery, and even asthma.

Wilson postulated that this suffering results from a deficit in the activity of the enzyme that converts T4 to T3 brought on by a physical or mental stress. This decrease of T3 in the organs causes a slowing of metabolism, reflected by a drop in temperature. In fact, what Dr. Wilson is describing and addressing is a state of cellular hypothyroidism that I discussed in Chapter 2.

Wilson also postulated that the decrease in the enzyme responsible for the conversion of T4 to T3 and the slowing of metabolism occur as a result of the stress and do not return to normal after the stress has passed. Therefore, despite normal thyroid levels in the blood, hypothyroidism remains as a residual effect of post-traumatic stress syndrome. In his book, Wilson recommends treating patients having these symptoms with a high dose of T3 and monitoring and adjusting the T3 dose based on basal temperature, rather than on thyroid testing.

Even if some of the patients diagnosed as having Wilson's syndrome are truly hypothyroid or do have cellular hypothyroidism, they should not be treated with such high doses of thyroid hormone as to make them hyperthyroid.

Treating patients indiscriminately with high doses of T3, failing to do thyroid testing, and adjusting the dose only according to basal body temperature is unacceptable even for thyroid specialists who have developed an expertise in the interaction between the brain and the thyroid. Actually, the best way to treat cellular hypothyroidism is making body cells healthier and removing the free radical burden as well as addressing the root cause of the cellular hypothyroidism (see Chapter 2).

Kathleen, a thirty-seven-year-old nurse, was referred to me by a friend of hers. Her amazing story illustrates how the mislabeling of suffering and inappropriate use of thyroid hormone can result in further suffering. When I saw Kathleen for the first time, she brought with her a pile of temperature charts and a sheet outlining a complicated protocol of thyroid hormone treatment based on checking basal temperature that had been given to her by a physician three months previously. The doctor had diagnosed Kathleen with Wilson's syndrome and told her to take T3 (Cytomel) three times a day. She was to adjust the Cytomel dose according to temperature readings taken three times a day. As long as her average daily temperature was lower than 97.8 degrees Fahrenheit, she was to increase her dose of Cytomel. She was guided during treatment by a manual for Wilson's syndrome.

Before she began having symptoms, Kathleen was experiencing tremendous stress at home dealing with a chronically ill husband and serious financial difficulties. Although her symptoms fit the description of Wilson's syndrome, they were all symptoms of depression as well. When given a very high amount of T3, Kathleen became severely hyperthyroid, which resulted in severe anxiety symptoms, hypomanic behavior, and irregular heartbeat.

I urge doctors who treat hypothyroidism and depression to monitor their patients with thyroid testing and not use doses of thyroid hormone that exceed what the body and brain need to function properly.

Correcting the Overactive Thyroid and Side Effects

If you've been diagnosed with an overactive thyroid due to Graves' disease, understanding the available treatments will allow you to work with your doctor in selecting the best option.

TREATMENT OPTIONS

The three major methods currently used to treat Graves' disease—administering antithyroid drugs, destroying a significant portion of the thyroid gland with radioactive iodine, and surgically removing a significant portion of the gland—address the consequences rather than the cause of the condition.[23] A potential new treatment target for Graves' disease in the future might be a medication that could block the effects of the thyroid-stimulating antibody (the antibody that causes the overactive thyroid) on the thyroid gland.[24]

ANTITHYROID DRUGS

Doctors may prescribe antithyroid drugs such as methimazole or propylthiouracil (PTU) for six months to two years (the average is one year) to maintain normal thyroid levels and perhaps achieve a remission. (You have achieved a remission if, after several months of treatment, you no longer require medication to maintain normal levels of thyroid hormone and TSH.) Antithyroid medications are picked up by the thyroid gland, where they inhibit the production of thyroid hormone. They also have an effect on the immune system, diminishing the autoimmune attack on the thyroid. In general, 30 to 50 percent of patients achieve a remission when they take one of these medications for at least six months to a year.[25] (Even if you achieve a remission, you are always at risk for having a relapse. Graves' disease tends to relapse more often in the spring and summer, according to research.[26]) Women in their reproductive years with mild hyperthyroidism and small goiters respond well to this form of treatment.

Methimazole lasts longer in the body, and you can take it as a single daily dose if you require 30 mg or less, whereas PTU should be taken three to four times a day. With either medication, experienced physicians can often maintain thyroid function in the normal range for as long as the treatment is continued.

Several common minor side effects may occur during treatment and often resolve spontaneously or after the patient switches to another medication. In some instances, the persistence of such symptoms requires stopping the medication. These side effects include:

- Itching
- Skin rash
- Hives
- Joint pains
- Fever
- Upset stomach
- Metallic taste

One of the adverse effects of antithyroid medications that often worries patients is agranulocytosis, a reaction in the bone marrow, which suddenly stops manufacturing white blood cells. This frightening complication, which occurs more frequently in the first three months of treatment, should not cause you undue anxiety because it is quite rare. One study showed that this complication occurs in approximately three to four of every one thousand people treated with medication each year.[27] Although physicians usually do not monitor your white blood cell count, it is safer if this is done each time you have your thyroid tested while being treated. If a sore throat, a mouth sore, or an infection occurs, you should report it to your doctor and have your white blood cell count measured. If the white cell count drops significantly, you need to stop the medication immediately. The low white blood cell count can result in a blood infection. Your doctor will often recommend isolation in a hospital room, antibiotics, and treatment with medications that raise your white blood cell count to appropriate levels.

Liver damage, another unusual complication of antithyroid medications, is rather serious and often occurs in the first few months of treatment as well. For this reason, your doctor will typically test your liver on a regular basis. If liver tests become abnormal, the medication should be stopped immediately.

Other serious, albeit rare, side effects from using antithyroid drugs include:

- Suppressed production of red blood cells in bone marrow (aplastic anemia)
- Low platelet count
- Inflammation of blood vessels (vasculitis), causing symptoms similar to lupus; may lead to kidney disease, arthritis, and life-threatening lung complications

If you have tolerated the medication well, you need to stay on it for at least eight to twelve months to give it a chance to produce a remission. During treatment, you need to be retested (by checking not only TSH but also free T4 and free T3) every two months and have your dose adjusted. Typically, the dose is gradually reduced as your requirement for the medication decreases and the activity of the disease slows down. At the end of the treatment period, most doctors tend to stop the medication abruptly to see whether you stay normal without it. With methimazole, I usually decrease the dose first by 5 mg daily until the patient has reached a dose of 5 mg per day; if thyroid levels remain normal on this low-dose regimen for a few months, I will further drop it to 5 mg every other day, then to 5 mg twice a week and even less before stopping the medication. Only if the TSH remains normal while you are taking 5 mg twice a week for at least two months should you stop taking the medication. Research has shown that when patients with Graves' disease are treated for six months with a protocol similar to the one I use and their blood tests are maintained at normal, 81 percent of them go into remission.[28]

If the TSH is not normal, you may become hyperthyroid again, and the vicious cycle will resume. If the TSH level becomes low even though thyroid hormone levels are normal, that means your gland still requires medication. In this case, the dose of medication will need to be increased to achieve normal levels again. At this point, you may want to proceed with an alternative treatment or continue the medication for another six-month period before you try stopping it again.

While you are being treated for hyperthyroidism, I urge you to take a mix of adequate amounts of antioxidants (such as ThyroLife Optima). Antioxidants will reduce your symptoms and other effects of hyperthyroidism on your body and will reduce immune system reactivity. For this reason you need to pay attention to your intake of antioxidants regardless of which treatment you are receiving for your overactive thyroid.

DESTROYING A SIGNIFICANT PORTION OF THE
THYROID WITH RADIOACTIVE IODINE

Another treatment method is to destroy a significant portion of the thyroid gland with radioactive iodine (radioiodine). This method is simple. You are given a small amount of radioactive iodine to drink. The amount is either fixed (10–20 mCi) or based on the size of your thyroid gland and its level of activity after you have had a radioactive iodine uptake test (see Chapter 7). This method is the preferred form of treatment for toxic nodules and multinodular toxic goiters. Doctors also find this method effective for treating nontoxic goiters that have caused pressure in the neck, including difficulty swallowing.[29] For patients with Graves' disease, this method should be chosen if you are unlikely to achieve a remission with medications or if you have experienced side effects from the medications. Doctors frequently recommend this method for men and people older than forty-five.

Also, your doctor will often prescribe radioactive iodine to treat your Graves' disease if, after a year or two of medication, your thyroid gland continues to be overactive. In general, this method is used if, after you have achieved a remission with medication, your thyroid becomes overactive again months or years after you completed the course of medication.

Even when radioactive iodine is chosen from the outset, some doctors prescribe an antithyroid medication for two months prior to the radioiodine treatment to bring your thyroid levels down to normal first. I often elect this last approach so that the patient improves—emotionally and physically—and has time to learn more about the condition and the treatment options. Using medications initially will also help determine whether your gland is responsive to medication. It will often prevent you from rapidly swinging from hyperthyroidism to severe hypothyroidism. You will be asked to stop the antithyroid medication two to five days before the radioactive iodine treatment and to restart the medication at smaller doses three to five days after the treatment. If the medication you have been taking is PTU, make sure that you are switched to methimazole three to four weeks prior to the radioiodine treatment. Recent research has concluded that PTU treatment causes the gland to become more resistant to radioiodine treatment.[30] Research has shown that methimazole treatment before radioactive iodine treatment does not affect the effectiveness of radioactive iodine treatment.[31]

The purpose of radioiodine treatment is to destroy enough of the thyroid gland so that the remaining part does not produce excess thyroid hormone. The destruction begins within days after the treatment and may continue over a period of several years. Many patients are led to believe that radioactive iodine rapidly destroys the entire gland, whereas most of the time it actually destroys only a portion. In fact, the amount of the thyroid gland destroyed with treatment varies from person to person because glands have different levels of sensitivity to the damaging effect of radioiodine. Very rarely do people become hyperthyroid again many years after treatment with radioactive iodine. One study showed that 55.8 percent of patients treated with radioactive iodine became hypothyroid one year after the treatment. But ten years after the treatment, 86.1 percent had become hypothyroid.[32]

Many doctors in the United States prefer this method because it is in general safe and effective. In many European countries and in Japan, doctors favor trying medications first. One treatment with radioiodine may not suffice. Nearly 30 percent of patients treated with radioactive iodine need to be retreated one or more times. It is important to select a dose of radioactive iodine that cures the excess thyroid hormone without having to administer additional doses. Young patients with very large thyroid glands, patients who have high thyroid hormone levels, and patients who are pretreated with antithyroid medications for more than four months are less likely to respond to low doses of radioactive iodine.[33] For these patients, a higher dose of radioactive iodine will be more effective.

This method should not be used if you are pregnant. If you are a woman of childbearing age, your doctor will typically order a pregnancy test prior to the treatment. This treatment should also be avoided in people having moderate to severe eye disease until the eye condition has become stable. It can cause or worsen eye disease in 15 percent of patients. For this reason, some doctors prescribe prednisone (a corticosteroid medication that slows down the inflammation in the eyes) for several weeks after radioactive iodine treatment, which may reduce the occurrence of eye disease.

Many people, when told about the option of radioactive iodine treatment, become concerned that it will cause long-term adverse health effects. However, radioactive iodine treatment has been used for more than fifty years, and there is no scientific evidence so far that the treatment causes thyroid cancer or leukemia. There is debate, however, about the increased risk of cancer of the stomach, hypopharynx, and esophagus. One study, for instance, concluded that the occurrence of stomach cancer may increase years after the treatment, particularly in younger people.[34] Because these concerns are not quite settled yet, it is perhaps safer to treat children and adolescents with medications first and consider radioiodine treatment for young people as a last resort. Unfortunately, many patients are treated with a much higher activity of radioactive iodine than they actually need to have their gland destroyed.[35] The higher-than-needed doses cause unnecessary radiation exposure for the patient, the family, and the public. High radioactive iodine activity also requires longer radiation protection for family members when you come back home.

Children born to women previously treated with radioactive iodine do not experience a significantly increased risk of genetic defects. Nevertheless, if you are treated with radioiodine, you should avoid becoming pregnant within six months after the treatment. It is not known, moreover, whether radioactive iodine received during the reproductive years will have any genetic or carcinogenic effects on future generations.

SURGICAL REMOVAL OF A SIGNIFICANT PORTION OF THE THYROID

Surgical removal of a significant portion of the thyroid gland (subtotal thyroidectomy) is not frequently used in the United States unless special circumstances exist. For example, for patients who choose not to take radioiodine and who have experienced reactions to medications, or have very enlarged thyroid glands and are concerned about eye disease, surgical removal of a part of the gland may be an option. Complete removal of the gland may relieve some of the symptoms in some persons suffering from thyroid eye disease. Another advantage of surgery is the rapid control of symptoms. The patient must be treated with medications (iodine and a beta-blocker) before the operation, however, to avoid complications such as thyroid storm that could develop as a result of surgery.[36]

I tend to recommend surgery for children and adolescents who have not responded to the medication or could not tolerate it. Surgery often cures the condition and prevents fluctuation of thyroid levels and its detrimental effects on mood and behavior. A pregnant woman treated with medication who experiences significant side effects can be treated with surgery during pregnancy.

If you decide to have an operation, choose a surgeon who has continued and proven experience with thyroid surgery. This is crucial because surgical removal of the thyroid can result in impairment of the voice and problems with low calcium due to damage to the parathyroid glands (four small glands right behind the thyroid that control calcium metabolism). To ensure the best outcome, choose a surgeon who has done at least ten to fifteen thyroid surgeries a year for the past two to three years. Ask about his or her track record. The procedure for Graves' disease is subtotal thyroidectomy, although some surgeons may recommend a total thyroidectomy for people with eye disease to help the eye problem. A total thyroidectomy, however, is more likely to cause complications such as low calcium and nerve damage. You also need to know that in nearly 30 percent of people who have a subtotal thyroidectomy, the thyroid gland will become overactive again in the future. If that happens, radioiodine treatment will be the best option. If you are planning to become pregnant right away, surgery may be the best alternative.

Surgical removal of the thyroid gland can also be performed with an endoscope through a small incision in the areola of the breast. The technique can also be used in patients with benign thyroid tumors or nodular goiters and even in patients with thyroid cancer. Endoscopic thyroidectomy is safer than conventional surgery and causes fewer complications to the recurrent nerve or the parathyroid glands.[37]

A new treatment that has been shown to be effective in curing hyperthyroidism is thyroid arterial embolization, a method that consists of blocking blood supply to the thyroid gland. Prior to this treatment, you need to have a selective arteriography to visualize the blood vessels that supply blood to the gland, and this is associated with some risk. Research, however, has shown that this treatment generally does not produce serious complications. If thyroid levels remain high after the embolization, you may end up requiring additional treatment with antithyroid medications; however, one study showed that of patients treated with interventional embolization, nearly two-thirds regained normal thyroid function after the treatment.[38]

Some patients with Graves' disease, frightened by the potential side effects of treatment, refuse the conventional treatments currently available and search for a holistic or naturopathic approach. There is, however, no nonconventional treatment that has proven to be consistently effective.

MAKING THE RIGHT DECISION
If you have just been diagnosed with an overactive thyroid due to Graves' disease, you should discuss the three treatment options with your doctor and get advice on which method to choose. Some patients are more comfortable than others with taking the responsibility for contributing to this decision. If you have significant eye disease, you should not rush into radioactive iodine treatment because that may worsen your eye problems.

If you have Graves' disease, your thyroid gland may also contain a nodule that could be cancerous. For this reason, prior to deciding which is the most suitable treatment for your overactive thyroid you need to have an ultrasound of the thyroid gland. It will determine whether your gland contains a thyroid nodule or not. One study found that 35.1 percent of 245 patients with Graves' disease who were evaluated by an ultrasound of the thyroid had a coexistent thyroid nodule. The striking finding in this research is that 3.3 percent of the patients studied also had thyroid cancer, which in more than half of them had already spread to lymph nodes or other areas.[39] In addition, research has shown that thyroid cancer may be not only more common in patients with Graves' disease but also more aggressive than in patients with normal thyroid glands.[40] For this reason, thyroid cancer should be detected as early as possible and should be treated aggressively in patients with Graves' disease. If the ultrasound does reveal a lump, a fine-needle aspiration biopsy should be done *before* you receive the radioactive iodine treatment, since this treatment will affect the results of any biopsy performed afterward. If a cancer is present, then the treatment for both the overactive thyroid and the lump should be surgery.

Some endocrinologists recommend the same treatment for all their patients suffering from an overactive thyroid due to Graves' disease. This explains why a patient seen by two or three endocrinologists may be given different opinions with respect to treatment. The method chosen should in fact depend on several factors, including your age, whether you are a woman in your reproductive years, whether your overactive thyroid is severe, and how long you have suffered from hyperthyroidism before the diagnosis was made. The size of your thyroid gland and whether you have significant eye problems are, as I explained, other factors that ought to be taken into account in making the decision.

Claire, like many Graves' disease patients having no knowledge of the condition, became confused during her first visit with the endocrinologist. She said:

I went to see this one doctor, but my first visit was not a good visit. He came in with this one little lab report and said, "Okay, you have Graves' disease. We need to start you on these pills, and you're going to take them every day." He then went on to say, "But it's not going to do any good, so we might as well forget that, and we'll go ahead and give you the radioactive iodine. Let me just go ahead and schedule that, and we'll get it done in two weeks." I didn't like that. I still didn't know what anything was. I went back to my husband's doctor and asked for another referral.

Claire had mild hyperthyroidism and a small goiter. She was treated with methimazole for one year by another endocrinologist and achieved a remission. She has been off medication for almost two years, and her thyroid function has remained normal. If she had gone ahead with the radioactive iodine treatment, she could have become immediately hypothyroid. To avoid receiving the wrong form of treatment, ask your endocrinologist for specific reasons why one option is recommended over another.

Adriana, a thirty-three-year-old accountant, suffered unnecessarily for more than a year because she did not receive the right form of treatment. By the time she was seen by an endocrinologist, she had a big goiter and had been severely hyperthyroid for about two years. She described her first encounter with the physician. "We talked about what forms of treatment were available. My understanding was that I had to start with medication to control the hyperthyroidism, and if that didn't work within a few years, I would be given radioactive iodine to destroy the gland, and if that did not work, we could resort to surgery." She left the endocrinologist's office with a prescription for PTU.

Adriana took the antithyroid medication for a year and a half but did not achieve a remission. Many patients like Adriana who have large goiters and severe hyperthyroidism at the outset do not achieve a permanent remission with medications and should be considered for more radical treatment, such as radioactive iodine, from the beginning. Adriana had to take five to six PTU pills three to four times a day and her thyroid levels rarely reached normalcy, whereas she could have been offered radioiodine treatment much sooner.

"My dosage went up and down all the time," she said. "I was adjusted so often it was like riding a roller coaster. I just felt like the physician did not understand me or how truly ill I was. There was a little improvement, but many of my symptoms persisted. It was like trying to put out a forest fire with a fire extinguisher."

If medications are chosen to treat your condition, you need to commit to taking them daily as prescribed. Otherwise, you will prolong your suffering and be more likely to experience lingering effects down the road. Agoraphobia in particular can make a person unwilling to take medications.[41] Agoraphobia is a form of anxiety disorder that may be triggered by hyperthyroidism, in which the sufferer becomes easily frightened and reluctant to leave home and face new people. If you have become agoraphobic or are experiencing other symptoms of an anxiety disorder, you are likely to do better with radioactive iodine treatment.

Many patients suffering from an overactive thyroid improve rather quickly when they are prescribed, from the outset, a beta-blocker such as propranolol (Inderal). I often prescribe propranolol at a dose of 20 to 60 mg four times a day for the first three weeks, then ask the patient to reduce the dose by half for another week or two while thyroid hormone levels are being brought down with antithyroid treatment. In Chapter 4, I explained how stress generated by thyroid imbalance can become self-perpetuating and how stress can affect the activity of Graves' disease. Reducing the stress and anxiety by using mind-body relaxation techniques is certainly effective. But you may also need to use medication to alleviate your anxiety symptoms. This will increase your chances of reaching a remission.

You need to know that whatever method is chosen, you could be disappointed. For instance, you may take medications for more than a year and find that you are not responding and have to try another method, or you may be treated with radioactive iodine and find six months or a year later that you need another radioactive iodine treatment. You must be prepared for such disappointments. Sometimes the initially chosen treatment simply does not work, and alternatives must be considered.

WORKING WITH YOUR DOCTOR TO AVOID WILD SWINGS

Whether you are being treated with medication or have received radioactive iodine treatment, fluctuations in thyroid levels can be expected. You need to work with your doctor, however, to minimize the occurrence of major, rapid swings. Major fluctuations can cause you to experience significant emotional and physical suffering, including anxiety, variations in energy level, anger, and mood swings. Emotional instability may alter your brain chemistry and make you more vulnerable to mental anguish even after your thyroid is regulated. If these fluctuations in thyroid function occur while you are being treated with medication because the dose has not been adjusted smoothly, you will typically experience frustration and despair and your symptoms will persist. Your initial hope of ending your suffering dissipates and is replaced by anger at the physician and feelings of being condemned to suffer.

To avoid major swings in your thyroid levels, make sure that you are retested six weeks after starting the medication. Then you need to be retested every two months. Each time the levels are normal during the course of treatment, I typically decrease the dosage to avoid the occurrence of hypothyroidism. This is the best way to avoid major swings in thyroid levels.

Some early studies showed that combining methimazole at a steady dose to block the thyroid gland with thyroxine to replace the deficit caused by the methimazole (called a block-replace regimen) increased the remission rate. You are given a high dose of methimazole (30 to 40 mg daily) in conjunction with thyroxine. The thyroxine dose will be adjusted to maintain normal thyroid test results. More recent studies, however, have not confirmed that the block-replace regimen leads to higher rates of remission. Although the block-replace regimen allows the maintenance of stable thyroid hormone levels throughout the course of treatment,[42] it is likely to cause more side effects from the high dose of antithyroid medication.

People treated with radioactive iodine may also suffer wild fluctuations, which can be minimized or prevented. Although many patients assume that they take the radioiodine cocktail, their gland is destroyed, and that's the end of the story, it does not happen that way. Radioactive iodine has an initial "blasting" effect on the gland, which lasts a few months, and an ongoing destructive effect, which begins at the time of treatment and could go on for years—often many years. But what complicates the matter further is that the sensitivity and vulnerability to the radioactive iodine differ from one person to another. This explains why, after treatment with radioactive iodine, the thyroid hormone levels may remain high over the following several months or may plunge to very low levels within a few weeks. Even if you become hypothyroid very quickly after the treatment, the gland may recover, and you can become hyperthyroid again, or you may stay hypothyroid. Research has shown that nearly 15 to 20 percent of people treated with radioactive iodine experience within the first six months a temporary hypothyroidism, which lasts several weeks.[43] Under these conditions, if your doctor starts you on high doses of thyroid hormone thinking that you have become permanently hypothyroid, you may easily become hyperthyroid a few weeks later when your gland has recovered some of its function.

This instability of thyroid levels for a few months after the treatment can take a toll on your physical and emotional health. I have even seen a few patients who experienced clear-cut cases of fibromyalgia following the brutal swings of their thyroid levels resulting from their treatment.

While your thyroid gland is being destroyed by radioiodine, you need to receive treatment for as long as is necessary to maintain normal or near-normal thyroid hormone levels. Hyperthyroidism could worsen for a few days after the treatment as a result of stopping the antithyroid medication. One woman who received radioactive iodine treatment said, "It was not explained that I would be more hyper- before becoming hypo-. I woke up in the middle of the night with terrible anxiety. If the doctor had just explained to me what would happen after treatment with radioactive iodine, maybe I would have felt less anxiety and emotion. I would have known why things happened."

Avoid taking high doses of antithyroid medications after radioiodine treatment. A small amount may help bring down thyroid levels while the radioiodine is working, but high amounts can add to the radioiodine's effect and make you plunge rapidly into a severely hypothyroid state. After you receive the radioactive iodine treatment, you need to be retested four weeks later so that your doctor can adjust your medication.

Treating Thyroid Imbalances During Pregnancy

I explained in Chapter 15 the importance of thyroid testing prior to conception and throughout pregnancy. This way, a potential thyroid imbalance can be detected early on, before you experience deleterious effects on your health and the baby's health. Diagnosing a thyroid imbalance, even minimal, prior to conceiving, and treating it with thyroid medication, will prevent infertility and miscarriage. It is estimated that 2 to 4 percent of women are found to be hypothyroid when tested during the first trimester of pregnancy. That being said, even if your tests are normal in the first trimester, you could become hypothyroid at any time during pregnancy. One way of predicting that you have a higher than normal chance of becoming hypothyroid during pregnancy is if you have a high antithyroid antibody level in the early stages of pregnancy. For this reason, I recommend that both TSH and antithyroid antibody levels be tested in the early stages of pregnancy. But even if you test normal, you may still become hypothyroid at a later stage of your pregnancy.

Detecting gestational hypothyroidism (occurrence of a new low-thyroid condition in pregnancy) will allow your doctor to intervene and prescribe the right amount of thyroid medication to achieve thyroid hormone balance. This is very crucial for your baby's health and for the prevention of the occurrence of potentially life-threatening conditions such as eclampsia.

If you have been diagnosed and treated with thyroid medication before becoming pregnant, I recommend that you get tested before conception. This will allow your doctor to fine-tune the dose of your medication so that your thyroid hormone levels are perfectly well balanced when you become pregnant. The best way to treat hypothyroidism during pregnancy is by using a levothyroxine medication to maximize the stability of thyroid hormone levels. However, taking a well-balanced T4/T3 combination treatment is an option. Regardless of the treatment you are receiving, I recommend that your TSH level be maintained between 0.6 and 1.7 mIU/L and that you receive frequent monitoring, every six to eight weeks. Pregnant women taking thyroid hormone for hypothyroidism often experience a significant increase in their thyroid hormone requirement, and researchers estimate that 80 percent of these women require an increase in the dose. This reflects both the increased need for thyroid hormone and the higher levels of the proteins that carry thyroid hormone in the bloodstream. Without proper thyroid balance, the pregnant hypothyroid woman has a higher chance of miscarrying or giving birth to a baby with congenital malformations.[44] Another possibility is that mental development of the fetus may be hindered, adversely affecting the baby's later intellectual growth.

When a pregnant woman is taking thyroid hormone for an underactive thyroid, she cannot rely on symptoms to signal whether her thyroid is well regulated. For this reason, periodic thyroid testing (every two months) is needed to ensure adequate thyroid levels throughout the pregnancy. Finding out that your levels are off while pregnant does not mean that they cannot be regulated quickly.

If you are pregnant and have an overactive thyroid caused by Graves' disease, you should be treated with antithyroid medications. If you were taking methimazole before becoming pregnant, your doctor might switch you to PTU because of the possibility that methimazole may cause in the fetus a rare congenital abnormality of the scalp called aplasia cutis.[45] There is considerable doubt about this complication occurring as a result of methimazole, but many doctors feel it is safer to use PTU during pregnancy. As the pregnancy progresses, the activity of Graves' disease slows down, and the dose of antithyroid medication must be gradually reduced so that thyroid hormone levels remain on the high side throughout the pregnancy. PTU crosses the placenta and can cause hypothyroidism in the fetus if the dose is too high. Frequent monitoring is highly important. I recommend that if you are pregnant and suffer from an overactive thyroid, you should be tested every month until delivery so that your thyroid levels are maintained at high normal with the lowest dose of medication. Toward the end of pregnancy, you may not need to take the medication any longer because the immune attack on the thyroid will have slowed down significantly. However, it has been estimated that approximately 70 percent of patients with Graves' disease who are in remission during pregnancy have a recurrence within the first year after delivery. To minimize the likelihood of recurrence of hyperthyroidism in the postpartum period, your doctor may advise you to continue medications at a low dose throughout pregnancy.[46]

If you have recurrence of hyperthyroidism after delivery, the medication frequently must be restarted or the dose increased to avoid high thyroid hormone levels.

Antithyroid medications are excreted in the milk, with PTU apparently present in lower amounts than methimazole. Nevertheless, research has shown that methimazole at a dose of 20 mg or less a day is safe for newborns.

Important Points to Remember

- Choose a doctor who is knowledgeable in treating thyroid disorders and who can also deal with your emotions.
- If you are diagnosed as hypothyroid, the dose of thyroid medication that you need to take initially will depend on how high your initial TSH level is.
- Optimize your thyroid hormone treatment by taking your pill before breakfast, and avoid taking it with medication that will affect its absorption.
- If you are treated for an underactive thyroid, once your thyroid tests have become normal, you need to be retested at least every six months.
- If you have an overactive thyroid, learn about the treatment options and discuss them with your doctor before making the decision. Learn about

side effects, too. No treatment is perfect. But choose a doctor who has expertise in treating Graves' disease.

- Work with your doctor to avoid major swings in thyroid hormone levels during treatment. These swings may be a bad experience for you and may cause you to suffer lingering symptoms after the imbalance is corrected.

18

CURING THE LINGERING EFFECTS
OF THYROID IMBALANCE

The negative effects of thyroid disease may not end after you have your thyroid imbalance adequately treated. You may continue to suffer annoying symptoms that can affect your quality of life, as well as long-term health consequences that can become quite serious down the road. In Chapter 22, I will detail a comprehensive program that will help you reduce or abolish these symptoms and long-term effects. In this chapter I will focus on some components of the program that will help counteract the common disturbing negative mental, cognitive, and cardiovascular consequences of thyroid disease.

If you have suffered a thyroid imbalance, your symptoms will typically resolve with adequate treatment. Sometimes, however, even after the physical and mental symptoms of hypothyroidism or hyperthyroidism have disappeared, you may still not feel like your old self. If your imbalance was severe or of long duration, moreover, you may continue to have emotional problems, anxiety, depressive symptoms, and even some residual cognitive deficits. As a result, you may not feel normal even though, technically and medically, you no longer have a thyroid imbalance.

Hyperthyroidism and hypothyroidism shake up your brain. Although you may recover completely if the imbalance is minimal and of short duration, a significant, long-term imbalance could affect your mind for a long time even after you've been properly treated. Thyroid imbalances can affect your brain chemistry in the same way as long-term abuse of alcohol or drugs! Yet your physician may not know about these lingering effects because they have not been widely publicized, discussed, or taught.

In this respect, conventional medicine has been unfair to thyroid patients with persistent symptoms. Because your doctor assesses whether you have been adequately treated for your thyroid condition by measuring blood hormone levels, he or she will look at the lab results and say, "Your thyroid test is normal; your symptoms are not due to your thyroid." Yet you may feel deep inside that your persistent suffering does have something to do with your thyroid. And you would be correct.

Imagine that your water bill has doubled in the past month and you suspect a leak in your house. You call the plumber, who inspects the pipes, sinks, and toilets. Finding no leak, the plumber says, "I can't do anything for you." But the outside pipe that runs from the meter to the house does have a leak. The plumber you called not only didn't see it but may even have believed it wasn't his or her job to deal with it. This situation is analogous to the aftereffects of thyroid disease. Often the symptoms are dismissed by the doctor treating the thyroid condition or the patient is referred to a psychiatrist because of the nature of the symptoms. Even though these symptoms are chronic, they may not fulfill the rigid criteria of mood disorders, so some patients are left further frustrated and misguided.

One of the most widely read endocrinology textbooks states, "Once thyroid hormone therapy is commenced, the recovery from the mental disturbances of hypothyroidism often lags behind the restoration of normal metabolism."[1] Typically, however, doctors fail to mention that the time lag may be quite long. This reality is haunting to the patient, family, and friends and confusing to many physicians.

From Depression to Lingering Anxiety and Stress

In hypothyroid patients, the most common residual suffering is the persistence of depression that was initially triggered by thyroid hormone deficit.[2] This kind of depression can take on a life of its own, unabated and untouched even after blood levels have returned to normal. A survey conducted in my outpatient clinic tells me that 25 percent of patients whose blood tests have become normal with thyroxine treatment have had persistent symptoms of depression. Many continue to be tired or exhausted and report that they have not returned to their "normal" selves. Hypothyroidism of long duration may also generate a situation similar to post-traumatic stress syndrome, in which the depression triggered directly or indirectly by the patient's thyroid condition affects his or her job or personal life in stressful ways that can become self-perpetuating and even overwhelming.

In some cases, the lingering depression and anxiety may remain unnoticed except for when it emerges every once in a while in response to new stresses. One patient, Rhonda, said, "After I got on a stable dose of thyroid hormone, the depression was better, but as soon as any stressors would enter into the picture, whether finances or trouble at my job, it would come back. As long as I wasn't stressed, and as long as my thyroid level was stable, I was fine."

Many patients with Graves' disease who have suffered from thyroid imbalance for quite some time without treatment become less emotionally tolerant and resilient after their overactive thyroid has been corrected than before the onset of Graves' disease. They may still feel angry and impatient, as well as depressed and anxious. Results of a survey published in the *Journal of Neuropsychiatry and Clinical Neurosciences* showed a significant persistent impairment in memory, attention, planning, and productivity in patients with Graves' disease long after their thyroid levels had become normal.[3]

Research from Sweden has shown that patients with Graves' disease have a lower quality of life fourteen to twenty-one years after they were treated for an overactive thyroid.[4] The patients had lower vitality and lower mood. The impairment of their quality of life and their mood disturbances occurred in the same way regardless of the treatment they received for their overactive thyroid. Another group of researchers in Germany showed that 35.6 percent of patients with Graves' disease who have had normal thyroid tests for more than six months after treatment of hyperthyroidism suffer from psychological distress and have high levels of anxiety, and 95.6 percent of them had clearcut depression.[5]

Why these symptoms persist is not clear. It is possible that hyperthyroidism, being a form of severe mental stress, can cause residual abnormalities in brain function, as has been shown in concentration camp survivors.[6] It is also possible that the lingering symptoms are related to brain cell damage caused by too much thyroid hormone, and this can make the patient unable to deal with stress the way he or she would without a thyroid imbalance.

Tiffany, who suffered from Graves' disease for two years prior to being diagnosed, had had stable thyroid tests for at least one year since receiving adequate thyroid hormone treatment. In a follow-up visit, she complained that she was no longer the same as she had been before her illness and was trying to find a reason for the way she was feeling:

> I got in the habit of being that way but not as bad as when I was hyperthyroid. I am more tolerant now, but I still have waves of anger. I feel like I live alone. It is quite possible that I am depressed.
>
> I have two nephews, and if I see them once a month, that's okay, and they only live six miles away from me. I never have been a big eater, but now I crave food, especially in the afternoon when I feel tense and tired. I'm generally a giving person, and now it's like I am not going to give anyone anything. Graves' disease has changed me.

Tiffany's stamina and energy levels are no longer the same as before her illness. Her case and others like hers raise many questions: Is she feeling different and low because she is missing a little T3 that her thyroid gland would normally have produced now that she is relying on T4 pills to maintain normal blood levels? Is a persistent chemical imbalance affecting her tolerance level, mood, and anger? If so, is this a residual, subtle chemical imbalance due to the flooding of brain cells by thyroid hormone when she was hyperthyroid? Or did the overwhelming effect of stress from the hyperthyroidism leave her with some form of post-traumatic stress syndrome? Or is it the immune system reactivity and its inflammation consequences related to autoimmunity that is perpetuating fatigue and lack of physical and mental wellness?

Whatever the exact cause of the depression and emotional instability that continue to haunt you, you will benefit from engaging in the mind-body program that I outline in this book and that I detail in Chapter 22, including relaxation, yoga, and exercise. By doing so, you will help yourself get over these changes, and you will help the tiredness, low coping ability, and concentration and memory impairments to subside. Tiffany's experience was typical. After a few months of following my mind-body program, her temper and tolerance level improved dramatically, while her thyroid levels stayed normal.

If your symptoms are severe, you are likely to be helped by antidepressants, such as selective serotonin reuptake inhibitors (SSRIs). In Chapter 20, you will learn how combining T4 and T3 for the treatment of your underactive thyroid may help you get rid of your lingering symptoms.

Using Mind-Body Techniques to Avoid Lingering Effects

Techniques such as meditation, music therapy, dance or movement therapy, yoga, or tai chi enhance the strength of your mind and its ability to master your body's functioning. Jon Kabat-Zinn, founder of the Stress Reduction Clinic at the University of Massachusetts Medical Center, has said, "Yoga does far more than get you relaxed and help your body to become stronger and more flexible. It is another way in which you can learn about yourself and come to experience yourself as a whole, regardless of your physical condition or level of fitness."[7] Through the mind, you can improve your overall wellness. Mind-body interventions, including relaxation, meditation, imagery, biofeedback, and hypnosis, have been used for several medical conditions.[8] I view them as efficient and practical ways to make the immune system less reactive and produce less inflammation in patients with autoimmunity. These practices will have a tremendous positive effect on your body image and self-esteem as well. They will also help your depression and may even help you with your communication skills. Mind-body techniques will improve the efficiency of other treatments and the quality of life in patients with mental suffering. They produce a physiological relaxation response that causes a release of nitric oxide, which lowers the effect of stress in our body and mind.[9] Mindful exercise (a combination of slow, graceful movements and peaceful mental imagery) is much more effective for women than for men in enhancing feelings of well-being. Choose the technique best suited to your lifestyle. For instance, because of time constraints, you may wish to combine an aerobic exercise program with music therapy.

Dr. David Brown compared the effect of an exercise-training program three times a week using moderate-intensity walking (65 to 75 percent of heart rate reserve), low-intensity walking (45 to 55 percent of heart rate reserve), low-intensity walking in conjunction with relaxation (from wearing a portable cassette player and headphones), and mindful exercise (tai chi) for forty-five minutes three times a week.[10] He showed that the use of mindfulness in conjunction with exercise has a greater effect on psychological well-being than just walking. In meditation and relaxation techniques, thoughts are structured and focused on a sound, word, prayer, or phrase. Negative thoughts are overridden by focused thinking. Such techniques are suitable for people suffering from lingering depression, anxiety, and chronic fatigue and for older people who may not be able to engage in vigorous exercise.

Tai chi, an ancient Chinese exercise, combines an aerobic type of exercise and relaxation and has done wonders for many of my patients. Tai chi will provide protection against cardiovascular disease and improve physical health. Scientific research has shown that tai chi will improve your mental health and emotional well-being and will reduce stress.[11]

If you suffer from lingering anxiety and panic attacks, meditation and biofeedback might be the solution. During biofeedback, sensors are applied to some areas of your body and connected to a device that detects and monitors body functions that are considered to be involuntary but which you can learn to control through practice.

Meditation has a major beneficial effect on your physical and psychological symptoms. It will lower anxiety, pain, and depression and will improve your self-esteem.[12] Mindfulness meditation, in conjunction with qigong movement therapy, can be of great help. It has been shown to be quite effective in the treatment of fibromyalgia.[13] Living mindfully and using meditation may be an important component in the treatment of residual effects of thyroid disease. But whether you choose biofeedback or meditation, do not forget your aerobic exercise.

For some people with other health problems that prevent them from exercising, guided imagery and art therapy can be helpful. In guided imagery, you focus on images or sensations that help you relax. Many believe that it can also enhance the strength of the immune system. It certainly helps relieve anxiety.

Self-help groups are an important mind-body resource that helps persistent sufferers cope better with their symptoms and speed up their recovery. Meeting as a group, expressing personal thoughts, and exchanging experiences with others have helped many people suffering from conditions ranging from obesity to alcoholism in which the mind, attitude, and behavior play an important role in the recovery process. These groups help you feel and see that you are not alone. I find it very helpful for thyroid patients to meet and discuss their symptoms and problems. You may also want to start practicing a mind-body technique with other patients from the group. To find out about local patient support groups, call one of the main thyroid patient organizations (see the Resources at the end of the book).

Counseling and Psychotherapy

Many thyroid patients need counseling and psychotherapy. Counseling can be designed to help you overcome your lingering suffering once thyroid tests have become normal. It may also help you resolve many of the personal and relationship issues generated by the thyroid imbalance. The inability to function as before and the relationship problems generate a feeling of loss similar to grief. You may feel that you have lost control of your life and are unable to regain the happiness that you enjoyed before the thyroid disorder. Counseling will help you come to terms with your loss and feel hopeful and optimistic about your life and your future.

Yet many doctors do not counsel their patients. Even in a primary care setting, only a third of patients suffering from depression who need counseling receive a maximum of three minutes of counseling per visit.[14] Many patients have already gone through a great deal of stress by the time they're diagnosed, and many will continue to deal with personal or job-related problems generated by the imbalance. These psychological issues need to be addressed, and a therapist can help you deal with them.

Supportive psychotherapy is needed most by patients with lingering symptoms of depression and anxiety. There are other practical methods of psychotherapy that can help. In behavioral psychotherapy, the therapist may focus on identifying what in your life is likely to trigger your symptoms. The aim is to help you understand and change the way you react to situations. In cognitive therapy, the therapist looks for patterns of thinking that are likely to cause symptoms. These methods do not address your unconscious conflicts, but they are aimed at correcting your symptoms. The therapy will help you regain your emotional balance, cope better with the stress, and strengthen your defense mechanisms so that you regain control. Behavioral/cognitive psychotherapy has been shown to be as effective as medication in the treatment of mild depression and anxiety disorder.[15] I find behavioral/cognitive psychotherapy extremely helpful for thyroid patients with residual symptoms, even when their thyroid imbalance has been properly treated.

You may also need marital or couples therapy. Ask for a referral from your primary care physician or endocrinologist, who will probably know of a few competent therapists who have developed a great deal of experience dealing with marital issues. The couples therapist may be a psychiatrist, a psychologist, or a psychiatric social worker.

Finally, psychodynamic psychotherapy, which focuses on addressing unconscious conflicts and resolving the root of psychological conflicts, may be necessary for patients whose thyroid imbalance unmasks deep-rooted psychological issues or who have psychological issues independent of the thyroid imbalance. Psychodynamic psychotherapy can be an expensive and protracted type of treatment, but it is the only way to address deeply rooted psychological problems.

Selecting the Right Antidepressant

If your residual emotional symptoms are overwhelming and you have not been able to break the vicious cycle of depression, stress, and anxiety while you are taking the right amount of L-thyroxine, you are likely to improve if you change your treatment to a combination of T4 and T3 (for details, see Chapter 20). However, that may not be enough, and you may benefit from taking an antidepressant. When you use an antidepressant, you need to educate yourself about its most common side effects and how often they occur. You also need to know that it takes time for an antidepressant to begin working. Many need at least six to eight weeks to elevate mood.

The currently available antidepressants include SSRIs, SNRIs, atypical antidepressants, tricyclic antidepressants, and monoamine oxidase inhibitors (MAOIs). Generally speaking, the most currently prescribed antidepressants are the SSRIs, the SNRIs, and the atypical antidepressants because of their effectiveness and also because of their lower adverse-effects profile. The accompanying table lists the most commonly prescribed antidepressants.

COMMONLY PRESCRIBED ANTIDEPRESSANTS

Drug	Trade Name	Common Side Effects
SELECTIVE SEROTONIN REUPTAKE INHIBITORS (SSRIs)		
Fluoxetine	Prozac, Sarafem	Drowsiness, headaches,
Sertraline	Zoloft	nervousness, insomnia, fatigue,
Citalopram	Celexa	sexual problems, sweating,
Escitalopram	Lexapro	weight changes, nausea, diarrhea
Fluvoxamine	Luvox	
Paroxetine	Paxil, Pexeva	
Vortioxetine	Brintellix	
Vilazodone	Viibryd	

Drug	Trade Name	Common Side Effects

SELECTIVE NOREPINEPHRINE REUPTAKE INHIBITORS (SNRIs)

Drug	Trade Name	Common Side Effects
Reboxetine	Edronax	Dry mouth, constipation, insomnia, sweating, tachycardia, urinary retention, dizziness
Atomoxetine	Strattera	Dizziness, dyspepsia, nausea,
Levomilnacipran	Fetzima	vomiting, decreased appetite
Desvenlafaxine	Pristiq	

SELECTIVE SEROTONIN REUPTAKE INHIBITORS AND SELECTIVE NOREPINEPHRINE REUPTAKE INHIBITORS (SSRIs + SNRIs)

Drug	Trade Name	Common Side Effects
Venlafaxine	Effexor	Drowsiness, dizziness, nausea,
Duloxetine	Cymbalta	appetite changes, constipation, dry mouth, insomnia, nervousness, sweating, change in blood pressure, muscle weakness

NOREPINEPHRINE-DOPAMINE REUPTAKE INHIBITOR

Drug	Trade Name	Common Side Effects
Bupropion	Wellbutrin, Aplenzin	Agitation, anxiety, insomnia, weight loss, nausea, dry mouth, sweating, seizures

TRICYCLIC ANTIDEPRESSANTS

Drug	Trade Name	Common Side Effects
Amitriptyline	Elavil, Endep	Drowsiness, dizziness, dry
Doxepin	Sinequan, Adapin	mouth, blurred vision,
Imipramine	Tofranil	constipation, urinary retention,
Nortriptyline	Pamelor, Aventyl	changes in sexual function,
Desipramine	Norpramin	increased heart rate, headache,
Clomipramine	Anafranil	low blood pressure, sensitivity to
Protriptyline	Vivactil, Triptil	sunlight, increased appetite,
Trimipramine	Surmontil, Rhotrimine	weight gain, nausea, weakness
Amoxapine	Asendin	

MONOAMINE OXIDASE INHIBITORS (MAOIs)

Drug	Trade Name	Common Side Effects
Phenelzine	Nardil	Drowsiness, dizziness, fatigue,
Tranylcypromine	Parnate	nausea, bowel habit changes, dry
Selegiline	Emsam	mouth, light-headedness, low
Isocarboxazid	Marplan	blood pressure, changes in sexual function, sleep disturbances, tremor, decreased urine output, weight gain, blurred vision, headache, increased appetite, sweating

Drug	Trade Name	Common Side Effects
ATYPICAL ANTIDEPRESSANTS		
Maprotiline	Ludiomll	Drowsiness, nausea, lethargy, anxiety, insomnia, nightmares, dry mouth, skin sensitivity, weight and/or appetite change
Trazodone	Desyrel, Oleptro	Drowsiness, dizziness, dry mouth, blurred vision, headache, nausea/vomiting
Mirtazapine	Remeron	Drowsiness, dizziness, seizures, mouth sores, dry mouth, sore throat, chills, fever, constipation, increased appetite, weight gain
Nefazodone	Serzone	Drowsiness, dizziness, vision
Lurasidone	Latuda	changes, clumsiness, light-headedness, itching, nightmares, agitation, confusion, constipation, diarrhea, dry mouth, flushing, headache, increased appetite, nausea, vomiting, edema, tremor, insomnia

Scientific studies have not yet compared the efficacy of the various antidepressants after blood levels of thyroid hormones have become normal with treatment. However, I typically use an SSRI first because side effects are less common with this class of antidepressants. The SSRIs have become the first choice to treat many forms of depression. These medications not only help with depression but can also be effective in obsessive-compulsive disorders. Even if you are not depressed but suffer from persistent emotional instability after correction of your thyroid imbalance, you will benefit from taking a small dose of an SSRI. The most troubling side effects of SSRI therapy are sexual dysfunction, weight gain, and sleep disturbances. Other side effects that will subside within two weeks are nausea and headaches. Nausea can be avoided by taking the medication with food. The most commonly used SSRIs include fluoxetine (Prozac), sertraline (Zoloft), and paroxetine (Paxil). However, in recent years, the newer SSRI escitalopram (Lexapro) has become quite popular. Escitalopram is the most selective of the selective serotonin reuptake inhibitors. It is more effective than the other SSRIs and its adverse effects are less common.[16] Escitalopram also starts working faster than other antidepressants.[17] If your depressive symptoms have completely resolved and you keep taking it, it will help prevent a recurrence of the depression. Escitalopram is also effective in treating generalized anxiety disorder. One of the advantages of escitalopram is that it causes fewer sexual side effects than the other SSRIs. Research has shown that 68.1 percent of patients who suffer from a sexual dysfunction when treated with an SSRI have an improvement in their sexual function when switched to escitalopram.[18]

Paroxetine is unique among the SSRIs because it also works on noradrenaline. It is quite effective in treating panic attacks, but the long-term results are better if you continue treatment for at least a year. The drawback of paroxetine is that it causes weight gain, sexual dysfunction, and difficulty reaching an orgasm in women. Paroxetine can also cause gastrointestinal side effects, irritability, headaches, and eating and sleeping problems.

Serotonin-norepinephrine reuptake inhibitors are increasingly favored over the SSRIs to treat a wide range of symptoms. The current trend, in fact, is to use SNRIs as a first-line treatment for depression simply because they are more effective on both the mental and physical symptoms of depression, including pain. The class of serotonin-norepinephrine reuptake inhibitors includes venlafaxine and duloxetine. These medications block the reuptake of both serotonin and norepinephrine. Research has shown that SNRIs are as effective as the SSRIs in treating anxiety disorders.[19]

Venlafaxine may work if one of the SSRIs has failed to give you the response expected. It might also work faster than the other antidepressants. Venlafaxine is certainly not my favorite antidepressant, as it causes adverse effects such as nausea, high blood pressure, sexual dysfunction, and withdrawal issues more often than duloxetine. You may experience withdrawal symptoms within hours of stopping or reducing the usual dose of venlafaxine. The problem is that this can affect your motor and coordination skills and cause you to have serious accidents. If you take venlafaxine, you need to adhere to a strict medication routine or not drive a car.

The extended-release form of venlafaxine (Effexor XR) is more effective and safer than the standard form of the drug. It is quite effective in the treatment of anxiety disorders, including social anxiety disorder, generalized anxiety disorder, post-traumatic stress syndrome, panic disorder, and obsessive-compulsive disorder.

Duloxetine in general is tolerated better and does not cause adverse cardiovascular effects. At a dose of 60 mg a day, it is effective in the treatment of major depression. The side effects are by and large mild, with minor adverse effects comparable to the other antidepressants.[20] Duloxetine also helps with pain and is effective in treating panic disorders.

Bupropion is another popular antidepressant. It has recently received much media attention for its usefulness in helping people stop smoking. This antidepressant increases your energy but can promote agitation, anxiety, insomnia, headaches, and, rarely, seizures. If you have a history of seizing, do not take bupropion. In August 2003, bupropion became available in the form of a once-daily extended-release medication, which makes it more practical to take than the older twice or three times daily dosing.[21] Bupropion inhibits reuptake of norepinephrine and dopamine neurotransmission and does not affect serotonin. Bupropion is an effective long-term antidepressant. Among all the antidepressants, bupropion has the lowest incidence of sexual dysfunction, weight gain, and sleepiness. It can be used in conjunction with other antidepressants.

The two antidepressants that work on your adrenergic system are atomoxetine and reboxetine. Atomoxetine (Strattera) has an antidepressant activity and works on the neurotransmitter noradrenaline. Research in children, adolescents, and adults has shown that atomoxetine is safe and well tolerated for the treatment of attention deficit hyperactivity disorder.[22]

Reboxetine is a selective noradrenaline reuptake inhibitor. It is an effective and safe form of treatment in patients with depression who have not responded to SSRIs.[23] Reboxetine is more effective at relieving anxiety, a symptom mediated by the noradrenergic system. Reboxetine also improves social adjustment. If you are treated with an SSRI and have not seen positive results, switching abruptly to reboxetine is usually well tolerated.

The atypical antidepressants are a group of medications that affect different combinations of neurotransmitters. In general, doctors turn to them if SSRIs are not effective. Trazodone and nefazodone are useful if the patient is suffering from insomnia. The insomnia can be effectively treated with doses smaller than the dose that would be needed to treat depression. A small dose of one of these two medications makes an SSRI work better.

Mirtazapine is a noradrenergic and specific serotoninergic antidepressant. It works well on anxiety symptoms and helps you with your sleep disturbances. It also prevents sexual dysfunction that frequently occurs with the use of SSRIs. I have found no use for mirtazapine in thyroid patients. It has potent appetite-promoting effects and often causes weight gain. Other side effects of mirtazapine are sedation, dizziness, dry mouth, and constipation.

In case the SSRIs, SNRIs, or atypical antidepressants do not work or you have had an adverse reaction to them, the next course of action would be a tricyclic antidepressant, such as amitriptyline or nortriptyline. Tricyclics are effective in treating depression and controlling panic attacks. Amitriptyline is quite effective in acute post-traumatic stress syndrome. If you are suffering from agitation and loss of appetite, doxepin will help. If you are sleeping too much, desipramine will have a stimulating effect. The most common side effects of tricyclics are weight gain, sedation, dry mouth, sexual problems, constipation, sensitivity to the sun, urinary retention, blurry vision, heartbeat problems, and dizziness when you stand up or sit down.

Nowadays tricyclic antidepressants have largely fallen by the wayside because they may cause many side effects. I have found that tricyclic antidepressants are most useful for the patient who has problems sleeping at night (often a patient with Graves' disease) and lingering depression with significant anxiety symptoms. Tricyclic antidepressants can be used instead of SSRIs during pregnancy and in the postpartum period when a woman is breast-feeding.[24]

Doctors now generally view monoamine oxidase inhibitors (MAOIs) as the last drugs to be considered for treating depression, although they can be helpful in atypical depression. Even though MAOIs are quite potent at alleviating depression, they are troublesome to work with, sometimes causing side effects such as sleep problems, high blood pressure, sexual problems, and weight gain. If you are taking an MAOI, you need to watch your diet and avoid eating many common foods, such as cheese and chocolate, that contain the chemical tyramine. The combination can trigger severe high blood pressure and other serious health problems.

Taking a monoamine oxidase inhibitor together with another antidepressant may cause "serotonin syndrome," characterized by agitation, diarrhea, involuntary muscle movements and muscle rigidity, trembling, high temperature, high blood pressure, and even seizures and coma.[25] Taking L-tryptophan or a tryptophan substitute in conjunction with an SSRI may lead to serotonin syndrome. Serotonin syndrome is due to very high serotonin activity in the brain stem and can be caused by the use of one or more serotoninergic drugs.

Lithium carbonate is a potent antidepressant used more commonly in bipolar disorders, especially manic-depression. For patients who do not respond to an SSRI or a tricyclic, some doctors add lithium to enhance the efficacy of the antidepressant. While taking lithium, you need to have your blood levels monitored to avoid toxic effects such as diabetes insipidus (which causes increased urination), high calcium levels, and kidney problems.

If in addition to depression you suffer from anxiety and insomnia, you should perhaps take medications that target these symptoms. This way, you will have a sense of well-being that will encourage you to continue the treatment. The SSRIs have become the medications of choice for anxiety disorders, though benzodiazepines, which work on the GABA system, are still widely used.[26] Because you may become addicted to benzodiazepines, you should use them only if an SSRI or SNRI has not cured your symptoms. You may, however, need a combination of an SSRI and a benzodiazepine, which is an effective and practical way of treating most anxiety disorders. The most commonly used benzodiazepines are Valium, Librium, Xanax, and Ativan. BuSpar, a nonbenzodiazepine antianxiety medication, is also quite effective. Adverse effects of antianxiety medications include sedation and lack of coordination.

In general, once you are started on an antidepressant, the treatment is continued for at least six months and, if necessary, extended for up to one to two years. Depression can come back even if you are taking an antidepressant medication, including all of the ones I've discussed here.

Less than half of patients suffering from major depression have complete resolution of symptoms when they take an antidepressant.[27] If you have improved significantly but continue to have residual symptoms or if you feel that you have issues with social adjustment or you are not fully functional, you remain at risk for having a recurrence of full-blown depression in the future. For this reason, you may need to both address the psychosocial issues that could have perpetuated your depression and discuss with your doctor the option of changing the antidepressant that you are currently taking or adding another antidepressant. When you combine antidepressants, these medications have a higher chance of achieving full results if the medications work on different neurotransmitter systems. Improving the serotonin and noradrenergic systems will give you the most benefit. This will speed up the response and help you be depression-free in the long haul. Popular combinations prescribed by psychiatrists are an SSRI with bupropion, an SNRI with an SSRI, an SSRI with a tricyclic, and the triad of bupropion, venlafaxine, and mirtazapine.

Even if your symptoms of depression have resolved, you may continue to suffer from fatigue. Research has shown that three out of four depressed patients who have responded to antidepressant treatment continue to suffer from fatigue.[28] Fatigue is one of the most disturbing residual symptoms of depression. It has to do with an imbalance of serotonin in certain areas of the brain. This imbalance can be counteracted by a medication that enhances dopamine, such as bupropion. It can also be corrected by graded aerobic exercise. To improve the residual fatigue, you could use cognitive interventions. Modafinil (Provigil) has also been shown to be effective in improving residual fatigue. As your energy improves, so will your cognition.

Herbs and Supplements for Lingering Symptoms

Tryptophan was used as a dietary supplement for a long time until it was banned in the United States in 1989 as a result of an outbreak of eosinophilia myalgia syndrome, which was related to the contamination of synthetic L-tryptophan from one manufacturer. It is now back on the market. L-tryptophan, which is a precursor for serotonin, has been marketed as an antidepressant in several countries. Research has shown that L-tryptophan supplementation in women improves mood and emotion as serotonin antidepressants do.[29] You may get tryptophan from deoiled gourd seed. One gram of protein derived from deoiled gourd seed contains 22 mg of tryptophan.[30] If you suffer from insomnia, tryptophan will help you sleep better. After the removal of L-tryptophan from the market in the United States, 5-hydroxy-tryptophan became a quite popular supplement, and no toxicity has been reported.[31] This supplement enhances serotonin in the brain and improves depression. It also promotes the secretion of melatonin.

You can also improve your anxiety symptoms and stress-related symptoms by taking the supplement glutamic acid, which regulates GABA. But too much of it can make you eat more, as mentioned in Chapter 10. Medications that enhance glutamic acid in the brain are useful to treat anxiety, obsessive-compulsive disorder, post-traumatic stress syndrome, generalized anxiety disorder, and social phobia.[32]

Quercetin, which is one of the major flavonoids in fruits and vegetables, has a great antioxidant effect. Quercetin also helps protect brain cells from free radicals and is highly recommended in thyroid patients.[33] I often recommend two herbal ingredients to improve thyroid patients' quality of life: *Rhodiola rosea* and spirulina. These are included in the thyroid supplement ThyroLife Optima.

Rhodiola rosea, or rose root, is a plant used in traditional medical systems in Eastern Europe and Asia. It has an enhancing effect on the nervous system, decreases depression, enhances your energy, and improves work performance.[34] Researchers call it an adaptogen because of its ability to increase resistance to physical, chemical, and biological stress. It is claimed to help prevent cancer and to protect against heart disease. *Rhodiola rosea* increases your ability to concentrate and it enhances your mental and physical power. *Rhodiola rosea* affects the hypothalamic-pituitary-adrenal system, the system that plays an important role in the reaction of the body to stress.[35] This herb typically provokes no adverse effects, and if you use it for a long time you will not become addicted to it.

Spirulina (blue-green algae) too has antioxidant properties that will help your thyroid condition. Experimental research has shown that spirulina effectively treats certain allergies, hyperglycemia, and high cholesterol. It helps the immune system and reduces inflammation. A diet rich in spirulina has been shown to reduce the degenerative changes in the brain of animals as they age.[36]

Saint-John's-wort improves depressive symptoms and works well in thyroid patients with lingering symptoms of low-grade depression.

Although we know little about the various constituents of many herbal products and their potential beneficial or detrimental effects on the thyroid, you ought to be aware that there could be such effects. For instance, the popular culinary herb thyme contains an essential oil that may reduce thyroid activity.[37] Thyme oil is found in mouthwashes and decongestants and used to treat tiredness, depression, digestion problems, and muscle aches and pains. A 1985 study of freeze-dried extracts of the common relaxant herb lemon balm (*Melissa officinalis*), which is used to treat viral infections, documented potential thyroid-related effects.[38] The extracts were shown to diminish the activity of thyroid-stimulating immunoglobulin, the antibody that causes overactive thyroid in Graves' disease.

More research is needed to determine which plant compounds affect the thyroid and whether plants might directly provide significant amounts of thyroid hormone, but in the meantime, if you are using herbs, do not abuse them. Many of their effects and side effects remain to be discovered.

The Persistent Cognitive Effects of Thyroid Imbalance

"I feel as if my brain aged by ten years," Cheryl told me during her first visit to my office. Cheryl, age forty-seven, suffered from an overactive thyroid that was undiagnosed for almost two years. After receiving radioactive iodine treatment, she became hypothyroid and was prescribed an adequate amount of thyroxine by her former endocrinologist. Although she maintained normal blood test results, she had continued to struggle with some impairment of her intellectual and cognitive abilities.

"My most significant problem," she went on to say, "is that I am unable to concentrate, even on trivial matters. It seems like I cannot process information and act on it as I used to. I forget words, or they elude me in a conversation. I would go into a room and not remember why I went in there. It would take me a few minutes, then I would sometimes remember."

A severe thyroid imbalance may cause a significant impairment in cognitive function, particularly memory and the ability to concentrate and to register and process incoming information. After the thyroid imbalance is corrected, these impairments often subside and treatment halts their progression. Some patients who experience a thyroid imbalance, however, continue to have a deficit in cognitive function after the thyroid imbalance is treated and corrected. The impairment of these functions may be more profound when the patient is afflicted at a young age.

In some patients, the cognitive deficit associated with prolonged and severe hypothyroidism may be more permanent with regard to memory and temporary with regard to general intelligence and concentration. Treatment also typically stops the progression of memory impairment, but if the thyroid hormone deficit remains untreated, cognitive impairment may worsen with time. Research has suggested that hypothyroidism could cause a direct and perhaps irreversible effect on brain structures, causing the memory impairment,[39] while other brain functions that rely on adequate amounts of neurotransmitters may be restored to normal.

Occasionally, patients previously treated for an overactive thyroid experience significant residual intellectual difficulty that impairs their ability to work. Dr. Hans Perrild, studying neuropsychological function in patients with a previous history of hyperthyroidism, found among his patients four who were granted disability because of a significant reduction in their ability to perform any work.[40] One study showed that patients whose thyroid function had been restored to normal and who were in remission were found to experience impaired cognitive functions more frequently than normal and more frequently than before they got sick,[41] even two and a half years after their last hyperthyroid episode. This suggests that people who are afflicted with hyperthyroidism that has lingered for some time may not be the same even ten years after correction of the imbalance.

Impairment in cognitive abilities due to hypothyroidism may range from minimal (detected only by standardized neuropsychological testing) to quite significant (noticeable to the person and close family or friends). In extreme cases, when brain structures are significantly affected by the thyroid hormone deficit, the impairment can even progress to dementia, particularly in older people.

How Thyroid Imbalance Causes Damage to the Brain: The Link with Aging

In a sense, Cheryl was correct to compare her suffering to an accelerated aging of her brain. As you get older, you become apt to suffer impaired cognition. You may have difficulty remembering names, keeping several things in mind at the same time, and processing information. You may have difficulty finding words, or you may slowly lose the ability to grasp details of what is going on around you.

Why do many people like Cheryl, after a severe thyroid imbalance, experience a deterioration of their cognitive abilities similar to what older people might experience over an extended period of time? Can untreated hypothyroidism lead to irreversible dementia? And does normal aging worsen the deterioration of your cognitive abilities if you experienced a long-lasting and significant thyroid imbalance? Recent advances in medical research in this field are revealing the answers to these questions. Research is also suggesting what we should do to improve intellectual faculties and prevent further age-related deterioration of the brain.

Thyroid imbalance of some duration can damage the brain in the same way aging does. With increasing age, the brain becomes more subjected to the adverse effects of free radicals, the toxic oxygenated compounds released during metabolism. These radicals gradually damage major components of the brain, including myelin, a protective layer (composed of protein and fat) that surrounds some types of nerve fibers and increases the efficiency of nerve transmission. Myelin in the brain is sensitive to the damaging effects of free radicals and becomes damaged by the buildup of free radicals.[42]

In patients with dementia, including Alzheimer's disease, homocysteine levels are high because of deficiency in antioxidants such as the essential polyunsaturated fatty acids, vitamin B_{12}, and folate. Homocysteine causes damage to the protective layer of cells in blood vessels and causes damage to the brain cells.[43]

Once myelin has been damaged by free radicals, it becomes more vulnerable to further damage as we get older. Scientists now know that damage to myelin is one of the most important factors that accelerate the aging of the human brain.

Thyroid imbalance can increase your risk of impaired cognition as you become older because it has the same ability as aging to damage areas of the brain that are essential for normal cognition.[44] When your thyroid gland is overactive, oxygen consumption increases, and the number of free radicals overwhelms the cells' ability to clear them from the body. With aging, the machinery in cells that is designed to clear these "bad guys" becomes less efficient. In essence, the oxidative stress resulting from too much thyroid hormone causes damage to our brain similar to aging. Long-standing hypothyroidism also has a damaging effect on many brain structures simply because thyroid hormone is essential for maintaining healthy brain cells. In fact, the development of these brain structures in the critical period of rapid growth during the fetal stage and immediately following birth also depends on normal thyroid levels.[45] During this time, thyroid hormone is essential for adequate formation of myelin. This explains why infants with congenital hypothyroidism suffer severe neurological problems and mental impairment.

How to Prevent and Cure Residual Cognitive Impairment

When Cheryl came to me with impaired cognition after a significant thyroid imbalance, she was more frightened than most such patients. Her mother and maternal aunt had just been diagnosed with Alzheimer's disease. She had learned that Alzheimer's disease runs in families and that she could become a victim of this condition in the future. But the health program that Cheryl now follows—which includes a well-balanced diet, antioxidant supplementation, hormone treatment, and control of her blood pressure—not only helped her recover from some of the cognitive deficits she endured but also will slow down the anticipated deterioration brought on by aging. Furthermore, it will help prevent Alzheimer's disease or slow it down if she becomes afflicted by it.

All of us should practice preventive measures to preserve a healthy, functioning brain and try to prevent the decline in cognitive abilities that occurs with aging. But if you have experienced a significant imbalance that left some residual deficits, you need to be more vigilant.

If you are predisposed to Alzheimer's disease or have a medical condition that could cause damage to your brain, a prolonged deprivation of thyroid hormone may accelerate dementia. Even if the damage caused by hypothyroidism is not severe, it may represent a setback. It will make you more vulnerable to developing dementia later in life. Long-standing depression and stress also cause deterioration of cognition.

Several measures are now recognized to help prevent further deterioration of brain function. The first step is to pay more attention to the many lifestyle factors that can affect your brain function. Supplementing your diet with adequate amounts of antioxidants and omega-3 fatty acids is one of the most important measures. Vitamin C, zinc, and vitamin E could prevent the damage and loss of brain cells due to the buildup of free radicals. Phosphatidylserine, a phospholipid, improves the communication between brain cells. It is a safe supplement that improves cognitive function.[46] You can safely take 400 mg a day in divided doses. Phosphatidylserine comes from several sources, including soy foods. (See Chapter 22 for more on antioxidants.)

You also need to reduce your risk of cerebrovascular disease and strokes, which are known to accelerate the dementia process. Atherosclerosis, or hardening of the arteries, typically increases with age. When this process affects the arteries in the brain, it can lead to poor blood supply, strokes, and ultimately loss of brain cells. Hardening of the arteries of the brain is a major factor in impairment of cognition and even dementia in older persons. Researchers have found that more than 50 percent of patients older than eighty-five had hardening of the arteries in the brain.[47] It is likely that many people with dementia, including those with Alzheimer's disease, have atherosclerosis as a contributing factor to their dementia.

If you suffer from a thyroid condition, you should control the vascular risks that could predispose you to hardening of the arteries and poor blood supply to the brain. To achieve this, you need to exercise and take antioxidant multivitamin supplements containing folate and vitamins B_6 and B_{12}. Controlling your blood pressure is essential. High blood pressure can damage blood vessels of the brain, heart, and kidneys. The longer your blood pressure stays high, the more damage it can cause. One study showed that patients already suffering from vascular dementia who received a treatment that lowered their blood pressure to an acceptable range experienced either an improvement in their cognitive deficit or a delay in the worsening of their dementia.[48] Research has also linked cardiovascular risk to accumulation of the amino acid homocysteine.[49] The B-complex vitamins just mentioned will help reduce the accumulation of homocysteine and lower your risk of having low brain blood flow.

You also need to lower your cholesterol and triglycerides by diet and medication if necessary. High LDL (bad) cholesterol is an important risk factor for cardiovascular disease in both men and women. Raise your HDL (good) cholesterol to more than 60 mg/dL by eating less fat and less cholesterol and by exercising. Lower your triglycerides by eating less sugar. Avoid alcohol if you have high triglyceride levels. Do not lower your cholesterol too much, however. Very low cholesterol can reduce brain serotonin, thereby causing depression and aggressive behavior. It can damage brain cells and cause impaired cognition as well. Try to keep your total cholesterol less than 200 mg/dL for the vascular benefit. However, do not have your cholesterol lowered excessively to avoid low mood and impaired cognition.

Several common health problems can act alone or in concert with others to precipitate or contribute to the development of cardiovascular disease (see the following list). Long-standing untreated hypothyroidism is one of these factors. Hypothyroidism can raise blood pressure, increase LDL cholesterol and even triglycerides, and lead to excess weight and thus a sedentary lifestyle. Even low-grade hypothyroidism has recently been shown to elevate LDL cholesterol. In Great Britain in the early 1970s, research already showed that people with Hashimoto's thyroiditis had a higher rate of cardiovascular disease even after exclusion of other risk factors, such as weight, high blood pressure, and high cholesterol.[50] Nowadays, it has become established that thyroid disease should be viewed as an important risk factor for cardiovascular disease. The reasons for this are the thyroid imbalance and the body inflammation related to immune system reactivity. Because of the high frequency of Hashimoto's thyroiditis and low-grade hypothyroidism in menopausal women, it is likely that thyroid disease contributes to the increase in frequency of coronary artery disease among menopausal women.

RISK FACTORS FOR CARDIOVASCULAR DISEASE
- High blood pressure
- High blood levels of cholesterol and triglycerides
- Smoking
- Diabetes
- Long-standing hypothyroidism
- Excess weight
- History of heart disease in other family members
- Sedentary lifestyle
- Metabolic syndrome
- High insulin/insulin resistance
- Menopause

For people who suffer from a thyroid imbalance and possible damages from its consequences, it is essential to pay serious attention to the other additive risk factors.

High insulin levels can result from eating too much refined sugar and from developing insulin resistance. This occurs in people who are capable of producing insulin but whose organs do not respond well to insulin, causing the hormone to work less efficiently. High insulin levels increase the vascular risk. They also promote the retention of salt in the body and cause narrowing of the arteries in organs. Because insulin does not work efficiently, patients with metabolic syndrome and insulin resistance have a tendency to develop diabetes; they also have hypertension and high fat levels in their bloodstream. The key here is to lose weight and to follow an eating plan low in simple sugars, animal fat, and dairy fat, and high in fiber (see Chapter 21). Vegetable oils such as olive, sunflower, and safflower should always be included in your diet.

The Mental Benefits of Estrogens

Serotonin is one of the brain chemicals that regulates mood and emotion. It also interacts with physiological functions, much like a hormone does. In women, constantly changing estrogen levels during the menstrual cycle cause serotonin levels to change as well. This explains how changes in estrogen levels can cause headaches, dizziness, and nausea, which are known to be effects of serotonin. Estrogens also combine with serotonin to affect bone density, vascular functions, and even the way the immune system works.[51]

In Chapter 14, I discussed the benefits of hormone replacement therapy in menopausal women and some of the controversies pertaining to the risks associated with the use of estrogen-progesterone treatment after menopause. Not as widely publicized, however, are estrogen's beneficial effects on mood and cognition. Scientific evidence for the use of estrogen not only to prevent impaired cognition but also to prevent and treat dementia is expanding. The loss of estrogen that occurs at menopause could be an important factor in the brain damage of Alzheimer's disease. Research suggests that estrogen has a protective effect in relation to Alzheimer's disease, reducing the risk by 29–44 percent.[52] Estrogens minimize the decline of cognitive functions, including the memory loss that tends to occur with aging. This has been shown only in younger postmenopausal women; however, if you are sixty-five or older, estrogens may promote dementia, according to the Women's Health Initiative Memory Study.[53]

Lack of estrogen after menopause is perhaps one of the reasons why dementia affects two to three times more women than men. Estrogen replacement improves several cognitive abilities of postmenopausal women not suffering from dementia—in particular, skills pertaining to verbal memory.[54] Estrogens stimulate brain cells to produce more of the neurotransmitter acetylcholine, which plays an important role in memory and cognition. Blood flow tends to decline after menopause, and estrogen replacement increases the blood flow in certain regions of the brain responsible for cognitive abilities. Estrogen treatment in postmenopausal women has a tempering effect on stress. A woman who takes estrogen produces less cortisol in response to stress and is therefore subjected to fewer of the deleterious effects of cortisol on brain cells and memory. During menopause, the effect of stress on the activation of your autonomic nervous system becomes more significant and bothersome, and estrogen attenuates the physical symptoms that occur as a result of the response of your autonomic nervous system.

Perimenopause is undoubtedly a transition period when you become at greater risk for depression. As you are becoming menopausal, your brain neurotransmitters change and will make you more vulnerable to depression and also to symptoms of menopause. If your depression is minor, estrogen may be all it takes to treat your depressive symptoms.[55] Research has shown that in menopausal women suffering from depression, the use of transdermal estrogen in conjunction with an antidepressant makes the antidepressant work much faster and more effectively.[56]

In young postmenopausal women, estrogen reduces anxiety and depression. It does so by increasing serotonin levels. Women who suffer from even minute thyroid hormone deficits in brain cells risk a worsening of depression by not taking estrogen. The lingering effects of thyroid imbalance in postmenopausal women may not go away unless your doctor implements a well-balanced sex hormone regimen. Thyroid hormone treatment by itself may not resolve the depression. Only when estrogens are added is the depression improved. In some women, adding a small amount of testosterone helps to improve both cognition and mood.[57]

The Circle of Wellness

The "Circle of Wellness" that I provide to my patients is a model that anyone can use to minimize cognitive deterioration with aging and to achieve and maintain optimal physical and mental wellness (see illustration, page 328). Patients suffering from thyroid imbalance should recognize the importance of early diagnosis to minimize any permanent residual damage to cognition. They should also make sure their thyroid remains in balance throughout their lives. Even that may not be enough. If a significant blow to the brain has occurred as a result of the imbalance, people should do everything they can to minimize other deleterious effects on the brain.

What some of my patients like Cheryl now know is that they need to take steps to preserve healthy brain structures as much as possible for the years to come. By failing to do so, they will place themselves at a much higher risk for further deterioration of their cognitive ability and possibly even dementia.

It is crucial for people afflicted with a thyroid condition to understand

CIRCLE OF WELLNESS FOR THYROID PATIENTS

Start:
Get diagnosed early.

For postmenopausal women, take
estrogen replacement therapy to:
• Improve cognition
• Prevent dementia
• Improve mood

Correct the imbalance promptly:
avoid a treatment roller coaster.

Avoid too much or too
little iodine, which causes
changes in thyroid function.

Maintain thyroid balance:
TSH = 0.5–2 mIU/L

Avoid lingering depression
and stress through:
• Stress management
• T4/T3 protocol
• Course of antidepressant
  if needed
• Counseling and
  psychotherapy

Take antioxidants and essential
free fatty acids to:
• Help thyroid hormone
  work efficiently
• Protect yourself from age-
  related brain damage
• Reduce autoimmune
  reactions and immune system
  reactivity
• Speed up your metabolism

Get support and understanding:
• From family
• From friends
• At work

Control blood pressure:
high blood pressure causes
vascular disease and
accelerates cognitive
impairment.

Control weight through:
• Mindful exercise
• Low-fat/high-protein,
  low-glycemic,
  high-fiber diet

Control cholesterol levels:
• High cholesterol causes vascular
  disease.
• Too-low cholesterol impairs
  cognition and causes depression,
  suicide, and violence.

that the more a thyroid imbalance alters brain function, the greater their chances of having some residual effects, such as not feeling as well as before. Fight these residual effects using my mind-body program, which can help you alleviate some of the emotional effects. The Circle of Wellness depicted above is an important component of the program.

Important Points to Remember

- If you've been successfully treated for a thyroid imbalance but have continued to be emotional, moody, tired, or exhausted, or have continued to have achy feelings throughout your body or other symptoms of an underactive thyroid, you are not alone! It is just the aftermath of the effects of the imbalance on your brain chemistry.
- To fight these symptoms, use mind-body techniques and aerobic exercise, maintain thyroid balance, and if necessary, use T4/T3 combination treatment and an antidepressant.
- The damaging effects of a severe thyroid imbalance on your brain may lead to impaired cognition and memory problems that resemble the effects of aging. You need to pay attention to your lifestyle, take antioxidants, lower your cholesterol, control your blood pressure, and avoid simple sugars.
- Pay attention to sex hormones if you are postmenopausal, and consider small amounts of androgens to improve your mood and cognition. You need progesterone if you have a uterus.

19

LIVING WITH
THYROID EYE DISEASE

Thyroid eye disease, formerly known as Graves' eye disease, is one of the most dreaded thyroid-related conditions because of its potential emotional, personal, and professional effects on a person's life. In the minds of many people, having Graves' disease is associated with having bulgy eyes. I should note, however, that at the most half of those with Graves' disease have bulgy eyes, and some people with Hashimoto's thyroiditis who have either normal or below-normal thyroid function may have this thyroid-related eye disease.

Support groups dealing exclusively with thyroid eye disease have formed in the United States and other countries to help patients understand their disease and cope with their suffering. Despite these organizations' efforts to help people become better informed about thyroid eye disease, fear generated by the unknown continues to be rampant among patients with Graves' disease. However, in less than 20 percent of patients with thyroid eye disease is the condition severe enough to require aggressive intervention. Technological advances in corrective surgery as well as other treatments have improved the prospects of these patients.

The Affinity Between the Eyes and the Thyroid

Eye problems range along a continuum from minimal to severe in thyroid eye disease.[1] If researchers did a diagnostic study, such as an ultrasound or a magnetic resonance imaging (MRI) of the eye orbits (bony sockets), they would find that more than 90 percent of people with Graves' disease have some involvement not of the eyes themselves but of the fat surrounding the eyes and the muscles that are responsible for the movement of the eyes. There is typically an enlargement of the muscles due to inflammation. Nearly 40 to

45 percent of people with Graves' disease have evidence of minimal involvement of the tissue surrounding the eyes but show no symptoms. Of the more than 50 percent remaining, the eye disease can range from mild to very severe.

Although thyroid eye disease is not a direct consequence of the thyroid condition, it occurs as a result of the immune system's having produced antibodies that target the eye muscles and structures situated around the eyes. The reason for the production of such antibodies in persons with thyroid disease is related to some molecular similarities in the tissues surrounding the eyes and the thyroid gland.[2] Because of these similarities, the immune system attacks the eyes as well as the thyroid. Therefore, the eye disease may be viewed as an incidental process occurring in autoimmune thyroid disease. Some patients, however, have eye symptoms even though their thyroid function is normal. In fact, nearly 10 percent of patients with thyroid eye disease have normal thyroid levels. In such patients, the eye disease progresses on its own and may be the only actual problem the patient experiences. A number of these people, when followed for months or years, may subsequently develop some kind of thyroid dysfunction, either hypothyroidism or hyperthyroidism.

Thyroid eye disease is more common in women than men simply because Graves' disease is primarily a woman's condition. Severe cases, however, tend to occur in older people and men.[3]

Thyroid eye disease may have one or more of three major components:

1. An inflammation of soft tissue that can affect the conjunctiva (a protective fine layer of mucosa normally covering the sclera of the eye and inner parts of the eyelids) and structures surrounding the eyes. This can cause redness, a sensation of sand in the eyes, increased tearing, and visible swelling around the eyes.
2. Swelling and increase in the volume of fat inside the orbit. This promotes excess pressure on the eyes and makes them protrude. Pressure on the optic nerve can also result in optic neuropathy (an inflammation and damage to the optic nerve) that can threaten vision.
3. Inflammation and loss of function in one or several of the four small muscles that are normally responsible for the movement of the eyes.

How a person reacts to being diagnosed with thyroid eye disease is affected to some extent by the timing of the onset of the eye problem in relation to the thyroid imbalance. The onset of thyroid eye disease could occur simultaneously with the onset of hyperthyroidism, or it could occur months or years before or after. People who have just been diagnosed with hyperthyroidism due to Graves' disease but who do not currently have the eye disease typically ask, "What about my eyes? Will I ever have bulgy eyes?" As is the case with most questions pertaining to thyroid eye disease, the physician's answer is often, "I don't know." If you have been diagnosed with an overactive thyroid due to Graves' disease, you need to educate yourself about what to watch for should you develop eye disease.

Some of the most important eye changes in Graves' disease are the retraction of the upper eyelids, resulting in a wide-eyed look (because more of the visible portion of the eye is uncovered when the person looks straight ahead) and infrequent blinking. The condition is also responsible for the upper eyelid's inability to smoothly follow downward movements of the eyes when the person is asked to look down (doctors call this "lid lag"). In addition, when the patient looks straight ahead without staring, one can see a white band of sclera (connective tissue) above the border of the cornea (the central colored circle of the eye). This retraction of the upper eyelid, resulting in the impression of staring and a widening of the eyes, frequently causes cosmetic concerns when it is noticed by patients or their family and friends. Appearance issues become an even greater concern when bulgy eyes develop, resulting from swelling in the fat tissue surrounding the eyes.

Other types of changes not only have cosmetic implications but also cause the patient significant discomfort. These include changes inherent to the inflammatory reaction of the soft tissue of the orbit, such as increased tearing, a feeling of having a foreign body in the eye, and a sensation of tense eyes. The eyelids become swollen and pockets of fluid form below the eyes, the conjunctiva becomes red, and blood vessels become apparent, as occurs in allergic reactions involving the eyes. This redness and blood congestion in the visible structures surrounding the eyes result in part from increased pressure within the orbits. In some patients, exposure to warm temperatures and radiation from the sun cause eye irritation and prevent them from engaging in outdoor activities during warm weather.

The most disabling symptom of the condition is double vision, resulting from inflammation and thickening of the eye muscles. Eye movement abnormalities may occur, the most common one involving the upward movements of the eyes. Finally, when the disease has progressed significantly, the protrusion of the eyes may cause the cornea to be exposed continuously even during sleep, thus making it susceptible to damage from foreign bodies. This may result in infection or perforation of the cornea, potentially causing loss of vision and even loss of the eye. Another dreaded effect is the compression of the optic nerve, which is likely to restrict vision. It is due to muscle swelling and enlargement as well as swelling of the orbit content.

The following lists summarize the symptoms of thyroid eye disease:

MOST COMMON SYMPTOMS
- Aversion to light
- Redness of eyes
- Protruding eyes

- Swelling of upper eyelids
- Blurred vision
- Watery eyes
- Sore eyes
- Gritty sensation in eyes
- Aches behind the eyes
- Dry eyes
- Poor night vision
- Eye pain when the person moves around
- Flashing lights

LESS COMMON SYMPTOMS
- Double vision
- Reduced sight in one eye or (more rarely) both eyes
- Reduced color brightness
- Swelling of lower eyelids

Which Comes First: The Eyes or the Thyroid?

Some Graves' disease patients initially develop symptoms of hyperthyroidism with virtually no eye symptoms. Months or years after their thyroid condition has been treated, however, eye symptoms such as bulging or irritation of the conjunctiva or even eye muscle malfunctioning may develop.[4] These symptoms may be attributed to other problems or may come as an unhappy surprise. Although you shouldn't become unduly alarmed about your chances of being afflicted with this condition in the future, you do need to learn about possible symptoms of thyroid eye disease.

Theresa, age forty-nine, had experienced no eye symptoms whatsoever in the twelve years since she had received radioactive iodine treatment for hyperthyroidism due to Graves' disease. Suddenly, she started having redness in her eyes, as well as puffiness, and her eyes began to bulge. Not suspecting that her eye symptoms were related to her thyroid condition, she went to see an ophthalmologist, who made the connection.

Theresa was devastated. She was also infuriated that no one had explained to her that this could happen even twelve years after the radioiodine treatment. "When I started having the eye problem," she said, "I was concerned about my appearance. The eyes were getting larger but were not grotesquely buggy at the beginning. I was aware of some eye changes, but I didn't know what they meant." Theresa was happy to hear that her eye disease was not severe. In fact, her eye condition later improved with treatment.

If eye disease occurs at the same time as the thyroid imbalance, the diagnosis is easy. The patient is frequently frightened, however, by the presence of eye problems. The fears are exaggerated because of the anxiety and loss of control or depression frequently generated by the thyroid imbalance. The loss of self-esteem that can be provoked by the thyroid imbalance is exacerbated by the appearance or functional impairment of the eyes and may make the thyroid patient feel unable to function mentally or physically.

In some patients, the onset of hyperthyroidism and eye disease is simultaneous, but hyperthyroidism symptoms are minimal, so the only discomfort experienced is related to the eyes. The suffering of such patients can be compounded by dismissal, misdiagnosis, or a lack of understanding, which could continue for a long time before doctors make the correct diagnosis and initiate treatment of the eye problems. The patient and even physicians frequently implicate allergies. Barbara Bush indicated in her memoirs that she attributed her eye symptoms to allergies for some time before she was diagnosed with Graves' disease.[5]

Paulette, like many patients with Graves' disease, suffered from eye symptoms but had no symptoms of a thyroid imbalance. She wandered from physician to physician for almost a year and was diagnosed with allergies even though she was experiencing worsening eye disease. She said:

> When I finally found out what was wrong with me, it had taken exactly one year and a lot of treatments at an allergy clinic that I was referred to. The doctor there who was giving me allergy shots kept telling me that my eyes were becoming red and itchy from allergies. I was told I was allergic to a lot of things, especially cats, but that was not my problem.

Although the patient and his or her immediate family may not notice the eye changes, strangers who see the person for the first time may notice these changes and even comment on them. Laura, the wife of a physician, suffered from undiagnosed hyperthyroidism due to Graves' disease for more than a year and was angry that her husband had failed to notice the changes that strangers immediately spotted. Laura said:

> People would ask, "What is wrong with your eyes?" Even people I didn't know. One day, someone took a close-up picture of me, and when I saw it, I was stunned. How could my husband have let me go to work like this? No wonder people ask me what's wrong with my eyes! Now I'm self-conscious about it.

Because few ophthalmologists are trained to recognize or manage thyroid eye disease, patients suffering from eye problems due to undiagnosed Graves' disease may remain undiagnosed for some time even when they are seen and evaluated by eye doctors.

Twenty-nine-year-old Elizabeth, an attractive, successful architect, was under the care of an ophthalmologist when she showed signs of thyroid eye disease. She was seeing the ophthalmologist to have a radial keratotomy, a surgical procedure involving the cornea and aimed at correcting myopia. She could not see as clearly as she had before and wanted to correct her focusing problem to eliminate the need for glasses. Prior to the scheduled surgery, Elizabeth started experiencing more symptoms in her right eye, which became swollen and developed a pocket. She said:

> It was like a water bubble. I could push it, and it was squishy. I could feel the pressure on it, and I started getting headaches. I thought maybe I had contracted an infection or the eyedrops had done it. I did not notice the eyelid receding, though my eye looked puffy and bruised. I told the ophthalmologist, "I know I'm scheduled for surgery, but my eye is doing something." He looked in my eye and saw no infection, so he recommended going ahead with the surgery.
>
> The surgery caused swelling for maybe two weeks. When I went back for my visit, I started complaining that my eye was drooping. I thought this was part of the recovery. He kept saying to come back for checkups. He kept saying this was not one of the reactions. I went to an ear, nose, and throat doctor, and he said he didn't know either.
>
> My face was distorting. All I could see in the mirror was that I was getting uglier every day.

For six months, Elizabeth went from doctor to doctor. A couple of eye doctors said the condition might be sinus-related. Finally, Elizabeth went to see an internist for other symptoms, and he suspected Graves' disease.

In Elizabeth's case, the ophthalmologist did not consider that her initial eye symptoms could be caused by thyroid eye disease. In fact, the eye surgery could have worsened the eye problem. Any trauma to the eye, including surgical trauma, may exacerbate or even trigger the autoimmune reaction to the eye in a patient with preexisting thyroid eye disease and may make eye problems worse.

The Diverse Effects of Thyroid Eye Disease

The onset of eye symptoms may have numerous effects on how you perceive your overall health and on job performance, lifestyle, self-esteem, and even mood. Research published in the *Archives of Ophthalmology* showed that thyroid eye disease may cause patients to have increased inner tension, more depression, lack of vitality, confusion, fatigue, and anger.[6] The impact on mood is worse if there are cosmetic changes, such as bulgy eyes. Elizabeth, for instance, had almost quit her architectural design job as a result of thyroid eye disease. Her eye disease manifested itself as a severe inflammation and bulging, but she did not suffer from eye muscle problems. Thus, she did not see double unless pressure in her eyes increased due to improper positioning of her head. Her suffering was due primarily to the swelling around the eyes and the pressure in her eyes, which affected her vision.

In some patients, thyroid eye disease does not cause inflammation or bulginess but primarily attacks the muscles that allow the eyes to move around smoothly. The resulting sudden onset of double vision is one of the most frightening manifestations of thyroid eye disease. The afflicted person may experience many difficulties during this time that will be compounded if doctors don't make a prompt diagnosis.

Mark, age fifty-four, had had a stable job for twenty-two years in the same company when he began suffering from anxiety, depression, and total turmoil in his life as a result of eye muscle malfunction. He did not experience any symptoms of swelling or inflammation around his eyes, however. Because double vision was the only symptom of an eye problem, physicians were searching for a neurological condition, and it took some time for the diagnosis of Graves' eye disease to be made.

Mark was unable to relax and began to experience sleeping problems. He became intolerant and irritable. His anger peaked when he realized he could not do simple things such as change a lightbulb or push a button. His wife said that he became a totally different person.

An ophthalmologist at a major medical school who saw Mark finally diagnosed the condition and initiated plans for treatment, which included eye muscle surgery and external radiation. Months later, Mark's functional ability returned.

Without adequate family support, patients with severe thyroid eye disease find it difficult to cope with the disease and its effects on functioning both at home and at work. Spouses and partners are often called on to play a major role in understanding the disease process and its treatment, as the person with the condition is frequently stressed by the situation and may not comprehend what the doctor is trying to explain. The spouse should be involved as much as possible in the case and, in turn, should reassure his or her partner about the outcome. This will minimize the anger and mood swings generated by the effects of eye disease. These feelings, which are also symptoms of thyroid imbalance, are exaggerated when eye impairment or disfiguration from thyroid eye disease occurs.

More Questions Than Answers

Once eye disease is diagnosed, the patient is usually faced with a situation in which answers may not be forthcoming because of uncertainty about the effectiveness of treatment and a lack of knowledge about the natural history of the disease. Many patients become frustrated and angry because they cannot get straightforward answers to such questions as:

- "What might happen later?"
- "Is it reversible?"
- "Could it be corrected totally without further damage to my eyes?"

Vanessa suffered from symptoms of thyroid eye disease for about six months before she was diagnosed. She had red, bulgy eyes and a fixed stare. After she was told that most of her eye problems were due to Graves' disease, Vanessa joined a thyroid support group to learn more about her condition. Her endocrinologist did not give her definite answers or provide her with literature describing outcomes and treatment options. The ophthalmologist to whom she was referred told her, "Let's wait and see." Attending thyroid support meetings helped her cope better because she found out that she was not the only one dealing with this situation. She said:

Nobody seems to have answers. In the support group meetings, I meet a lot of people who have been misdiagnosed for a lot of years.

At first, before going to the support group, I was so bitter and angry. It's a disease to be angry at. It's like righteous justification. We should be angry for having to go through this. Some of the people I see are so disfigured it makes me want to cry. I say, "That could be me in a year or two."

I think now I'm willing to fight, though I still don't understand this complicated disease. I now realize that I was not really in tune with my health until it became bad.

The lack of adequate and reassuring information contributed to Vanessa's anxiety when she saw other people disfigured from Graves' disease. Only after her endocrinologist explained to her that, in general, only a small percentage of people afflicted with thyroid eye disease reach a severe stage did she feel better. Vanessa said, "Talking with my husband and other patients with Graves' disease helped me to cope better with this. Now I don't feel as awkward and different as before. Most of the time, I just feel that I have an eye disease, and I am hopeful it will get better."

Promising Treatments for Thyroid Eye Disease

Graves' patients view thyroid eye disease with dread, and unfortunately, some people afflicted with severe eye disease may find their personal and professional lives significantly affected and become depressed. Such patients can take comfort in the following information:

- Having Graves' disease and even thyroid eye disease does not necessarily mean that your eye condition will become severe, disfiguring, or disabling. In only 5 to 10 percent of patients with thyroid eye disease is the condition severe enough to warrant aggressive treatment interventions.

- Many patients with Graves' disease–related eye changes will experience a spontaneous improvement or near resolution of those changes over time; only a small percentage (nearly 20 percent) may have worsening eye disease, and even then, it could subsequently improve on its own.[7]

- Generally speaking, from the time the eye disease begins, a worsening or progression of the eye symptoms may occur over a period of six to twenty-four months.[8] After this initial period (often referred to as the hot phase), the eye symptoms often remain stable for a period of one to three years. Later, many patients experience a gradual improvement and often an incomplete resolution of the symptoms. For instance, one study showed that lid retraction disappeared in 60 percent of people several years after the beginning of the eye problems[9] and that eye muscle problems improved in 38 percent of patients. Bulgy eyes, however, tend to persist: less than 10 percent of people with bulgy eyes will have an improvement in the condition without receiving treatment. This has to do with the increased amount of inflamed fat inside the orbit that cannot regress spontaneously.

- For those with significant eye changes, several treatments can improve or even correct the most severe eye effects. When such patients understand from the outset that the treatment process may be lengthy, it helps to minimize frustration, anger, and despair. It is also important for patients to be confident that treatments are available, not only to prevent loss of vision and to restore and maintain normal eye function but also to correct cosmetic disfigurement.[10]

For example, eyedrops that counteract the effect of the increased retraction of the eyelid are often quite helpful. Increasing the humidity in the home and in the work environment will help alleviate the dryness of the eyes caused by constant exposure to air and sunlight as a result of the retraction of the lid. Prisms can be used to correct double vision. It is helpful for patients to wear sunglasses when outdoors and to use artificial tears (methylcellulose 1 percent solution) during the day, as well as emollients to lubricate the eyes at bedtime. You also need to tape your eyelids at night to prevent dryness and exposure of the cornea. I often recommend that my patients elevate the head of their bed or use two or three pillows to reduce swelling and double vision upon awakening in the morning.

For upper eyelid retraction, cosmetic upper eyelid surgery, performed when the patient's thyroid imbalance has been corrected and normal thyroid function has stabilized, provides excellent results when done by well-trained specialists. This problem can also be treated with injection of botulinum toxin type A (Botox). Often, a single injection corrects the problem. This form of treatment seems to be safe and effective; however, it may rarely cause double vision.[11] You can receive this treatment while waiting for a surgical procedure, such as orbital decompression or eye muscle surgery. Some patients also may require blepharoplasty, which is the removal of excessive amount of eyelid, or removal of orbital tissue that hangs out from the orbit.

For patients experiencing discomfort (a sensation of having sand or dirt in their eyes) and disfigurement from soft tissue inflammation around the eyes, a more aggressive treatment is needed. It consists of either a course of corticosteroid drugs, external radiation treatment to the orbits, or surgery to decrease the swelling in the orbits. An experienced ophthalmologist may recommend one or more of these treatments after performing a complete and thorough evaluation. In general, for patients having pain or severe inflammation around the eyes, a course of corticosteroids is the most effective form of treatment. Corticosteroids are powerful and effective immunosuppressive medications that act by slowing down the release of inflammation chemicals in the body. Corticosteroids can be administered intravenously or in the form of prednisone pills. The intravenous form might be more effective, but the oral treatment continues to be the most popular and is given initially as 60 to 80 mg of prednisone a day for two to four weeks. You may notice some reduction in the inflammation within one or two days. Then the dose can be gradually reduced by 2.5 to 10 mg each week over a period of several weeks if the eye symptoms do not flare up. You may need steroid treatment for a total of three to twelve months. The corticosteroids seldom improve the bulgy eyes or muscle problems, however, and are beneficial mostly in the active or "hot" phase of the eye disease. Another medication that can also be helpful is cyclosporine, with or without corticosteroids. However, steroids are by and large more effective than all other immunosuppressive medications, including cyclosporine. Newer medications currently used to treat autoimmune disorders and cancer, such as rituximab, adalimumab, and teprotumumab, may potentially have a role in the treatment of thyroid eye disease.

Patients who experience worsening bulginess but no major inflammation and those who have significant functional impairment of the eyes are generally treated with external radiation given in several sessions over two weeks. After external radiation, two-thirds of patients have a noticeable if not dramatic improvement in the soft tissue swelling.[12] The improvement is often noticeable as early as six weeks after treatment, and after three months, the eyes may be much less bulgy. Inflammation of the optic nerve also improves after external radiation. Although external radiation does not help with eye muscle dysfunction, it is often recommended before eye muscle surgery.

External radiation usually produces significant improvements and is especially helpful when the optic nerve is affected by the swelling. Some patients who are initially treated with corticosteroids but fail to improve may be given external radiation as well. Orbital radiation improves soft tissue changes in 80 percent of patients treated with this method. The best results are seen when corticosteroids and external radiation are used together. This combined treatment promotes a more rapid improvement in the swelling of soft tissue, eye muscle movements, and vision.[13] However, radiation combined with corticosteroids does not improve the bulging. Corticosteroids and/or orbital radiation are best used when active inflammation exists.

Nearly one-third of patients who require corticosteroids, radiation, or both will also need some form of surgery, either decompression surgery, eyelid correction, or eye muscle surgery. Surgery to remove portions of the bony walls of the orbit and decrease the pressure existing in the orbits may be recommended for cosmetic reasons or because vision is affected. The surgery improves bulginess of the eyes as well as vision. It will allow your cornea to be more protected and will help optic neuropathy. In fact, the surgery may be indicated even if you do not have bulgy eyes; optic neuropathy occurs more frequently in patients who do *not* have bulgy eyes simply because the pressure that builds up inside the orbits in such patients is much higher on the optic nerve. Orbital decompression surgery is performed when drugs and radiation have failed to achieve an improvement. In general, surgery is more effective when the activity of the disease has slowed down. When surgery is performed during the hot phase of the eye disease, it is more often complicated by double vision.[14] An indication of activity of the eye disease is when there is inflammation and redness of the eyes. Make sure you stop smoking before having such procedures, since smoking negates the benefits of the surgery.[15]

Eye muscle surgery is delicate and may be needed if you have persistent double vision. Note that in general, orbital decompression should be done before muscle surgery because muscle surgery may cause swelling that worsens the bulginess of the eyes. Strabismus surgery will allow you to have single vision. This means that it will improve vision when you look straight ahead and when you read. However, after surgery, you may continue to have double vision when you look to the side or upward. If you have this residual problem, it does not mean that the surgery is not considered successful.

Because of the lack of specific treatments to cure thyroid eye disease and completely eliminate the autoimmune attack on the eye, patients afflicted with thyroid eye disease continue to be treated with these unpleasant methods. The good news is that, by and large, these treatments achieve significant cosmetic and functional improvements. The assurance that help is available should serve to dispel much of the fear and anxiety that patients experience upon being diagnosed with thyroid eye disease.

How to Ensure the Best Possible Outcome

Patients with Graves' disease, with or without eye disease, often ask what they can do to prevent or stabilize their eye problems. The answer is: anything that has been shown to reduce immune system reactivity and to reduce any potential negative effect on the eyes should be done.

First, any thyroid imbalance should be corrected as promptly as possible. Researchers have clearly shown that thyroid imbalances promote a worsening of eye symptoms.[16] Severe hyperthyroidism may be associated with a higher risk of having more severe eye disease. In addition, occurrence of hypothyroidism during the treatment of Graves' disease may cause a worsening of eye symptoms. The reason for this is that thyroid hormone imbalance, even minimal, can make the immune system more reactive and attack the structures surrounding the eyes. Therefore, both thyroid specialists and patients must ensure that normal thyroid function is maintained throughout the course of treatment, especially in those patients with more severe eye disease. A block-replace regimen, utilizing an antithyroid medication such as methimazole (which seems to have a beneficial effect on an autoimmune attack) in conjunction with levothyroxine (so that the patient has a stable, normal thyroid function), may help stabilize thyroid levels during the hot phase of thyroid eye disease. This regimen, administered for the first year to patients with moderate to severe eye disease, will help prevent the deleterious effects of a thyroid imbalance on the eye disease.

In addition to keeping your thyroid levels as well balanced as possible, you need to take all the measures known to reduce your immune system reactivity. I cannot emphasize enough the importance of taking appropriate amounts of selenium, as research has clearly shown a correlation between low selenium levels and the presence of thyroid eye disease. Selenium will lower the production of inflammation chemicals by the immune system. Other antioxidants that I detail in Chapter 22 are also of tremendous benefit to help you keep your eye disease as quiescent as possible. As I indicated in Chapter 17, the use of antioxidants in conjunction with the antithyroid medication methimazole enhances the chances of remission of Graves' disease. Research has shown that taking antioxidants results in improvement of mild to moderately severe thyroid eye disease.[17] Vitamin D deficiency also can worsen the severity of your eye problems, so it is essential to take the needed amounts of vitamin D to keep your levels of this important vitamin in an excellent range. I also recommend that you stay diligent about not eating the foods that you are sensitive to, in order to minimize inflammatory effects on your eyes.

Second, for patients with significant eye disease, destroying a portion of the thyroid gland, by exposing it to radioactive iodine, should be avoided the first year until the eye disease is more stable. This is because radioactive iodine treatment can exacerbate the eye disease by enhancing the autoimmune attack on the tissue surrounding the eyes. Instead, it is advisable during this critical period to use an antithyroid medication to counteract the effect of hyperthyroidism and potentially diminish the autoimmune attack.

Even if you have mild eye disease, you may experience worsening eye changes after radioactive iodine treatment. Research has shown that among patients with minimal or no eye disease, 15 percent had appearance or worsening of eye disease two to six months following the radioactive iodine treatment.[18] Often, the eye changes that occur after radioactive iodine treatment are temporary. However, in some patients, the changes may persist. To prevent the worsening of eye disease, your doctor may prescribe prednisone for approximately three months. Corticosteroid treatment, in my opinion, is helpful if you had to be treated with radioactive iodine for your overactive thyroid and if you have significant eye disease but could not be treated with medications because of adverse effects, for example. In this situation, corticosteroids will prevent you from having a further worsening of the eye disease.[19]

As we saw in Chapter 4, stress is a major trigger of Graves' disease and of the autoimmune attack responsible for hyperthyroidism.[20] Although not much has been written about the effect of stress on thyroid eye disease, it is inconceivable that stress could affect the thyroid condition but not the eyes. Extensive research suggests that the mechanism and the underlying trigger are the same for both eye disease and the thyroid condition. Thus, people with even minimal thyroid eye disease should learn as much as possible about how to cope with stress effectively. The thyroid condition and the eye disease, themselves sources of stress, may overburden the patients, who can then easily lose control due to worrying and functional impairment. Again, strong support is crucial to help patients cope with the stress. People afflicted with thyroid eye disease need to educate themselves quickly, and learning about the promising treatment options that are available should serve to reinforce their sense of optimism. Remember, a positive attitude can promote a successful outcome.

Research has shown that smoking may make thyroid eye disease worse.[21] The negative effects of smoking are primarily related to increased inflammation of the eye. Thyroid specialists and ophthalmologists urge patients with Graves' disease to quit smoking. Such an emphasis on the adverse effects of smoking generates a great deal of anxiety among Graves' disease patients. For those who cannot quit smoking while experiencing the effects of an overactive thyroid, I suggest wearing suitable glasses that can protect their eyes from the detrimental effects of smoke. As soon as thyroid levels become normal, every effort to stop smoking should be made.

Despite the fact that we do not yet have a cure that entirely eliminates the root of thyroid eye disease, Graves' disease patients afflicted with eye problems need no longer resign themselves to despair and disability. A good understanding of their condition and the availability of effective treatments have changed the outlook for patients suffering from this condition. If you have thyroid eye disease and require treatment, ask your physician to refer you to an ophthalmologist with expertise in this field. You are likely to find the help you need in most institutions affiliated with medical schools.

Important Points to Remember

- Severe eye problems occur in less than 20 percent of patients with Graves disease.
- Thyroid-related eye disease is the result of an immune attack on the structures surrounding the eyes, including fat and muscle. The immune attack can cause inflammation of the soft tissue, swelling of the fat that leads to protrusion of the eyes (exophthalmos), and inflammation and dysfunction of the eye muscles responsible for the movement of the eyes.
- Many patients have spontaneous improvement of their eye disease over time.
- Several treatments are currently available to correct cosmetic disfigurement, inflammation, exophthalmos, and eye-muscle problems.

20

MY T4/T3 APPROACH

A few years ago, I was invited to a Christmas party at the home of a friend. Although I had known Alan for several years, I had never met his wife, Jennifer. When I arrived at the party, I noticed immediately that Jennifer had bulgy eyes, a symptom of the overactive thyroid condition Graves' disease. Not only did her eyes protrude, but she also appeared depressed and withdrawn. She didn't mingle easily and often snapped at her husband throughout the evening, clearly quite unhappy that she had to be at this party.

Later, I learned from Alan that Jennifer had been diagnosed with Graves' disease two years earlier. What had driven her to seek a doctor's help were her anger, extreme anxiety, and wild mood swings, which were taking a toll on their marriage.

Alan also explained that her emotional problems hadn't completely disappeared after her thyroid condition was treated. In fact, she never went back to "being herself." As a result of the treatment of her overactive thyroid, Jennifer had become hypothyroid and was receiving thyroid hormone treatment in the form of synthetic thyroxine (T4). Several physicians told her that her thyroid hormone levels were normal and there was nothing more they could do for her. One even suggested that she go see a counselor. Jennifer did take a course of an antidepressant but stopped the medication after three months, when she realized that it had produced no significant improvement in the way she felt.

Later, when I took over Jennifer's care, she gradually returned to normal through an innovative treatment program that corrected the brain chemistry imbalance resulting from her thyroid condition. The program included the practice of a relaxation technique, but more important, it involved a dramatic change in the nature of her thyroid hormone treatment, from the use of a T4-only drug to a protocol I've devised that combines synthetic T4 (levothyroxine) and T3, the most potent and biologically active form of thyroid hormone. I believe that this protocol holds tremendous promise for a large number of people who, for whatever reason, are suffering from an underactive thyroid and need thyroid hormone treatment. I regard this new T4/T3 treatment as a state-of-the-art treatment for hypothyroidism and a viable alternative to the most widely accepted current medical approach, which has been to prescribe T4, a portion of which is then converted to T3 by bodily organs, including the brain.[1]

"I think that there are a lot of women like me," Jennifer told me, "who have to deal with the problems I faced every day without ever realizing that an effective treatment exists. And that's too bad, because thyroid conditions can totally alter not only your personality but your physical appearance, and Lord knows that's a tough burden to bear in today's society."

Lifting the Cloud

It was quite obvious from the symptoms Jennifer described that while suffering from a glandular disorder, she had gone through an unpleasant journey of disturbed mood and emotions that were never validated for her. Jennifer told me recently:

> Before I started on the new T4/T3 treatment, I was constantly wondering, Is this what it's going to be like for the rest of my life?
> Since then, the cloud has lifted. I'm once again able to process things in my mind normally and quickly. I have had, I would say, a 95 percent improvement in my symptoms. The tingling in my hands and feet is not as bad. I retain water less than before. I have more energy. I've gone back to work. I'm more outgoing and have a brighter outlook. I'm finally reclaiming myself. I really feel good, and I have hope!

When I began my career in the field of thyroid disease, my goal in treating patients with an underactive thyroid was to help them reach and maintain normal blood levels of thyroid hormones and TSH, the pituitary hormone that regulates thyroid gland function. I still remember those days when I faced countless patients who had achieved this goal but who nevertheless continued to complain of tiredness, dry skin, an inability to function, and other symptoms. I would vehemently reply to their complaints, "These problems are not from your thyroid." Although I was puzzled by these persistent symptoms, I felt in a way that I had accomplished my job. More often than not, when I searched for coexistent conditions, my efforts were in vain. My frustration continued to build, and I felt ineffective at providing the answers and cures that many of my hypothyroid patients were expecting of me.

In those early days, doctors began to be concerned about bone loss and osteoporosis in people being treated with too much thyroid hormone. Early treatments used desiccated animal thyroid. It is natural and provides both thyroid hormones (T4 and T3), but not in a composition close enough to what humans need to achieve appropriate and stable levels of these hormones.[2] The result was often daily surges of blood levels of T3 out of proportion to the normal pattern of human blood levels. Such patients were also at risk for significant bone loss. As many physicians did at the time, I switched to the newest treatment for hypothyroidism whenever possible: I took these patients off the desiccated thyroid and put them on synthetic T4.

Surprisingly to me, this was seldom entirely successful. Once switched from these natural T4/T3 tablets to T4 tablets, patients complained of sluggishness, decreased memory, impaired concentration, and a host of other symptoms. This was in spite of having reached normal blood levels of thyroid hormone and TSH. In fact, seldom was I able to convince a patient to remain on levothyroxine: they all wanted to go back on the old pill.

Because of these observations, I quickly came to realize that there must be a role for some form of T4/T3 combination therapy in many patients with underactive thyroid. Isn't this the reason why many doctors continue to prescribe desiccated thyroid to their hypothyroid patients? Isn't this the reason why medications combining T4 and T3 such as Nature-Throid and Westhroid have been manufactured for years? These combinations, however, have not been widely prescribed by conventional doctors since the 1970s, primarily because they also result in abnormal surges of T3 levels in the bloodstream. What levothyroxine-treated patients were missing was some T3, in the right amount and close to how the human gland produces it.

Adding T3 in the treatment of hypothyroidism is beneficial because the body and mind depend on this most potent form of thyroid hormone, which is also the main form of the hormone that works in brain cells. Therefore, even a minute T3 deficit, which may be present in many patients taking levothyroxine as a thyroid hormone replacement, may impair a person's functioning. It is also true, however, that one person missing a minute amount of T3 may be symptom-free, whereas another person may experience some effects.

Though pharmaceutical companies have tried to combine the two hormones, the results have not duplicated nature. In humans, 20 percent of T3 needed by the body is produced directly by the thyroid gland. The correct replacement is usually judged by monitoring what the pituitary senses and releases (TSH). But as we come to a better understanding of the complex chemistry and regulation of thyroid hormones in the body, we realize that these regulations in the pituitary gland, the brain, and other organs are somewhat different. The assumption was that by giving only T4, doctors could normalize thyroid hormone levels in the body. This turns out not to be true in all cases. By giving patients only T4 to normalize TSH, some still miss a small amount of T3 that is normally provided by the thyroid gland. It is possible that even though blood test results are normal and the conversion of T4 to T3 within organs is taken into account, some form of brain or perhaps even "general body" hypothyroidism, due to lack of T3, still exists. Having a normal TSH level does not necessarily mean that your brain and organs are receiving exactly the amount of T3 needed. Obviously, understanding what is missing in the brains and bodies of my hypothyroid patients became a prime concern.

I knew that T3 works as an antidepressant but that the doses used conventionally by psychiatrists were far higher than the physiological replacement doses (see Chapter 9). I also knew that the persistent suffering of treated hypothyroid patients is often of two kinds. Many people continue to suffer from symptoms of low metabolism. They have difficulty losing weight, and they complain of hair loss, dry skin, brittle nails, muscle cramps, and a host of physical symptoms. These symptoms indicate that the body is not receiving exactly the right amount of T3 from the conversion of T4. Many people suffer from some degree of depression, also probably due to some extent to low T3 in the brain. Some of the lingering effects of thyroid imbalance, discussed in Chapter 18, may be related to minor deficits of T3 in the brain.

This line of thinking brought all patients who required T4 treatment under the same umbrella, even those who had Graves' disease like Jennifer and those who had their thyroid gland surgically removed because of another thyroid disorder. The purpose of the treatment is to duplicate very closely how much T3 the brain and body require for normal functioning.

When T4 Simply Does Not Do It

Whether your underactive thyroid has been caused by Hashimoto's thyroiditis, as a result of the treatment of Graves' disease, or as a result of surgical removal of the gland, you may continue to suffer from symptoms of low thyroid if you have been prescribed T4 only for your condition. Research conducted in Norway showed that patients treated with T4 alone continued to have lower quality of life, depression, anxiety, and short memory.[3] Even though the patients improved with T4-only treatment, they did not necessarily feel as well as before they became hypothyroid, even after six to eight months of treatment. As I indicated in Chapter 18, research has shown that patients with Graves' disease continue to have significant mood, emotional, and cognitive symptoms, even years after the treatment of the overactive thyroid, and despite having normal thyroid tests with thyroxine treatment. You may have a TSH in the optimal range but your T3 level remains on the low side. One study comparing 85 patients treated with T4 only to 114 normal people without thyroid disease and who had similar TSH levels found that T3 levels were much lower in the patients treated with T4.[4] In this research, the patients who were treated with T4 had biological evidence of hypothyroidism demonstrated by low levels of sex-hormone-binding globulin (a protein produced by the liver that reflects thyroid hormone effects in the body). Research performed on rats who were made hypothyroid by surgical removal of their thyroid glands has shown that to restore normal T3 levels in the tissues of the animals, the animals needed excessive amounts of T4.[5] All this body of evidence clearly shows that in many patients with underactive thyroid, T4 alone is not adequate to reach and maintain perfect T3 levels in their blood and in their organs.

A teacher named Priscilla taught me the extent to which her cognitive impairment and symptoms were the result of the small amounts of T3 that she was missing. Her experiences illustrate the fact that administering thyroxine to replace what a normal gland produces and delivers to the brain and body does not duplicate nature. The conversion of synthetic T4 to T3 simply does not yield the T3 needed even when the pituitary TSH has become normal.

Priscilla had a complete thyroidectomy for a large goiter. She was given T4 for her hypothyroidism and reached normal blood levels of thyroid hormones and TSH. Prior to the thyroidectomy, Priscilla had no symptoms. She had been happy and energetic, but her problems started weeks after the surgery. In her words:

> I just couldn't seem to get the correct dosage. One doctor thought I was going through depression. He never really could get the dose straightened out either. I couldn't seem to get well. The doctors told me that everything was normal, although I certainly didn't feel normal. I was losing hair, I was nervous, I wanted to do destructive things. I thought I was crazy.
>
> It was an effort even to drive to a doctor's appointment. Unless I had the directions written down, I couldn't remember how to get there. Or I didn't feel like I could do it unless my husband came along, and I had been very independent before then. I became very scattered and couldn't stay focused on anything. Even in the house, it would be difficult to decide on which things to throw away and which things to keep. Everything would just seem to be a big mess. I was very disorganized.
>
> I had been teaching for twenty-five years, but it got to the point where I couldn't remember where I put files, and I couldn't remember what it was I wanted to do next. I'd become annoyed or upset with colleagues and just explode at times.

After removal of her thyroid gland, Priscilla's doctor gave her the exact amount of T4 needed to achieve a normal TSH level. But despite normal blood tests, she was missing a small amount of the active form of the hormone T3. As with low serotonin in the brain, this triggered depression, which became self-perpetuating.

The small deficit in T3 had caused Priscilla's dry skin, puffiness, and low metabolism. When I changed her T4 treatment to T4/T3 combination regimen, her emotional and physical symptoms rapidly resolved. Whereas most antidepressants take six to eight weeks to become effective, many people begin to notice an improvement in the way they feel as soon as one week after starting the T4/T3 treatment. Priscilla described the improvement in her symptoms as follows:

> On the combination treatment, I was better able to handle situations. I could once again deal with children and colleagues at school. My emotions became more stable. I have been able to face challenges in life, and I've been able to challenge myself—taking classes, for example. I've noticed a big difference in how I feel about myself, how I dress and do my makeup—things I was letting go because it was such an effort. I enjoy exercising again and want to do extra activities and go places.
>
> Before T3, I felt like I was outside of myself, sometimes even just watching what's going on and not being able to figure out why I couldn't be part of it. I feel like this new treatment has put me back in touch with me, a person who's creative and energetic—the person I was before. I have a lot more self-esteem and self-control.

Priscilla's case has taught me that part of the problem when people rely on the T4 pill to obtain normal amounts of T3 in their body and brain is that the T4 pill simply does not provide the correct amount of T3 needed for normal functioning.

You Need the Right Combination

While searching for the right amounts of T3 to be combined with T4 for my patients, I realized early on that each person needs a different amount, which depends not only on the total amount of thyroid hormone required by that particular patient but also on the patient's symptoms and on whether he or she has depression, anxiety, and/or residual physical symptoms. Some patients require between 5 and 10 mcg of T3 a day to achieve the best symptom relief. Other patients, however, may require as little as 2 or 3 mcg a day. There is no magic amount of T3 that will work for all people. The amount of T3 needed should be quite close to the amount that a normal thyroid gland produces each day. But if you are suffering from symptoms of depression, the amount of T3 may need to be slightly higher without causing you to have excessive levels of T3 in your system. In essence, your doctor needs to find the ratio of T3 to T4 that will make you feel at your best without causing undue adverse effects. T3 in the right amount and in the right ratio can provide you with miraculous changes in the way you feel, but too much T3 not only will make you not benefit from the treatment but also can generate other symptoms, such as worsening anxiety, worsening depression and fatigue, rapid heartbeat, and palpitations. The T3 is best taken twice a day (before breakfast and at 2:00 P.M.) to avoid abnormal surges in T3 levels. You can get the T3 by taking a combination of low doses of desiccated thyroid (such as Armour Thyroid) or low doses of Nature-Throid (a combination of synthetic T4 and T3), in addition to an appropriate amount of synthetic thyroxine if needed. But again, this may or may not work in your particular case. You can get the T3 from the synthetic T3 Cytomel; however, T3 levels typically rise and fall within a few hours of taking Cytomel.

Another alternative that I have found quite effective and safe is the use of compounded slow-release T3 to be taken once a day along with L-thyroxine one hour before breakfast on an empty stomach. When you take compounded slow-release T3, you will not experience major surges of T3 in your system, and your T3 levels will be steady and in a very good range for more extended periods of time during the day than if you took the short-acting synthetic T3.[6] Some patients, however, will benefit from taking the slow-release T3 twice a day.

Whatever combination treatment your doctor has chosen for you, you need to make sure that both thyroid hormone and TSH levels remain normal and stable. Treating persistent sufferers with T4/T3 combination mimics closely what a normal thyroid gland provides to the body and the brain. You need to monitor your TSH level, and your T3 should be measured two to three hours after you take your morning dose of thyroid hormone to make sure you are not overmedicated with T3.

The release of the first edition of *The Thyroid Solution,* where I detailed the benefits of T4/T3 combination in the treatment of hypothyroid patients with residual symptoms, coincided with the publication of the first research showing that Cytomel in conjunction with T4 does improve mood and cognition in hypothyroid patients.[7] Even though the design of this research was not perfect, I was excited to see the results of this study. Since then, however, over ten more research studies have appeared in medical journals evaluating the effect of T4/T3 combination treatment in patients with hypothyroidism, and some of them have failed to demonstrate any benefits.[8] For this reason, a large number of doctors continue not to accept that T4/T3 can help a great number of hypothyroid patients suffering from residual low mood and fatigue despite having normal blood tests on T4 alone. In my opinion, however, no research so far has been conducted adequately enough to provide evidence that the T4/T3 combination is not beneficial for patients with lingering symptoms. The quality of the published research is so poor that it should not have been published to start with. Most of the studies suffered from a wide range of flaws in their design. The number of patients was in general too small, and the selection of patients studied was often inappropriate. As I explained earlier, not all patients with underactive thyroid have residual symptoms of low mood and fatigue, yet the patients included in research were not selected to evaluate these residual effects. The other major problem with the published research has to do with the dose of T3 used. Most studies used a fixed amount of T3 for all patients irrespective of the total amount of thyroid hormone needed and irrespective of their symptoms. As mentioned earlier, T3 in the right amount and right proportion works, but the dose has to be tailored to your needs. Too much of it not only will not relieve symptoms but can bring on new symptoms and even adverse effects. Also, in the published research, when patients were switched from T4-only treatment to T4/T3 treatment, their thyroid status might have been slightly changed, which could have affected results of the research.

Clearly authorities in the thyroid field who teach doctors about ways of treating thyroid disease need to conduct very thorough and meticulous research before reaching the verdict that this treatment has no benefits.

"I Feel Beautiful Again"

Erin, a forty-four-year-old woman, had been diagnosed with hypothyroidism five years previously and had also had a hysterectomy. Despite numerous adjustments of her T4 dose, she did not feel as good as she would have liked. Her symptoms had progressed, and three years ago she got to a point at which she could no longer function. Because she continued to suffer from tiredness, trouble concentrating, and a host of other symptoms, her physician kept increasing the dose of thyroid hormone to make her feel better. Erin had no energy and had tingling in her hands that the doctors could not explain. She said:

> One doctor kept telling me that there wasn't anything wrong. He would tell me that I was fine, I think because he really didn't know what to do. I got to the point where I thought there was something terribly wrong with me, although I had no idea what it was. I could feel that my body and my mind were not functioning properly for my age.
>
> At one time, the doctor said I was hypoglycemic and put me on six little meals a day. It still didn't improve the way I felt.

Like most patients suffering from the lingering effects of a thyroid imbalance, Erin did not even suspect she might be depressed. But when I asked Erin about her symptoms, she confessed that she had most of the symptoms of depression. In addition, she had a lot of undue anger and became very irritable. "I went through a period where people would ask me a simple question, like 'Do you like my new haircut?' Instead of politely saying they looked nice whether they did or not, I would say something like, 'You know, it doesn't suit your face shape,' or 'It's horrible and makes you look bad.' Then I would be embarrassed at what had come out of my mouth."

Erin no longer suffers from depression or anger. Her physical symptoms have resolved since she started taking the right amount of T3 in combination with T4. It took two adjustments in the amount of T3 that she needed to feel at her best. She said:

> Now I'm happier and more stable. I feel like I have a life again. I have more energy. I am not angry. I don't think I'm depressed at all. I'm able to do stuff for other people that for a long time I couldn't do. For a while, I couldn't give of myself, and now I'm much more involved in my church and in social activities.
>
> As far as my relationship with my husband, he loves this change because I'm back to being my normal self again. I greet him with a smile and want to know about his day. Before, I wasn't able to do even that. I think I was so wrapped up in my own problems that I couldn't think about him. Now, we are back to where we sit down and we have our talks and spend time together.
>
> At work, I'm more able not to be angry when the telephone rings at the wrong time or things don't work out as planned. I don't get as frustrated as I did.

As a result of this protocol, Erin lost ten pounds when she first started. Her skin felt better, and she stopped losing hair. The swelling around her face and her bloated look went away. "When I look in the mirror," she says, "I feel beautiful again. This treatment totally revolutionized my life."

Some patients with an underactive thyroid are treated with high doses of desiccated Armour Thyroid taken as a single daily dose. These patients go through periods of high T3 levels in the brain for a long time and typically experience a withdrawal syndrome once the desiccated thyroid is stopped and replaced by levothyroxine. In such patients, if one uses the combination of levothyroxine and T3, as explained before, symptoms of brain hypothyroidism—including tiredness, exhaustion, and depression—often resolve. This approach has allowed me to successfully switch many patients from desiccated thyroid to a more physiological regimen combining the right amounts of T4 and T3.

The T4/T3 Protocol for Fibromyalgia

T4/T3 treatment is clearly the best thyroid hormone treatment for patients who suffer from fibromyalgia caused by an underactive thyroid (hypothyroid fibromyalgia).

As I explained in Chapter 13, people suffering from euthyroid fibromyalgia have a problem with thyroid hormone not working efficiently. They may not be producing enough T3 in their organs. For this reason, the ideal treatment for patients with an underactive thyroid who also have fibromyalgia should include T3. In fact, the only way I can achieve normal tissue thyroid hormone levels in patients with hypothyroid fibromyalgia is to use a T4/T3 combination therapy.

Michelle was one of the many patients who suffered from fibromyalgia that I successfully treated with T4/T3 combination therapy. She was thirty-seven years old when she started feeling tired and noticing hair loss and brittle nails. She gained weight and was feeling sleepy. Gradually, she began suffering from pains in her shoulders, the middle of her back, and her arms. She eventually started going to doctors when her symptoms worsened.

For four years after Michelle was diagnosed with an underactive thyroid, she continued to suffer from many symptoms that clearly indicated fibromyalgia, despite receiving an adequate dose of thyroxine. Here's how she described these symptoms:

> The pain in my shoulders at the top and right in the middle of my back was severe enough to wake me up in the middle of the night. I couldn't sleep because my joints hurt all the time. I was taking eight Advil a day, and they didn't help. I was exercising, which only seemed to make it worse. Sometimes the pain would shoot down my back, and I'd have tingling in my fingers, and sometimes it would come down my arm or up my neck.
>
> I had a friend who thought it was arthritis, and that's when I went to a series of specialists. After three years of going to them, one doctor told me I had back problems. He gave me a neck brace, and I received physical therapy three times a week for three weeks, and that didn't do any good. Another doctor told me that I probably had bruised some muscles in my back due to stress. One doctor told me that it was probably marital problems and stress.
>
> Finally, I went to another doctor, who, within five minutes, was touching the tender points in my back and my shoulders and took some X-rays and diagnosed me with fibromyalgia.

When I saw Michelle, she was taking L-thyroxine for her underactive thyroid. Instead, I prescribed a T4/T3 combination treatment using small doses of T3 given three times a day. Not only did the lingering symptoms disappear, but her fibromyalgia also improved dramatically. Michelle also started practicing a relaxation technique and receiving massage therapy. Michelle said:

> When I was just being treated with the T4 for my thyroid, I got to the point where I could hardly drag myself out of bed, and I really didn't want to be so-

cial anymore. Within a few weeks of starting on the T4/T3 protocol, I began to recognize a remarkable difference in the way I felt. I no longer wanted to sleep twenty-four hours a day. I could get up and function like a normal person. I no longer suffered from joint pain and body aches. That was exciting to me because I had felt so bad for so many years, I didn't think I would ever feel good again.

Michelle had suffered from hypothyroid fibromyalgia. Even in patients with fibromyalgia who have normal thyroid tests and have not experienced an underactive thyroid, this treatment may be beneficial. Remember, part of the problem may be an inefficiency of thyroid hormone. The body and brain need plenty of T3 to overcome this inefficiency. Administering T3 in appropriate amounts will not result in thyroid hormone excess and will provide more consistent and stable levels of T3 throughout the day.

T4/T3 in Conjunction with Antidepressants

Thyroid hormone pharmacotherapy may help many people suffering from depression who have a brain deficit of T3 not completely corrected by Prozac and the other selective serotonin reuptake inhibitors (SSRIs). The initial success I've had with T4/T3 treatment in people who have been prescribed antidepressants for lingering depression that resulted from a thyroid imbalance is astonishing. T3 has an almost miraculous effect on the brain chemistry. The beauty of this treatment is that blood levels of T4, T3, and TSH stay within the normal range.

As discussed in Chapter 18, it is not unusual for hypothyroid people to experience depression and require an antidepressant. Later, however, when their blood tests have been normal for some time, attempts to stop the antidepressant may cause the depression to return or become worse. In some patients, the antidepressant alone is not enough. When the patient is switched from T4 to the T4/T3 combination, the depression is resolved. It is as if the SSRI was not working properly because the brain chemistry mix was missing a small amount of T3 that was not being provided by the T4 pill.

Pat, a thirty-two-year-old pharmacist, recalls being diagnosed with hypothyroidism when she experienced a major depression that required hospitalization. She had had a previous episode of depression twelve years earlier when she was in college and broke up with her boyfriend. Her psychiatrist put Pat on Prozac along with thyroxine, and she regained normal thyroid function four months later. She continued to have low-grade depression and anxiety, however, despite taking the maximum dose of Prozac and enough thyroid hormone to maintain normal blood levels.

Like most patients with residual suffering, Pat found the solution in the T4/T3 combination treatment. When she came to see me, she wondered whether it was her thyroid that was causing her depressive symptoms to persist. Adding T3 to her T4 treatment in conjunction with the Prozac transformed her mood and energy spectacularly. Again, it is likely that the Prozac-levothyroxine treatment was not fully effective in curing the depression because Pat had a T3 deficit in her brain.

The small amount of T3 given in divided doses does not typically cause T3 levels in the blood to rise above the normal range. Nevertheless, before switching to a T4/T3 combination treatment, make sure that your doctor checks you for heart problems. That's because patients with heart disease may have heart rhythm problems or other heart complications that could be adversely affected by even minimal increases in the levels of T3. I do not advocate using this combination treatment in patients who are at increased risk of heart disease, notably older patients. Combine this protocol with a relaxation technique, diet, and exercise, and use the questionnaires provided in Chapters 5 and 8 before and during treatment so you can assess how well you are doing on this treatment program.

No longer do my patients with persistent symptoms who are being treated with T4 and have normal blood tests leave my office with the verdict that nothing else can be done for their suffering. My patients who had been taking desiccated thyroid now receive a treatment that allows them to feel better without having to accept bone loss as the price.

In my patients with lingering depression, standardized tests of depression show marked mood improvements after T4/T3 therapy. Scores for anxiety symptoms and cumulative physical thyroid-related symptoms go down, reflecting the change from a tired and disconnected person to a happy, symptomless one. One of my many patients who no longer needed Prozac and Zoloft after being switched to T4/T3 treatment told me, "I have not felt this way for God knows how long! Every day I think that this is going to stop working. I have great fears. But it has not. God bless you for bringing my life back together. Nothing worked for me ever before!"

Important Points to Remember

- Hypothyroid patients treated with T4-only drugs may suffer lingering effects because they're missing the right amount of T3, the most potent form of thyroid hormone as well as the main form that works in brain cells.
- Switching from T4 treatment to the T4/T3 combination regimen can begin to resolve emotional and physical symptoms, including depression, as soon as a week after the treatment is started.

- T4/T3 combination therapy may help maintain normal thyroid levels and improve symptoms in people suffering from persistent cases of fibromyalgia.
- Patients with underactive thyroid treated with T4 and an antidepressant for residual depression and fatigue improve tremendously when switched to T4/T3 combination therapy. This treatment can phase out antidepressant therapy.

21

THE THYROLIFE DIET FOR SUCCESSFUL LONG-TERM WEIGHT LOSS AND HEALTHY METABOLISM

Over the years I have seen hundreds of frustrated patients with thyroid-related weight gain problems who have tried many popular diets and failed to achieve their weight loss goals. They either initially lost weight and quickly gained it back or failed to lose any, all because of their intractable weight loss resistance and sluggish metabolism.

The reason thyroid patients have a hard time losing weight with popular diets, such as the Paleo diet, is because most of them only focus on one fundamental, such as low carbohydrate intake or high protein intake, while ignoring the other important ones. Yet, as I explained in Chapter 10, patients affected by thyroid disease are haunted by a high level of body inflammation, insulin resistance, and leptin and thyroid hormone inefficiency, leading to a slowing of metabolism and abnormal appetite and food cravings. An effective weight loss eating plan needs to take into account how metabolism-regulating hormones work in the body. Any diet that does not take into account the fundamentals that keep your hormonal system harmonious becomes an imbalanced diet and will not be conducive to long-term healthy weight loss. If you want to boost leptin and thyroid hormone efficiency and lower insulin resistance and inflammation, it is crucial to follow an eating plan that combines high protein intake, high fiber intake, and low-glycemic-index properties with the avoidance of metabolism-damaging and immune-system-agitating saturated and trans fats. For years I have suggested to anyone with weight gain issues that they combine these fundamentals. Following an eating plan that respects all these principles has allowed thousands of people, whether they have a thyroid problem or not, to lose weight efficiently and healthily, and keep it off for good. The ThyroLife Diet that goes along with my comprehensive thyroid mind-body program is an immune-system-friendly version of my weight loss diet, the Protein Boost Diet (consult my book *The*

Protein Boost Diet [Atria, 2012]).[1] In addition to boosting your metabolism and curbing your appetite with the right combinations of foods, the Thyro-Life Diet focuses on avoiding foods that irritate your immune system or promote the production of inflammation chemicals that impair and deregulate the harmony of your metabolism-regulating hormones. Another important guideline of my diet is the avoidance of environmental toxic chemicals that may have been contaminating your foods up until now.

The Seven Guidelines of the ThyroLife Diet

1. **Select high-quality protein sources.** Eating meals reasonably high in good quality proteins is the backbone of my diet.[2] Proteins contain essential amino acids that your body cannot manufacture on its own; you can only get them from foods. These amino acids boost the efficiency with which leptin and thyroid hormone help burn fat in the mitochondria. The most potent metabolism-energizing amino acids are leucine, isoleucine, and valine—branched chain amino acids (BCAAs) found in beans, lentils, quinoa, fish, and meats.[3] Methionine and L-arginine are also essential amino acids, but not of the branched chain category, and have powerful metabolism-boosting effects that lead to fat loss.[4] Foods rich in methionine include eggs, dairy, beans, turkey, fish, shellfish, and soy. Other amino acids have the ability to reduce cravings and reduce anxiety (lysine, taurine, and tryptophan).[5] For this reason, on my diet you will be eating combinations of favorite proteins at each meal to obtain an optimal amino acid profile that will make your thyroid hormone, leptin, and growth hormone work at peak efficiency.

2. **Low-glycemic-index meals.** I became an advocate of a low-glycemic-index diet when I realized that many of my patients were unable to lose weight unless they ate low-glycemic-index meals and reduced the amount of simple sugars in their diet.[6] How high your blood sugar goes up in response to a particular food or meal defines the glycemic index of that food or meal: the higher the rise, the higher the glycemic index. To design a low-glycemic-index meal, you first need to pick foods that are not loaded with simple sugars. Simple sugars, including refined sugars and fructose, cause glucose to enter the bloodstream faster and produce a higher rise in blood sugar, which in turn will trigger a much higher insulin spike. In addition, you need to focus on always combining foods containing carbohydrates with foods high in protein and fiber to keep the glycemic index as low as possible. By doing so, you will be less likely to accumulate extra fat and have insulin and leptin resistance. It also helps to recognize that your body has the ability to metabolize sugars much more efficiently during the

daytime than in the evening or at night, when you are sleeping.[7] For that reason, it is important to minimize carb consumption at dinnertime in order to prevent a significant insulin rise at night.[8] This will help leptin, thyroid hormone, and growth hormone work more efficiently at burning fat. In general, foods containing complex carbohydrates that are rich in fiber and protein, such as whole grains, quinoa, barley, nuts, and legumes, have a lower glycemic index than foods rich in simple sugars such as white bread, sweet corn, and white rice.

3. **Avoid fruits and drinks high in fructose.** In Chapter 10, I explained why and how consuming fructose or high-fructose corn syrup (HFCS) can damage your metabolism and induce insulin resistance, inflammation, and metabolic syndrome. I cannot emphasize enough the importance of paying attention to fructose and avoiding fruits rich in it, such as oranges, bananas, and pineapples. Definitely avoid foods and soft drinks with added HFCS. This additive has become ubiquitous in packaged foods such as deli items and canned baked beans.

4. **Avoid saturated fats and trans fats.** Anyone with a weight gain problem should avoid eating trans fats and saturated fats.[9] If you have an autoimmune thyroid condition and your immune system has become unstable, you should be quite rigorous in avoiding these immune-system-irritating foods.

5. **Consume at least 30 grams of fiber a day.** Consistently eating meals rich in fiber is an extremely important fundamental of my diet. Not only are fiber-rich foods loaded with antioxidants and other micronutrients that help your metabolism and immune system, but in the right amounts they have direct benefits on blunting appetite, reducing a meal's glycemic index, and reducing insulin resistance.[10] On my diet, you will be eating a mix of soluble and insoluble fiber, both of which will give you fantastic weight loss benefits.[11] For instance, soluble fiber, when it swells up in the stomach, will make the hunger hormone ghrelin go down, also speeding up your metabolism. Insoluble fiber, found in many of my favorite vegetables, helps you get rid of toxins through the GI tract. My diet requires that you eat at least 30 to 35 grams of fiber every day, with 5 to 7 grams at breakfast, 10 to 15 grams at lunch, and 10 to 15 grams at dinner. Paleo diet and other diets that do not respect this important fundamental are clearly insufficient and imbalanced diets, making them ineffective in the long term.

6. **Eat only immune-system-friendly foods.** As I explained in previous chapters, autoimmunity may be the underlying cause of your thyroid condition. This means that inflammation promoted by immune system

reactivity has certainly contributed to your weight gain. You need to be aware of the foods that irritate your immune system and cause it to produce metabolism-damaging inflammation chemicals.[12] Follow the food combination fundamentals of my diet and be diligent about eliminating any food your immune system is sensitive to. As I indicated in Chapter 10, the most common offenders in thyroid patients are gluten and dairy-containing foods, although you could be sensitive to anything—beans, cauliflower, asparagus, even almonds.

7. **Eat organic as much as possible.** In Chapter 2, I explained how environmental toxins can affect the function of the thyroid gland and lower the efficiency of thyroid hormones in your body. Many of these toxic chemicals also disrupt the immune system by being toxic to immune system cells and promoting a buildup of free radicals inside cells.[13] A lot of commercially grown produce is contaminated with high levels of pesticides, fungicides, and insecticides, which negatively affect the efficiency of metabolism-boosting hormones.[14] While scientific research has not yet fully proven that these toxins cause serious health consequences for the population as a whole, people with underlying autoimmunity problems are more likely to suffer from inflammation and its metabolic consequences. For this reason, I recommend choosing organic foods as often as possible and trying to avoid foods contaminated by toxic chemicals. If you eat dairy products, I recommend choosing organic low-fat and non-fat milk, cheese, and yogurt, as non-organic products may contain hormones that can affect your metabolism. Genetically modified products are more likely to be contaminated by toxic chemicals such as pesticides, so if you have an autoimmune thyroid condition, I recommend reducing or avoiding genetically modified products.

The ThyroLife Diet Protein Sources

To make your meal plan as efficient as possible at helping you burn fat, you need to select and combine protein sources that will provide the best mix of amino acids to boost leptin and thyroid hormone efficiency, while avoiding the protein sources that are most likely to make your immune system react and impair your metabolism. You should also avoid protein sources that are especially high in calories or potentially contain environmental chemicals that disturb your metabolism, such as tuna, which is frequently contaminated with mercury.

The three main protein sources of the ThyroLife Diet are seafood (including fish), poultry and lean meat, and vegetarian sources such as legumes and gluten-free grains.

Favorite Seafood	Favorite Poultry and Lean Meat	Favorite Vegetarian and Immune-System-Friendly Proteins
Tilapia, mahi mahi, catfish, flounder, haddock, Atlantic cod, bass, sole, wild salmon, trout, crab, shrimp, mollusks, herring, sardines	Beef liver, turkey, chicken (breast), veal, goat, game meat	**Legumes:** Lentils, fava beans, chickpeas, soybeans and soy derivatives (tofu, soy milk, tempeh), black beans, lima beans, navy beans, and other beans
		Gluten-free Grains: Quinoa, brown rice, amaranth, teff, buckwheat, oats

Although some dairy protein sources could be alternatives, I recommend avoiding or minimizing the consumption of dairy products made from cow's milk as much as possible. Sensitivities to dairy can develop over time, because thyroid patients' immune systems can become challenged by casein and whey, the two main protein components in dairy, as well as by other substances found in dairy products. I have found that patients with autoimmune thyroid disease are less likely to be sensitive to dairy products made from goat's milk. I have also found it possible to have a sensitivity to dairy even if your sensitivity test does not reveal it.

Quinoa, lentils, and the beans I have listed in the table above contain exceptional amino acid profiles that promote weight loss and curb appetite while giving you high amounts of fiber that help to reduce a meal's glycemic index.

The ThyroLife Diet Meal Plan

For you to get the right amounts and proportions of the different food categories at each meal, follow the meal plan outlined below. The recommended amounts are for a well-balanced diet that provides 1200–1500 calories a day, which is somewhat restrictive for most people with weight gain problems. However, you may adjust the caloric intake based on your basal metabolic rate and daily physical activity. You can do so by either reducing or increasing the protein portions. Once you have achieved your weight loss goal, you can increase caloric intake while continuing to follow the same meal fundamentals. Use the designated food category amounts (proteins, vegetables, fruits, and fats) to create meals with the optimal nutrition profile. Learn to eyeball proper portion sizes.

I recommend eating select fruits at breakfast and lunch *at the end of the meal* to avoid spiking glucose levels early in the meal, which can increase appetite. Avoid added sugars and saturated fats.

Including good fats is an important fundamental of the ThyroLife Diet. For each meal, systematically use one portion of any of the good fats listed below, as these are essential for optimal health and metabolism and make this diet a metabolism-boosting Mediterranean diet.[15]

- Healthy oils (olive oil, etc.) and nut butters: 1 teaspoon
- Nuts: 2 walnuts, 4 hazelnuts, 2 pecans, 6 almonds, 7 peanuts, or 7 pistachios
- Seeds: pine nuts, pumpkin, sesame, and sunflower seeds: 2 teaspoons; chia seeds: 2 teaspoons; flaxseed: 1 tablespoon
- Nut milks: 1 cup
- Avocado: ⅛ of whole
- Olives: 5

You may want to slightly reduce the amount of fat if your main protein is high in fat, such as salmon.

If you are sensitive to gluten, you need to avoid any whole grain that might contain gluten, such as wheat, bulgur, rye, barley, couscous, wheat bran, wheat germ, and whole-grain pastas. Even if testing does not reveal that you have a sensitivity to gluten, it is better to avoid these foods or at least eat them much less often than quinoa, brown rice, amaranth, and teff.

BREAKFAST MEAL PLAN

Protein Sources	+	Vegetables	+	Fruits	+	Good Fats
3–4 oz. fish or lean meat (see vegetarian alternatives below)		1–1½ cups		1 cup berries (or alternatives)		1 portion (see above)

LUNCH MEAL PLAN

Protein Sources	+	Vegetables	+	Fruits	+	Good Fats
1 cup legumes or gluten-free grains (cooked) + 3–4 oz. seafood or lean meat (see vegetarian alternatives below)		1–1½ cups		1 cup berries (or alternatives)		1 portion (see above)

DINNER MEAL PLAN

Protein Sources	+	Vegetables	+	Fruits	+	Good Fats
½ cup vegetarian protein + 6–8 oz. seafood or lean meat (see vegetarian alternatives below)		4 to 5 cups		None		1 portion (see above)

I recommend that you select seafood, particularly fish, over lean meat and poultry as a non-vegetarian protein at least four days a week. Although it is best to select one of the favorite seafood, poultry, or lean meats listed in the table on page 361, you can on occasion eat other fish and lean meats.

At lunchtime, the vegetarian protein (legumes or gluten-free grains) is an important component of the diet for its desirable amino acid profile and high fiber content.

VEGETARIAN PROTEIN ALTERNATIVES

You may replace at any meal (less often at dinnertime) 2 ounces of lean meat protein or fish with a vegetarian protein:

- Beans, lentils, quinoa, chickpeas, or brown rice = ⅓–½ cup
- Soy milk = ⅓ cup, tofu (extra firm or firm) = ½ cup
- Edamame = ½ cup
- Gluten-free cereals = ½ cup
- Whole-grain gluten-free bread = 1 thick or 2 thin slices

You may also, at any meal, substitute dairy protein for 2 ounces of lean meat or fish if you are not sensitive to dairy. Even if you do not have dairy sensitivity, I still recommend eating less of it. The amount of dairy protein that will replace the 2 ounces of lean meat or seafood is:

- Cottage cheese, plain low-fat or nonfat yogurt = ½ cup
- Ricotta or feta cheese = ¼ cup
- Goat cheese = 1 ounce

You may also substitute 3 egg whites for 1 ounce of lean meat or fish.

For breakfast and lunch, you may substitute ¼ cup unsweetened whole grain cereal or oatmeal and ¼ cup soy milk or 1 cup of almond milk (unsweetened) for 1 cup berries.

With respect to vegetables, the ones that are high in fiber, and relatively high in protein, and not loaded with fructose include:

- Broccoli
- Cauliflower
- Asparagus
- Brussels sprouts
- Mushrooms
- Okra
- Yellow squash
- Zucchini
- Chives
- Watercress

These vegetables will give you tremendous health and metabolism benefits. The amounts of vegetables provided in the table on pages 362–63 are for the vegetables that I just listed. That being said, I encourage you to mix these with other vegetables that do not contain significant amounts of protein, such as cucumbers, cabbage, mustard greens, collard greens, celery, kohlrabi, lettuce, bok choy, radicchio, spinach, eggplant, and banana peppers. Although I do not advocate avoidance of any vegetables, I recommend that you eat artichokes, kale, turnips, sprouts, beets, seaweed, shallots, fennel, string beans, carrots, snow peas, and butternut squash in a more limited amount as they may contain higher amounts of fructose.

Although the best fruits are berries, you may replace 1 cup berries with ⅓ cup papaya, 1 medium star fruit, 2–3 small limes or lemons, ½ large grapefruit, ½ medium kiwi, or 1 medium apple, pear, or peach. Many other fruits may contain higher amounts of fructose and should be avoided.

When you prepare your meals, I encourage using metabolism-beneficial spices such as hot peppers, black pepper, curcumin, garlic, cinnamon, and ginger root. These spices and herbs have potent antioxidant properties, reduce inflammation, and reduce insulin resistance. Spices such as annatto, cumin, oregano, sweet and hot paprika, rosemary, and saffron have some antioxidant properties as well.[16]

Tips for a Successful Weight Management Program

1. **Do not skip any meals.** Skipping meals will raise levels of your metabolism-slowing hormone, ghrelin, which can make you feel hungrier, possibly causing you to lose control over your food choices at a later meal.[17] Research has also shown that if you have ready-to-eat cereal, cooked cereal, quick breads, or fruits and vegetables for your breakfast—that is, items that include fiber—you will be less likely to have weight problems than if you skipped breakfast or ate meat and eggs instead.

2. **Eat a high-fiber, protein-rich midafternoon snack consistently, and a midmorning snack whenever possible.** This concept has been adopted in France, where people take the *goûter,* a snack eaten in the afternoon. A study has shown that people who no longer ate a *goûter* had a significant increase in weight. Eating four or five times a day will reduce your insulin levels, improve insulin and leptin efficiency, and lower your cholesterol and triglyceride levels.[18]

3. **Try to eat at the same time of day every day.** The idea is to synchronize your meal intake with the cellular clock of your body parts. This will optimize your body's metabolic functions. Equally important is to abstain from eating for at least three hours prior to bedtime, to maximize fat burn at night when you are asleep.[19]

4. **Drink plenty of water throughout the day.** Water is necessary both for hydration and for detoxing purposes, both of which are essential for optimal metabolic functions. But avoid drinking excessive amounts of water in the evening so that you will not disturb your sleep by waking up to urinate.

5. **Beware of high-calorie drinks loaded with simple sugars.** Soft drinks, beverages with added sugar, fruit juices, and alcoholic beverages all increase your calorie intake but will not make you feel full. Avoid consuming high-fructose corn syrup, used in many soft drinks; this can cause weight gain and damage to the metabolism. Milk has always been considered a healthy beverage; however, it is rich in lactose, which is a sugar. You need to be careful with respect to the amount of milk that you consume.

6. **When you dine out, pay attention.** A recent survey conducted in the United States has shown that we tend to eat out more often than in previous years.[20] Eating out tends to promote weight gain because of the types of foods you end up eating—high amounts of animal fat and simple sugars—and because restaurant portions tend to be large. Choose foods that get you as close to the food combinations of the ThyroLife Diet as possible.

7. **Minimize or avoid processed foods.** These can contain preservatives, artificial sweeteners, dyes, and a wide variety of additives that can disturb the efficiency of metabolism-regulating hormones. Also, minimize exposure to highly toxic metals such as mercury, a common contaminant of many fish such as swordfish, king mackerel, grouper, tile fish, orange roughy, tuna, halibut, snapper, and Spanish mackerel. Avoid the flavoring agent monosodium glutamate (MSG), as it contains very high amounts of glutamate, a molecule that has been shown to have a potentially damaging effect on the appetite center in the hypothalamus, which will make you hungrier and increase cravings.[21]

8. **The way you prepare your meals is important.** The preferred ways of cooking meats and fish are baking, roasting, and broiling. An alternative is grilling, but definitely avoid frying. For vegetables, I recommend steaming and boiling. Make sure you do not overcook your vegetables as this will deplete them of essential micronutrients.

9. **Make sure you get seven to eight hours of sleep daily.** Correct any sleep issue that can affect your metabolism (see Chapter 10).

10. **Improve the way you manage stress.** Stress has a twofold effect: it has a major impact on your leptin level and efficiency, and it can also cause impulsive eating. To help you overcome these effects, try a mind-body technique such as yoga or tai chi. This will help you lose weight and maintain the weight loss you have achieved.[22]

11. **If you are suffering from stress-related eating and uncontrollable food cravings, try a cognitive behavioral approach.** This technique entails monitoring and recognizing what stresses you out, adjusting your response to those specific stressors, and figuring out what you could be doing differently in response.[23] Increasingly, weight loss programs utilize this approach, which focuses more on the physiological health impact of weight problems rather than on weight loss per se. The thought that weight will have a detrimental effect on your health will motivate you to continue with your weight loss efforts. Research has shown that such cognitive behavioral programs promote weight loss, improve emotional well-being, and reduce the distress associated with dieting. They also encourage activity and fitness, and improve quality of life.

12. **Increase your calcium intake.** Animal research has shown that calcium affects metabolism in fat cells. A high amount of calcium in your diet increases the breakdown of fat.[24] High calcium intake has more metabolic benefits when you also consume high amounts of branched-chain amino acids, found in high amounts in fish, meats, mushrooms, vegetables, brown rice, beans, nuts, lentils, beef liver, and chickpeas, all favorite protein sources of the ThyroLife Diet.

13. **Increase your intake of omega-3 fatty acids.** Omega-3 fatty acids help speed up your metabolism and have a protective effect against cardiovascular disease.[25] (See Chapter 22 for more information on omega-3 fatty acids.) They will also reduce hunger.[26]

14. **Take adequate amounts of critical minerals, vitamins, and antioxidants.** Several vitamins and antioxidants are being touted for their ability to enhance metabolism and help with weight loss.[27] These micronutrients will reduce and prevent the accumulation of free radicals that could slow down your metabolism. While many minerals, vitamins, and antioxidants are essential adjuncts for any weight loss diet to be effective, I do not believe that just taking a good mix of minerals,

vitamins, and antioxidants will make you lose weight unless you also follow the eating plan outlined above and engage in regular exercise. Zinc, selenium, and chromium have a significant impact on your weight. For instance, low zinc levels correlate with obesity, and zinc has been used by nutritionists in the treatment of obesity.[28] Selenium affects metabolism at every level; you cannot lose weight efficiently without taking plentiful amounts of selenium.[29] Chromium, an essential nutrient, makes insulin work more efficiently and will help you lose weight more efficiently and keep the weight off.[30] Research has shown that in a weight management program, obese men who took chromium lost 11.7 pounds over a ten-year period, while men who did not take chromium lost only 6.1 pounds over the same span. Vitamin C also affects your metabolism and has been shown to be inversely related to body mass.[31] People who have adequate vitamin C intake burn 30 percent more fat during moderate exercise than people who are low in vitamin C. If you have vitamin C deficiency, you will have a hard time losing fat while dieting. In Chapter 22, I will provide a comprehensive list of all the minerals, vitamins, antioxidants, and other micronutrients that help rid you of the free radical burden, reduce inflammation, and help you lose weight by improving insulin, leptin, and thyroid hormone efficiency. These are the same micronutrients that will provide the best support for the immune system while reducing its reactivity. That, in turn, will reduce the inflammation chemical burden in your body.

15. **Take a probiotic supplement.** Depletion of the good bacteria in the GI tract is quite common in the general population, and it is almost universal in people with weight gain issues and thyroid disease. An imbalanced ratio of good and bad bacteria agitates your immune system and will promote inflammation in your body, increase your food cravings, and affect your food choices. All these factors can contribute to weight loss resistance. To overcome these negative consequences, you need to take a well-balanced mix of good bacteria (probiotics). In Chapter 22, I will give you specific recommendations for the types and amounts of probiotics that I encourage you to take on a daily basis, not only for the weight loss benefits but also for reducing immune system reactivity.

Supplements, Herbs, and Medications for Weight Loss

Throughout my career in thyroid disease and caring for thyroid patients struggling with weight problems, I very rarely recommended a pharmaceutical drug for weight loss. I have always believed that restoring the balance of metabolism-regulating hormones through a good diet while addressing the root causes of weight gain in thyroid patients is the best path toward successful weight loss. Several weight loss medications that affect appetite centers and/or fat burning have been developed but ultimately pulled off the market, such as sibutramine, because of their adverse effects. Some of the most common currently available medications that could potentially be useful in managing your weight gain include:

- **Orlistat.** Blocks the enzyme responsible for breaking down ingested fat, keeping it indigestible and excreted from your body along with your stools. Side effects include more bowel movements than usual, oily stools, less control over bowel movements, and gas with discharge.
- **Contrave (naltrexone plus bupropion).** A combination of naltrexone, an opiate antagonist, and bupropion, an antidepressant. Both work together on the brain by reducing your appetite and, consequently, the quantity of food you consume. Side effects include vomiting, constipation, difficulties sleeping, nausea, mouth dryness, and an increase in sweating.
- **Belviq (lorcaserin).** A serotonin receptor agonist that acts on the brain and makes you better able to control your appetite. Side effects include constipation, headaches, dry mouth, nausea, dizziness, and feelings of exhaustion.
- **Saxenda (liraglutide).** A substance that is similar to a naturally produced hormone that helps control digestion, blood sugar, and insulin levels. Side effects include constipation and diarrhea, nausea, loss of appetite, low blood sugar, dizziness, sluggishness, and tiredness.
- **Phentermine.** A sympathomimetic amine that acts on the brain and leads to appetite suppression. Side effects include increased irritability, nausea, vomiting, dizziness, mouth dryness, difficulty falling and staying asleep, constipation, and diarrhea.
- **Qsymia (phentermine plus topiramate).** A combination of phentermine and topiramate, an anticonvulsant drug. Both work together by reducing appetite and/or increasing bodily energy output. More research is needed to figure out the exact mechanism of how they work together. Side effects include difficulty falling and staying asleep, drowsiness, constipation, dizziness, and mouth dryness.

If you have PCOS, whether diagnosed in your early reproductive years or at a later age, you may benefit from taking a drug called metformin, which improves insulin sensitivity and is commonly used in non-insulin-dependent diabetes. The usual dose is 500 mg taken twice a day. Research has shown that taking metformin in conjunction with following a weight loss eating plan results in long-lasting weight loss.[32]

Alternative medicine practitioners commonly recommend several herbs that may help you lose weight. However, well-conducted scientific research is lacking to prove that these herbs are effective for weight loss, and the doses claimed to be effective for weight loss have not been standardized. Some of these herbs may be toxic when taken in excessive amounts. The following list gives you the best of the most popular ones.

COMMON NAME	SCIENTIFIC NAME
Saint-John's-wort	*Hypericum perforatum*
Garcinia cambogia	*Garcinia gummi-gutta*
Yerba maté	*Ilex paraguariensis*
Sand plantain	*Plantago psyllium*
Asian ginseng	*Panax ginseng*
Aloe vera	*Aloe vera*
Ginkgo	*Ginkgo biloba*
American ginseng	*Panax quinquefolius*

Other supplements have been studied more extensively. Pyruvate, for instance, has the best evidence to support its weight loss benefits in overweight people.[33] Glucomannan, a dietary fiber supplement, can help you lose weight by giving you a sensation of fullness, making you feel less hungry. The usual recommended dose is 600–1,000 mg taken with 8 ounces of water prior to a meal three times a day. Fiber-rich weight-loss supplements are likely to work by reducing ghrelin levels, which in turn curbs appetite and makes fat burn easier.

My favorite natural weight-loss helpers include:

- **Relora.** A patented extract from *Magnolia officinalis* and a proprietary extract from *Philodendron amurense,* Relora helps with stress-related eating and anxiety. It seems to work on countering the effects of cortisol on the body and mind, and can help give you more restful sleep, crucial for many thyroid patients.
- **Garcinia cambogia.** This suppresses appetite and lessens fat accumulation.
- **Raspberry ketones.** They have been touted for several metabolic benefits, including the stimulation of fat tissue to produce adiponectin, a hormone that has powerful effects on fat burn.
- **Yerba maté.** This herb has a high polyphenol content and tremendous antioxidant properties, which support fat burning when you follow my diet.
- **Chromium.** As I've said, chromium improves insulin sensitivity and is crucial for optimal metabolic functions.

- **Green tea.** Helps speed up metabolism, reduce fat formation, lower the absorption of fat, and reduce triglyceride levels.[34] High caffeine intake also promotes weight loss, as caffeine increases the breakdown of fat.[35]
- **Turmeric.** Turmeric (*Curcuma longa*) is one of my favorite natural ingredients to fight inflammation and support the immune system. In my opinion, all thyroid patients who suffer from significant immune system reactivity and/or weight gain issues should take this wonderful supplement continuously, without interruption. I typically recommend 50 to 150 mg daily. A plant in the ginger family, turmeric has been used to treat everything from stomach pain and heartburn, to colds and fevers, and has even been included in cancer treatments. Besides being a wonderful antioxidant, it helps calm the immune system by reducing bodily inflammation.[36] Turmeric is important for thyroid support and thyroid hormone efficiency in your body, helping boost your metabolism.
- **Alpha-lipoic acid.** This is one of the most powerful antioxidants and plays a major role in metabolism and fat burning. I always include it as part of the antioxidant mix for my thyroid patients in order to enhance their thyroid health and speed up their metabolism.
- **Grape seed extract.** Traditionally used as alternative medicine in the Mediterranean since the times of ancient Greece, grape seeds have a high concentration of vitamin E, flavonoids, linoleic acid, and oligomeric proanthocyanidin complex (OPC), a polyphenol with strong antioxidant properties. Resveratrol is another powerful polyphenol found in grape seed extract that shows promising metabolic benefits for people with weight problems. It relieves inflammation and oxidative stress associated with being overweight. Grape seed extract has been shown to reduce swelling and help people with poor blood circulation and other cardiovascular diseases.[37]
- **L-tryptophan.** An essential amino acid important for bodily functions, L-tryptophan increases serotonin and melatonin in the body. It has been used in alternative medicine to help promote appetite reduction and sleep.

The weight loss benefits of these ten natural ingredients become even more effective when they are taken together. Use them as an adjunct to my weight loss program. You can take them as separate dietary supplements or find them available as a mix in the ThyroLife Body Slim supplement.

Improper Use of Thyroid Hormone for Weight Control

Unfortunately, some weight loss centers continue to prescribe thyroid hormone without preliminary thyroid testing to people suffering from fatigue and weight gain issues. This practice could be very dangerous for patients with heart disease or who tend to be emotionally unstable. Frequently, the doses that are prescribed exceed what a normal thyroid gland produces. And while overweight people who are given high doses of thyroid hormone and also placed on a low-calorie diet experience greater weight loss than those on a diet alone, the consequences can be quite detrimental to their physical and mental health.[38] Moreover, the weight loss is temporary and unhealthy.

Some weight loss supplements may contain high amounts of thyroid hormone. People who took Enzo-Caps, a nonprescription diet pill allegedly made from "natural food products" of papaya, garlic, and kelp, became hyperthyroid. Analysis of the Enzo-Caps showed that these supplements were high in thyroid hormones T3 and T4.[39] Several years ago, a hundred women from various areas of Japan became hyperthyroid as a result of taking a weight-reducing pill, Basetsuper, that also contained thyroid hormones.[40] A third of these women experienced psychiatric problems as a result of the excessive amounts of thyroid hormone. Two of these women were admitted to a mental institution because their doctors believed they had become addicted to the weight loss pill. I therefore urge you to pay attention to exactly what you are taking when you attend a diet clinic or decide to use supplements for weight control.

The Exercise Program That Will Help You Lose Weight Efficiently

All weight-loss programs incorporate exercise to increase calorie burn and improve the chances of weight loss.[41] However, it is not how long, how much, or how often you exercise that determines how efficient the exercise program is. There is a misconception that the longer you exercise, the more fat you will burn. It is not uncommon to see people exercising for an hour and a half or two hours without seeing any results. The main reason is that the exercises they use put their body under major stress but are not necessarily able to boost their metabolism efficiently. When it comes to exercise, like anything else, it is all about balance.

You may think that the calories your body burns by exercising is what helps you lose weight. This is true to some extent. But if you engage in a structured program that combines aerobic exercises with high-intensity interval training (HIIT) and the right muscle workouts (focusing on core muscles while not ignoring the other muscle groups), you will burn much more fat overall. A balanced exercise program such as the Protein Boost Diet 20/10 exercise program, extensively detailed in my book *The Protein Boost Diet,* will make you continue to burn extra fat even hours after you have completed the exercise. This has to do with the release of hormones into your bloodstream that have the ability to boost your metabolism and make the fat-burn-boosting hormones leptin and thyroid hormone work more efficiently.

THE FUNDAMENTALS OF THE 20/10 EXERCISE PROGRAM
- A total of 30 minutes of daily exercise
- 20 minutes of daily aerobic exercise, alternating HIIT exercises in the form of walking, running, swimming, or biking with regular aerobic exercise
- Daily 10-minute muscle workouts that include five repetitive exercises focusing on specific muscle groups, with a special focus on core muscles

Combining the 20/10 exercise program, designed with the help of a national exercise expert, with the ThyroLife Diet and all the other steps I have outlined in this book will make your weight-loss easier, more effective, and long-lasting.

Important Points to Remember

- The ThyroLife Diet follows high-protein-intake, high-fiber-intake, and low-glycemic-index principles along with elimination of immune-irritating foods.
- On the ThyroLife Diet, the combinations of foods you select for your meals are important components of the diet.
- The ThyroLife Diet is conducive to healthy weight loss because it is designed to boost efficiency of the hormones that make you burn fat even at rest.
- While following the well-structured eating plan and paying attention to the foods you are eating, focus on important weight loss tips detailed in this chapter that will help you achieve your weight loss goals.
- One of the most important tips for successful weight loss is to take the right supplements to help improve the efficiency of metabolism-boosting hormones.

22
MY THYROID
MIND-BODY PROGRAM

Treating a thyroid condition with medications to restore and maintain thyroid hormone levels in a perfectly normal range is obviously necessary. However, thyroid medications alone are not sufficient for most patients. You also need to focus on continuously supporting the health of your thyroid gland and the health of your immune system, and on maximizing the effectiveness of thyroid hormone at performing its bodily functions. Unfortunately, many healthcare professionals do not focus on the health of the immune system, the root cause of your problem, or on the overall health of the thyroid gland. To achieve your health goals, overcome the many consequences of immune system reactivity, and reduce the health risks of thyroid disease, you need to follow a lifestyle that includes eating healthy foods, taking the right supplements, following an exercise program, and practicing relaxation techniques. In addition, you need to address your sleep issues, any other hormonal imbalance, coexisting depression, and other possible autoimmune conditions you may have. All of these steps are important for you to reach and maintain optimal physical and mental health. While some doctors may lead you to believe that regular monitoring of thyroid hormone levels and making adjustments in drug dosages is all you need, you have seen for yourself throughout this book that a combination of therapies is a must to deal with all the effects thyroid disease has on body and mind.

We've seen the role of stress in triggering and perpetuating thyroid disease. But lifestyle factors also influence the likelihood of you developing a thyroid condition, including your diet and whether or not you exercise. To some extent, these factors also determine how severe and consequential a thyroid disorder will be. Your genes may make you susceptible to developing a thyroid condition, but whether or not you actually develop one and the severity of its effects depend on how you live your daily life.

It is certainly easier to prevent the onset of an autoimmune attack on the thyroid than to treat autoimmunity once the attack has occurred. But even when thyroid autoimmunity and thyroid hormone imbalances have already occurred, you can minimize and even halt some of its adverse effects on your health by following a thyroid-friendly lifestyle. Any such lifestyle must take into account other health conditions that you have and any other medications you are taking that can contribute to the mental and physical effects of thyroid disease.

For instance, if you have an underactive or overactive thyroid, your risk of developing cardiovascular disease becomes much higher. And even if the thyroid imbalance is corrected with treatment, the elevated risk may haunt you your entire life. Patients treated for Graves' disease suffer from more hospital admissions with cardiovascular disease than people with healthy thyroids. According to research, patients with Hashimoto's thyroiditis who are older than fifty are three times more likely to be admitted to a hospital for a heart problem.[1] What puts thyroid patients at a higher risk for cardiovascular disease probably has to do with imperfect thyroid levels while being treated. The increased risk also has to do with a high level of body inflammation generated by the immune system as well as by the effects of depression, stress, overweight, and sleep issues on the cardiovascular system.

The Ten Pillars of My Thyroid Mind-Body Program

Years ago I realized that thyroid patients needed more than just medication, so over the years I have developed an increasingly comprehensive and multi-faceted treatment program. If I didn't address their stress issues, sleep problems, other hormonal imbalances, nutrition, and exercise routine, and if they didn't take their supplements, I was unable to restore their overall well-being. To be able to reach and maintain real thyroid wellness, you need to embrace the following ten components of my comprehensive thyroid mind-body program.

1. **Keep your thyroid hormone levels perfectly well balanced with the right thyroid medications at all times.** Work with your doctor to have the doses of T4 and T3 medications appropriately adjusted based on your symptoms and blood tests. I recommend that you choose a health-care professional who specializes in thyroid disease, is attentive to your symptoms and concerns, and is open to using a medication program that could include the combination of T4 and T3 that fits your needs. You need to know that deviation from perfection in your thyroid hormone levels will affect your well-being, your metabolism, and the reactivity of your immune system.

2. **Balance other hormonal issues.** I have already explained the interrelationship between menopause, immune system reactivity, thyroid disease, and changes in metabolism. Many perimenopausal and menopausal women who suffer from thyroid disease cannot reach thyroid wellness unless they address their hormonal deficiencies or imbalances with the right type of hormone replacement therapies. Similarly, many women with polycystic ovary syndrome and thyroid disorder need to address their hormonal imbalances in order to break the vicious cycle of immune system attacks on the thyroid, body inflammation, and weight issues. You may be suffering from growth hormone deficiency or other pituitary issues in addition to your thyroid problem. If you have lingering symptoms, these medical conditions need to be considered in order for you to get the right diagnosis and treatment.

3. **Proper nutrition.** Paying attention to what you eat and don't eat and respecting the important guidelines of the ThyroLife Diet will help you manage your weight efficiently. It will also help support your immune system and boost the efficiency of thyroid hormone in your body.

> **Main Benefits of the ThyroLife Diet**
> Weight management
> Cholesterol control
> Decrease in autoimmune reaction
> Mood enhancement
> Reduction in cravings

4. **Minimize food sensitivities.** Being aware of which foods your immune system is reactive to and avoiding these foods is an important component of my thyroid mind-body program. Ignoring this component will affect the intensity of the immune system attacks on your thyroid and can make you more vulnerable to other autoimmune attacks on different body parts. It will also worsen your body inflammation, make you gain weight, and make you unable to lose weight even when dieting. Eating the foods that you are sensitive to can cause fatigue and other annoying symptoms that affect your quality of life. You need to pay particular attention to gluten sensitivity, which you may have even if your gluten antibody testing is negative. There are several methodologies for food sensitivity testing (see table, page 376), but I found that methods using antibody testing, such as those provided by Cyrex, Meridian Valley, and Alletess, are more reliable. There is no perfect method for testing food sensitivities, but testing will give you a basis for eliminating the foods that are affecting you the most.

Food Sensitivity Testing	Technique Used
Alletess Medical Laboratory	IgG, IgE, IgA, ELISA
Cell Science Systems—ALCAT	White blood cell count and size
Meridian Valley	Combination IgG and IgE ELISA method
Great Plains Laboratory	IgG with candida, IgE
Oxford Biomedical Technologies	Mediator release test (mediator release corresponds to volumetric changes in neutrophils, monocytes, eosinophils, and lymphocytes)
Cyrex	IgG and IgA, proprietary QC2 method
ImmunoLabs	IgE solid phase chemiluminescent immunoassay
Revive Life	Vega Test, an EAV acupuncture technique testing device
Skin prick test	IgE

5. **A good supplement program.** An important pillar of the thyroid mind-body program is to take daily supplements that include minerals, vitamins, antioxidants, and other micronutrients to support the immune system (see below). Many of these micronutrients help reduce the free radical burden in immune system cells. They also help in preserving healthy thyroid cells as well as making thyroid hormone work more efficiently in the body. The supplement program for thyroid patients also includes specific probiotics in adequate amounts to rebalance bacterial flora in the gut. Probiotics in thyroid patients have many benefits, but the most significant one is the lowering of immune system reactivity and its consequences, something that is extremely beneficial for individuals suffering from autoimmune thyroid disease.

6. **Address your sleep issues.** Good-quality sleep is a must for reducing immune system reactivity and having stable thyroid function. It is also essential for healthy metabolism and brain functions. Sleep disorders can induce metabolic syndrome and affect your cardiovascular health. Research has shown that patients with thyroid disease who also have sleep apnea have a higher incidence of cardiovascular disease than people who do not have a thyroid disorder. This means that you need to pay a lot more attention to the quality of your sleep. If you have insomnia, sleep deprivation, sleep fragmentation, or sleep apnea, it is extremely important to treat these conditions so that your thyroid medications will work efficiently.

7. **Take a stress management approach.** As I explained in previous chapters, stress and the perception of stress make the immune system react on your thyroid and at the same time produce more inflammation chemicals, causing instability in your thyroid levels and promoting

metabolic changes that affect your weight and overall health. Use the relaxation techniques that work best for you, such as meditation, yoga, or tai chi. Getting support from family and friends is quite important. I recommend that you establish and follow a stress management routine tailored to your needs.

8. **Diligently follow the 20/10 exercise program or another well-balanced exercise program that combines aerobic exercise and muscle workouts.** This is crucial for optimizing weight loss, supporting cardiovascular health, and improving overall mood and perception of stress.

9. **Address depression and anxiety.** If you are suffering from depression or anxiety unrelated to your thyroid condition, it is important that you get help from counseling, psychotherapy, and/or appropriate antidepressant medications.

10. **Address cardiovascular risks.** Because thyroid patients have a higher risk of having cardiovascular disease down the road, you need to be even more vigilant about having your high cholesterol and high blood pressure adequately treated, since these issues are known to independently increase the risk of cardiovascular disease. An unresolved weight problem clearly has a greater impact on your cardiovascular health than it would for a person without thyroid disease.

The diagram highlights the main components of my mind-body program.

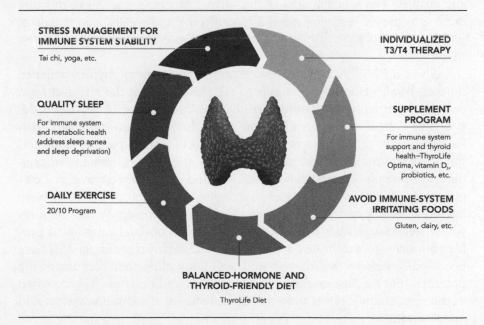

STRESS MANAGEMENT FOR
IMMUNE SYSTEM STABILITY

Tai chi, yoga, etc.

INDIVIDUALIZED
T3/T4 THERAPY

QUALITY SLEEP

For immune system
and metabolic health
(address sleep apnea
and sleep deprivation)

SUPPLEMENT
PROGRAM

For immune system
support and thyroid
health–ThyroLife
Optima, vitamin D₃,
probiotics, etc.

DAILY EXERCISE

20/10 Program

AVOID IMMUNE-SYSTEM
IRRITATING FOODS

Gluten, dairy, etc.

BALANCED-HORMONE AND
THYROID-FRIENDLY DIET

ThyroLife Diet

Healthy Nutrition, Healthy Life

What to eat and not eat has become an obsession in our society. For some people, dieting is one way to control weight. For others, eating the right foods is a way to prevent disease. Many people also try to select foods that promote a stable, happy mood.

In Chapter 10 I explained how and why thyroid patients often struggle with weight problems. I also emphasized that if you have a thyroid imbalance, the best diet to follow to overcome your weight is the ThyroLife Diet, a high-protein, high-fiber, low-glycemic-index, low-saturated-fat diet that takes into account immune system reactivity (see Chapter 21). As with other major health conditions, including coronary artery disease, high blood pressure, diabetes, and cancer (all leading causes of death in the United States), thyroid disease and its consequences can be prevented or minimized by proper nutrition. The ThyroLife Diet is also the most suitable eating plan to prevent or temper an autoimmune attack on the thyroid.

Research has shown that a high-protein, low-fat diet helps prevent the occurrence of autoimmune disease. Such a diet also appears to slow down the progress of autoimmune conditions.[2] Eating too much fat will harm your immune system and help precipitate an autoimmune attack on several organs, which could include your thyroid. A diet high in protein and fiber and low in fat and simple sugars helps you control your cholesterol and blood pressure and helps prevent damage to your brain from poor blood supply and strokes. The fundamentals of the ThyroLife eating plan make this diet quite effective in reversing metabolic syndrome and weight gain trends in patients with polycystic ovary syndrome, often associated with Hashimoto's thyroiditis.

Given the high rate of depression and anxiety among thyroid patients, no diet, however healthy, that fails to take into account the effect of food on mood can truly be thyroid-friendly. The functioning of the brain depends to a great extent on what you eat. A low-glycemic-index diet, rich in high-quality proteins containing high levels of essential amino acids and other anxiety-reducing amino acids such as tryptophan, lysine, and arginine, improves your mood, relieves anxiety, and reduces food cravings. Low-glycemic-index meals rich in essential amino acids often prevent you from having annoying symptoms and low mood after you eat. My diet requires you to get enough fiber while benefiting from an optimal amino acid profile conducive to weight loss and anxiety relief. Many thyroid patients have been led to believe that they should avoid soy altogether because of the potential (but media-exaggerated) effect on thyroid function. Yet soy eaten in the right amount offers tremendous benefits for the immune system and metabolism.

A soy-based diet (high in fiber and protein), like that traditionally eaten by the Japanese, is good for your mood and cognition. Soy has a beneficial effect on cholesterol and triglyceride levels and lowers cardiovascular risks. While there has been some concern that soy may impair thyroid function, research has shown that soy foods do not seem to slow thyroid function in people who have a normal thyroid gland and who get an adequate amount of iodine.[3] But if your gland is somewhat compromised and your iodine intake is not optimal, eating large amounts of soy foods daily for several weeks may make your gland become slightly underactive. Because of these potential thyroid effects as well as the possible effects of phytoestrogens on mood and cognition,[4] try to limit soy-based foods to three or four servings a week.

Avoid regularly eating large amounts of raw foods containing goitrogens, substances that can impair the manufacture of thyroid hormone (see Chapter 2). Heat neutralizes goitrogens, so it is usually quite safe to eat them when they are adequately cooked.

The Essential Dietary Fats

Fats in the body serve as a source of energy, but that's hardly their only function or even their most important one. Certain fats play roles in bodily processes as diverse as producing hormones and promoting intelligence (about 60 percent of the brain consists of fat). Your thyroid also needs specific kinds of fats to work properly. Like other parts of the body, however, it doesn't need the most common kinds of fat that most people eat, such as saturated fatty acids and trans fats.

The essential fatty acids are the fats that you may not be providing in adequate amounts to your thyroid and the rest of your body. Essential fatty acids play a crucial role in the structure of cell membranes, the formation of various hormone-like substances in the body, proper functioning of the cardiovascular system, and other aspects of health. They're called essential because the body cannot manufacture them on its own: they have to be supplied by foods or supplements. Essential fatty acids are polyunsaturated and classified in a number of groups, the best of which are the omega-3s and the omega-6s. The chief omega-6 essential fatty acid is called linoleic acid, and the chief omega-3 essential fatty acid is alpha-linolenic acid. Omega-6 fatty acids, by and large, promote inflammation, irritate the immune system, and temper the benefits of omega-3 fatty acids. For optimal immune system health, it is imperative that you keep the ratio of omega-3 to omega-6 around 2:1.

Omega-3 fatty acids play a major role in the structure and functioning of the brain, and low levels are associated with depression. In infants, omega-3 fatty acids affect brain and vision development. Omega-3 fatty acids help prevent certain aspects of cardiovascular disease, particularly at the level of blood vessel supply in the brain. Lack of omega-3 fatty acids will affect renewal of membranes in the brain and will accelerate aging of the brain, contributing to dementia (including Alzheimer's disease) and depression. Increased consumption of alpha-linolenic acid improves symptoms of attention deficit disorder. An analysis of research published in the *Journal of Affective Disorders* has determined that omega-3 fatty acids are quite helpful for the treatment of depression in adults.[5]

Main Benefits of Omega-3 Fatty Acids
Decrease in autoimmune attacks
Mood benefits
Cardiovascular system benefits
Maintenance of cell membrane integrity
Weight benefits

Two omega-3 free fatty acids have attracted the most attention for their health benefits: eicosapentaenoic acid (EPA) and docosahexaenoic acid (DHA). EPA and DHA are conditional essential omega-3 fatty acids, that is, they can be produced by the body as long as adequate amounts of alpha-linoleic acid are available. However, for the body to produce these two omega-3 fatty acids, high levels of cellular energy are required. For this reason, do not solely rely on your body to produce them in the right amounts. EPA has significant anti-inflammatory effects; DHA, a bigger molecule that can be produced by the body from EPA, is essential for brain health. The primary dietary sources of these two essential fatty acids are various deep-sea fish, such as mackerel, albacore tuna, salmon, herring, and sardines. Eating the flesh of these oily fish or taking fish oil supplements such as cod liver oil, shark liver oil, and halibut liver oil helps prevent heart disease. Animal research also suggests that a diet rich in EPA can prevent the occurrence of lupus-like autoimmune disease.[6] It also likely helps prevent autoimmune attacks on the thyroid. Some doctors advocate using EPA in the treatment of rheumatoid arthritis and psoriasis because of its tremendous immune system benefits. The known beneficial effects of fish oil are expanding to include the prevention of various types of cancer, such as colon cancer. I believe that taking omega-3 fatty acid supplements is a must for all thyroid patients, considering their effects on the immune system, mood, and the cardiovascular system. Omega-3 fatty acids enhance satiety, reduce food cravings, and make you burn extra fat more efficiently. They also help thyroid hormone clear fat from your liver. In essence, omega-3 fatty acids have the ability to reduce insulin resistance, lower your triglyceride and cholesterol levels, and improve the efficiency of the metabolism boosting hormone leptin. It is unlikely that you will get the right amount of omega-3 fatty acids even if you follow a healthy, well-balanced diet such as the ThyroLife eating plan and include omega-3-rich foods in your meals. For this reason, I recommend that you take, on a daily basis, a supplement that includes EPA (600 mg) and DHA (400 mg) in order to achieve and maintain excellent levels of those essential substances.

Antioxidants: Optimizing Thyroid Health and Immune System Support

About two thousand years ago Hippocrates said, "Let food be your medicine and medicine be your food." The body's cells need oxygen to function properly, but the result of oxygen intake is the production of free radicals, which are toxic to cells. A buildup of free radicals produced from bodily metabolism has the propensity to weaken the immune system and the body's ability to fight disease. Free radicals damage cells and their surroundings. An excess of free radicals can severely damage genes and as a result can promote cancer. Antioxidants are important for anyone with or without thyroid disease. However, if you have an autoimmune thyroid condition, not paying attention to your vitamin and antioxidant status will eventually lead to further damage of your thyroid gland, worsening of the immune system attacks on your body, and systemic body inflammation. Having inadequate levels of antioxidants in your body parts will also make thyroid hormone less efficient at fulfilling its functions, leading to serious adverse metabolic effects and negative health consequences.

Antioxidants are natural compounds that have the ability to bind and neutralize free radicals in the body. Antioxidants in the diet minimize the buildup of these "bad guys," preventing them from damaging important cellular components. In fact, antioxidants can help prevent cancer, and some of them—such as beta-carotene and vitamins C and E—help prevent thyroid cancer.[7] Adequate antioxidant intake also slows premature aging. This can help your thyroid, too, as advancing age leads to a cellular deficit in zinc and selenium, which may result in lower thyroid hormone action.[8] In Chapter 2 I discussed the importance of certain minerals (iodine, zinc, copper, selenium, and iron) and vitamins (vitamin A, vitamin E, and vitamin C) necessary for optimal thyroid gland function. However, other minerals, including manganese, chromium, molybdenum, magnesium, vanadium, and several other vitamins and antioxidants, are needed for optimal thyroid health. And even if you do not have a thyroid disorder, you need to take adequate amounts of these minerals and antioxidants to maintain proper functioning of your thyroid.

The benefits of antioxidants in thyroid patients are more than just supporting thyroid gland function. See the table that follows:

Main Benefits of Antioxidants
Optimization of thyroid health
Prevention of thyroid damage
Reduction of autoimmune reactions affecting the thyroid
Increased efficiency of thyroid hormone
Weight control
Mood and cognitive enhancement
Prevention of degenerative damage and dementia
Decrease in cardiovascular risk
Decreased risk of thyroid cancer

Unfortunately, you may not be able to get enough of the vitamins and antioxidants you need even if you follow a well-balanced diet. Most fruits and vegetables that you buy at the supermarket reach your table several weeks to a few months after harvest. Because the vitamins and antioxidants in fresh foods are unstable, the time lag between harvest and consumption reduces the amounts of these essential nutrients, as do processing and cooking. In particular, the selenium content of foods is easily lost during processing, storage, and cooking. As a result, many of us are deficient in vitamins and antioxidants.[9]

Another common cause of vitamin and antioxidant deficiency is an infection of the stomach by *Helicobacter pylori,* the most common bacterial infection in the world. Nearly 30 percent of the population in developed countries, and up to 80–90 percent of the population in developing regions have *H. pylori* infections, which are associated with stomach ulcers. This infection may make you deficient in iron, vitamin B_{12}, folic acid, vitamin E, vitamin C, and beta-carotene. This same infection may also contribute to the triggering of autoimmune thyroid disease.

Thyroid imbalance itself can make you become deficient in antioxidants. It can promote excessive production of free radicals, overwhelming the cells' ability to neutralize them. This free radical excess leads to the progression of degenerative diseases. Research has shown that when the thyroid is overactive, the consumption of oxygen is higher, leading to an accumulation of free radicals that are toxic to cells.[10] Antioxidant supplements such as vitamins C and E and mixed carotenoids help cells clear these damaging oxidants and might prevent cellular damage in many parts of the body, including the muscles.

If you are treated for an overactive thyroid due to Graves' disease, supplementation with vitamins C and E, beta-carotene, and selenium will make antithyroid medications work faster and help your thyroid levels become normal more quickly.[11]

Selenium plays a major antioxidant role in our system. The thyroid gland requires selenium to manufacture adequate amounts of thyroid hormone. Selenium has been shown to have a preventative effect against many conditions such as cancer, inflammatory disorders, thyroid dysfunction, cardiovascular disease, neurological disorders, aging, infertility, and infections. It also has an immune-enhancing effect. Researchers have noted a decline in blood selenium levels in many European countries,[12] which could account for the escalating prevalence of cancer and cardiovascular disease in the Western world. Various bacteria in the natural environment and in our bodies require selenium to survive. Therefore, when certain bacteria pollute the environment, they will consume the selenium that would otherwise be available to humans, creating a deficiency of this trace element essential for proper thyroid functioning.

Selenium is also important for the functioning of certain parts of the brain. It affects chemicals with some hormonal activity and neurotransmitters in the brain; therefore, selenium seems to affect mood and cognition in humans and behavior in animals.[13]

For thyroid hormones to work properly in body cells, adequate supplies of selenium are essential. Selenium is a crucial component of the enzyme that converts T4 to T3 in the body.[14] Without it, T3 cannot be produced in the right amounts, making your body hypothyroid even though blood levels are normal. Thus, adequate selenium intake is essential for thyroid hormone to regulate the function of various organs and for slowing down the effects of aging. Selenium deficiency causes muscle damage and lowers muscle performance partly because the damaging effects of free radicals on the muscles are no longer blocked.

Selenium is also important in modulating the immune system. Selenium deficiency decreases the function of our immune system and makes viral infections more likely. Selenium deficiency also promotes autoimmune attacks on the thyroid. Taking selenium protects against autoimmune thyroid disease. If you have Hashimoto's thyroiditis, taking selenium will reduce the inflammation in your thyroid and will lower your antithyroid antibodies.[15] Not only does a deficiency in selenium make the immune system attack your thyroid, but your gland is further damaged by free radicals. Low selenium increases the risk of thyroid cancer. Too much selenium can also damage your thyroid. Selenium taken in doses of 100–150 mcg daily is adequate enough to provide significant antioxidant activity.

Zinc is another important micronutrient that is essential not only for the thyroid gland to produce adequate amounts of thyroid hormone but also for thyroid hormone to work more efficiently in our body. Zinc plays a role in the functioning of the immune system, and people with a deficiency are more susceptible to autoimmune disease and infections.[16] Because zinc affects serotonin uptake in the brain and thus mood and behavior, it is now being viewed as an antidepressant. Research has shown that in major depression, zinc levels are low.[17] If you have a thyroid imbalance, even corrected with treatment, and you continue to suffer from low mood, I urge you to take adequate amounts of zinc as well as other antioxidants that affect brain neurotransmitters.

Both hypothyroidism and hyperthyroidism can make you deficient in zinc. However, the deficiency in zinc is more significant in hyperthyroidism, as too much thyroid hormone causes excessive waste of zinc in the urine. Zinc is also low in people with thyroid cancer.

Consuming adequate amounts of vitamin C is crucial for your overall health. Vitamin C is unequivocally the most important water-soluble antioxidant. Research has shown that it is safe to take up to 1,000 mg of vitamin C a day. This will help with brain function—including cognition—and mood. Vitamin C is essential in neurotransmission.[18] In fact, the nerve endings contain the highest amounts of vitamin C of any structure in the human body. Vitamin C reduces the risk of neurodegenerative disorders, such as Alzheimer's disease. It also has beneficial effects on your immune system.

Vitamin C is essential for your adrenal glands to produce cortisol, and for your gastrointestinal tract to absorb nutrients such as iron. It also protects you from the deleterious effects of heavy metals (such as cadmium) on your thyroid. Vitamin C reduces inflammation and makes the cells that cover the inside of blood vessels work more efficiently. The cardioprotective benefit of vitamin C has to do, to some extent, with its involvement in clearing your body of the blood-vessel-damaging amino acid homocysteine. The buildup of homocysteine is associated with diseases such as atherosclerosis, glaucoma, and high blood pressure, among others. If you lack vitamin C, your homocysteine level goes up, increasing your risk of heart disease. Having a high homocysteine level will also make you more susceptible to depression. In fact, research has been able to correlate depression with the risk of heart disease. In addition to vitamin C, folic acid and vitamin B_{12} are required for reducing the buildup of homocysteine in your body. If you are deficient in folic acid, you will also end up having a high homocysteine level, potentially affecting your mood and cardiovascular health. Knowing that thyroid imbalance is strongly associated with elevated homocysteine levels, you need to make sure that your thyroid hormone levels are consistently well-balanced with medications, and you need to take adequate amounts of folic acid. Foods rich in folic acid include leafy greens and legumes. I believe that you should not exclusively rely on nutritional sources of folic acid and recommend you take folic acid as a dietary supplement (roughly 200–500 mcg of folic acid daily). However, you need to make sure that you do not have methylene tetrahydrofolate reductase (MTHFR) gene mutation. If you do, instead of taking folic acid, you should supplement with L-methylfolate (i.e., Quatrefolic®), the active form of folic acid that your body can use. MTHFR gene mutation causes the body to be deficient in an important enzyme necessary in the process of converting folate and folic acid to its active form. It is the active form of folic acid that helps with the breakdown of the blood-vessel-damaging homocysteine. About 30 to 40 percent of the white population in North America has the MTHFR gene mutation, although the figure may be even higher for the entire population. A deficiency of the methylation enzyme also leads to the buildup of toxic environmental chemicals such as cadmium, lead, or arsenic that enter our body through our food and water. These toxic elements eventually disturb the functioning of the immune system and worsen autoimmunity. They can also promote the occurrence of cancer. There is indication that the MTHFR gene mutation might be more common in patients with autoimmune thyroid disease, but research has not been able to provide an unequivocal association so far. If you have this mutation, you will need to be even more cautious about the environmental contaminants that can exacerbate autoimmunity (see Chapter 3).

Taking adequate amounts of the right form of folic acid not only protects your cardiovascular system but also supports your mood. Folic acid is essential for the manufacture of neurotransmitters and affects mood independently of your thyroid levels. If your thyroid imbalance has been corrected with treatment, you may continue to have symptoms of low-grade depression because you are deficient in folic acid. You are also likely to respond better to an antidepressant if you supplement with folic acid.[19] Folic acid also improves cognitive function, including memory and concentration.

Equally important, vitamin B_{12} is a vitamin that can affect your mood and cognition. As many as 10 to 20 percent of older people have some level of vitamin B_{12} deficiency that could contribute to the decline of their cognitive function.[20] One of the most common causes of vitamin B_{12} deficiency in thyroid patients is pernicious anemia, caused by the lack of a substance normally produced by the lining of the stomach and required for vitamin B_{12} to be absorbed in the gut. If you have pernicious anemia (see Chapter 7), a dietary supplement taken by mouth will not help raise your vitamin B_{12} levels and you will need to take vitamin B_{12} in the form of a sublingual troche or weekly intramuscular injections.

If you have a thyroid disorder, you also need to increase your consumption of vitamin B_6 (pyridoxine) and vitamin B_1 (thiamine). Pyridoxine is important in the conversion of tryptophan to serotonin in the brain. Low vitamin B_6 can exacerbate depressive symptoms. Research has shown that vitamin B_6 is quite effective in the treatment of premenopausal women who suffer from depression.[21] Depression related to hormonal issues will respond to the addition of vitamin B_6.

Deficiency in certain B vitamins can affect your cardiovascular health and cognition because it leads to high homocysteine levels, as folic acid deficiency does.[22] If you are low in vitamin B$_6$, your C-reactive protein (a marker of inflammation) will be high, which reflects a higher cardiovascular risk.

Thiamine deficiency causes damage to brain and endothelial cells and can promote depression. If you have neuropathy caused by too much thyroid hormone, thiamine deficiency may be contributing to the problem.

Vitamin A is required for the body to convert T4 to T3 in appropriate amounts. Too much preformed, animal-derived vitamin A can build up to toxic levels in the liver. However, plant-based vitamin A precursors such as beta-carotene and other carotenoids are nontoxic and among the most potent antioxidants found in foods.

Vitamin E supplementation helps repair oxidative damage caused by a thyroid imbalance. Vitamin E can lower the risk of coronary artery disease and strokes, in part by preventing oxidized LDL cholesterol from damaging blood vessel cells. Vitamin E lowers the risk of prostate cancer and helps with fertility. It also supports the thyroid. Research has shown that the majority of men and women in the United States do not meet the current recommendations for vitamin E intake.[23]

Vitamin E also regulates mood. Blood levels of this vitamin are lower in people with depression, and vitamin E deficiency may be part of the problem. This substance is essential in nerve membranes as well.

A population-based study in people over sixty-five showed that supplementation with vitamin E protects against cognitive impairment and dementia in older people.[24] Dietary vitamin E may also have a protective effect against Parkinson's disease. All thyroid patients need to take the right amount of vitamin E to preserve cognitive function.

Your vitamin E intake should not exceed 400 IU per day, and perhaps the ideal intake should be in the range of 150–200 IU per day. Research published in *Preventive Cardiology* has shown that people who take too much vitamin E have an increased rate of coronary artery calcification, which may predispose people to coronary artery disease.[25] As you can see, vitamin E is important, but an excess of it is detrimental to the heart.

For a long time, the emphasis has been placed on alpha-tocopherol, one of the eight components of vitamin E (called isoforms), ignoring the "minor" tocopherols. However, recent research has uncovered unexpected beneficial effects of the minor tocopherols, such as gamma-tocopherol.[26] The effects of the other tocopherols may not have anything to do with their antioxidant properties, but rather reflect their ability to reduce inflammation and slow down cancer growth. Gamma-tocopherol has a greater beneficial effect than alpha-tocopherol as far as the prevention of certain types of cancer and heart attacks. Levels of alpha-tocopherol and gamma-tocopherol in the thyroid tissue of patients with papillary cancer are low.[27] The mistaken impression that alpha-tocopherol is the only form of vitamin E that we should be concerned about may lead people to becoming depleted of gamma-tocopherol, losing its great benefits to health and prevention of cancer.

Coenzyme Q10, also called ubiquinone, is a vitamin-like substance. It is crucial in the generation of energy in the cell and is also viewed as an antioxidant. Your levels of coenzyme Q10 typically become low if you have a thyroid imbalance. This has something to do with poor mitochondrial functioning. If you have congestive heart failure and hyperthyroidism, coenzyme Q10 will improve your cardiac function. After the age of thirty-five or forty, our body begins to lose the ability to produce coenzyme Q10 from food, making deficiency more likely. Stress, infection, and poor eating habits all contribute to low levels of coenzyme Q10. Coenzyme Q10 is an important supplement for thyroid patients since it slows down degenerative disorders of the brain. It is also recommended for Parkinson's disease and other brain conditions. Research has shown that levels of coenzyme Q10 in thyroid tissue are low in patients with Graves' disease and thyroid cancer,[28] suggesting that low levels may make these diseases more likely. An adequate daily coenzyme Q10 intake is 25–50 mg.

Alpha-lipoic acid is another important antioxidant that increases your glutathione levels and helps clear damaging free radicals. It also makes vitamins C and E work more efficiently.

You also need to pay attention to your magnesium intake. Magnesium is one of the most widespread elements on earth and is found in many foods. However, you can easily become depleted of magnesium if you consume too much alcohol or are sweating a lot during exercise. Magnesium deficiency can promote muscle cramps and weakness as well as cardiac arrhythmias and high blood pressure. Adequate magnesium intake will also increase bone mineral density. Magnesium supplementation has been shown to have a beneficial effect on coronary heart disease.[29] Magnesium is available in different preparations, but magnesium citrate may be superior to the others. I recommend that you take 200–300 mg of elemental magnesium a day.

FOODS RICH IN ESSENTIAL NUTRIENTS

Selenium: whole grains, wheat germ, mushrooms, cabbage, garlic, egg noodles, soybeans, Brazil nuts, walnuts, cashews, lean beef, tuna, eggs

Zinc: seafood, lean beef, turkey, wheat bran, whole grains, soybeans, green vegetables, ginger, dairy, nuts

Beta-carotene: kale, carrots, butternut squash, spinach, cantaloupe, broccoli, asparagus, pumpkin, liver, lettuce, apricots, papaya, oranges, peaches, apricots, tomatoes, kiwi, watermelon

Vitamin C: red peppers, cauliflower, broccoli, peas, kiwi fruit, leafy green vegetables, lemons, white potatoes, orange juice, parsley, cabbage, Brussels sprouts, melons, strawberries, tomatoes

Vitamin A: milk, eggs, liver, apricots, cantaloupe, pumpkin, squash, turnip, carrots, plums, watermelon, plantains, peas, oatmeal, broccoli, spinach

Vitamin E: whole grains, wheat germ, almonds, soybeans, corn, sunflower seeds, liver, vegetable oil, leafy green vegetables, asparagus

Riboflavin (vitamin B$_2$): Brazil nuts, almonds, whole grains, wild rice, wheat germ, dairy, eggs, green vegetables, avocados, chicken, turkey, lean pork, meats, salmon, asparagus, okra, olives

Thiamine (vitamin B$_1$): whole grains, brown rice, soy, peas, fish, lean meat, dried beans

Niacin (vitamin B$_3$): sweet potatoes, cabbage, tomatoes, mushrooms, lentils, asparagus, leafy greens, eggs, nuts, salmon, tuna, beef, chicken, Cornish hen

Vitamin B$_6$ (pyridoxine): chicken, turkey, roast beef, trout, potatoes, nuts and seeds, peanut butter, lima beans, wheat bran, oatmeal, liver, green beans, bananas, carrots

Folic acid: whole grains, green peas, broccoli, avocado, leafy greens, turnips, Brussels sprouts, okra, citrus fruits, shellfish, legumes

Vitamin B$_{12}$ (cobalamin): meat, poultry, eggs, dairy products, beef liver

How much of the various vitamin and antioxidant supplements should you take every day? The following list summarizes my recommendations:

OPTIMAL DAILY SUPPLEMENT LEVELS
- Vitamin A (as beta-carotene and mixed carotenoids): 2,000–4,000 IU
- Vitamin C: 100–200 mg
- Vitamin D$_3$ (cholecalciferol): 1,000 IU (many patients require higher amounts)
- Vitamin E (from mixed tocopherols): 150–200 IU
- Vitamin K$_2$: 20–50 mcg
- Thiamin (vitamin B$_1$): 5–15 mg
- Riboflavin: 5–15 mg
- Niacin (vitamin B$_3$): 15–20 mg
- Vitamin B$_6$ (pyridoxine): 20–50 mg
- Folate (preferably as L-methylfolate): 300–800 mcg
- Vitamin B$_{12}$: 30–50 mcg
- Biotin: 250–500 mcg
- Pantothenic acid: 6 mg
- Iodine: 120–200 mcg
- Magnesium: 150–250 mg
- Zinc: 15 mg
- Selenium: 150 mcg
- Manganese: 2–4 mg
- Chromium: 100–300 mcg
- Molybdenum: 20–60 mcg
- Vanadium: 20–40 mcg

You can take these vitamins, minerals, and antioxidants as individual supplements or in a well-balanced combination such as ThyroLife Optima, which includes additional potent anti-inflammatory and immune-system-soothing ingredients such as quercetin, L-glutathione, alpha-lipoic acid, lyco-pene, curcumin, and para-aminobenzoic acid.

If you are suffering from an overactive thyroid, I recommend that you take the vitamins and antioxidants even when your thyroid levels are high. If, on the other hand, you are hypothyroid, it is probably safer to start taking the supplements when your levels have become normal or close to normal.

Why Do You Need to Pay Attention to Your Calcium Intake?

People with thyroid disorders may be at risk for bone loss, osteopenia, and osteoporosis. Your risk is even greater if you are menopausal and have had too much thyroid hormone in your system, either from an overactive thyroid or as a result of thyroid hormone overmedication while being treated for hy-pothyroidism. The risk of bone loss can be quite significant, particularly if you are female and Caucasian, if you have a family history of osteoporosis, or if you are diabetic. If you have been treated with high amounts of a thyroid medication, particularly desiccated thyroid (Armour Thyroid), or other T4/T3 combination medications that contain high amounts of T3, you can be certain that it has contributed to some bone loss. Many patients do not get enough calcium in their diet, especially those who need to follow a low-fat diet, are sensitive to dairy, or are lactose intolerant. Yet calcium is crucial not only for bone health but also for many bodily functions. For instance, low calcium intake correlates with weight gain issues, and calcium supplementa-tion has been shown to facilitate weight loss.[30] I highly recommend that you evaluate how much calcium you get from your diet and take calcium supple-mentation as needed.

MAIN BENEFITS OF CALCIUM SUPPLEMENTATION
• Helps with bone health
• Helps immune system functions
• Helps with cardiovascular health
• Helps boost your metabolism and weight loss efforts

The Recommended Dietary Allowance (RDA) of calcium provided by the Institute of Medicine is 1,000 mg for both men and women and should be slightly higher (1,200 mg) for women between the ages of fifty-one and sev-enty. However, research indicates that excessive amounts of calcium may be associated with an increased risk of cardiovascular disease. For this reason, before you decide on whether you should take calcium in the form of a sup-plement, I recommend that you check the calcium content in the foods that you eat and in the multivitamin mix that you may be taking. I definitely rec-ommend that you take a multivitamin that is calcium-free so you can easily manage your daily intake of calcium in the most judicious way. If you do not eat dairy, you are probably consuming somewhere between 200 and 300 mg of calcium daily. If that is the case, you probably need to supplement somewhere around 750–1,000 mg of calcium a day, in divided doses, depending on your age, osteoporosis risk, and menopausal status, keeping in mind that your total calcium intake should not exceed 1,500 mg a day. Make sure you drink plenty of water during the day to avoid the constipation that can be caused by calcium supplements. And, again, make sure you take your calcium supplement at least four to five hours after taking thyroid hormone medication.

Probiotics

Probiotic supplementation is as important as taking antioxidants when you suffer from a thyroid condition such as Hashimoto's thyroiditis or Graves' disease. I recommend probiotics because gut health and bacterial balance in the GI tract are strongly correlated with immune system health.[31] I also recommend probiotics because inflammation, as I explained in Chapter 10, contributes to slowing of metabolism and affects food cravings. Since thyroid patients often struggle with weight gain issues, they cannot counteract all the negative consequences of immune system reactivity, thyroid hormone imbalance, and body inflammation without taking the right types of probiotics.[32]

Main Benefits of Probiotics
Help reduce inflammation in the GI tract and elsewhere in the body
Help thyroid patients, especially those suffering from autoimmune thyroid disease,
reduce the production of inflammation chemicals by the immune system
Help fight autoimmunity (multiple sclerosis, rheumatoid arthritis, lupus, etc.)
Help anyone suffering from irritable bowel syndrome
Help with weight loss management by making metabolism-boosting hormones work more
efficiently and reducing stress-related food cravings

There are many probiotic formulas on the market, but few of them provide a select mix of the best bacteria to help fight autoimmunity while reducing inflammation and weight loss resistance. After extensive research, I have identified seven of the most potent and beneficial bacterial strains that fulfill the needs of thyroid patients. I recommend selecting a probiotic mix that contains all of these strains, such as Probiotic 7-7 (21–42 billion CFU per day). The following strains are the ones I recommend you take in balanced amounts:

- *Lactobacillus rhamnosus.* Has the ability to stimulate mucosal immunity and protect from intestinal infections. Helps the immune system fight against pathogenic intestinal and urinary tract bacteria. Shown to make GABA, a brain neurotransmitter involved in reducing anxiety, work more efficiently, helping you improve mood and reduce stress-related cravings.

- **Bifidobacterium longum.** Powerful at preventing the growth of harmful bacteria. Helps boost immune system functions. Helps lower cholesterol and reduce symptoms of lactose intolerance. Also touted as having anti-cancer benefits. Because of its substantial benefits for the immune system, it helps in reducing allergies and inflammation associated with autoimmune diseases such as Crohn's disease.
- **Lactobacillus acidophilus.** Produces acidic substances that prevent harmful bacteria from growing. Also produces lactase, which converts lactose into simple sugars; this is helpful in reducing lactose intolerance, a common condition among thyroid patients and an aggravating factor that increases immune system reactivity. Many commercially available probiotics are made up predominantly of *Lactobacillus acidophilus*. Although this strain is beneficial to your gut bacterial balance and immune system, taking it alone may not provide all the needed benefits for auto-immunity and body inflammation.
- **Lactobacillus plantarum.** Naturally found in the human gut, this strain has beneficial effects on reducing the severity of gastrointestinal inflammation, and helps reduce allergies to foods such as soy. Because of its local gastrointestinal effects, this strain is likely to help with different kinds of food sensitivities.
- **Streptococcus thermophilus.** Commonly found in yogurt, this strain helps to reduce nitrites, harmful chemicals that can promote cancer and disturb the functioning of the immune system. Can help in preventing immune system agitation triggered by dairy because of its ability to break down casein, one of the main proteins in dairy.
- **Bifidobacterium bifidum.** Helps in maintaining regular bowel movements and optimal performance of the digestive tract while also supporting immune system function.
- **Bifidobacterium lactis.** A powerful strain that reduces intestinal inflammation and makes it harder for undigested molecules to enter your bloodstream, which can provoke food sensitivities and even leaky gut syndrome. Also helps in supporting the immune system and reducing immune system reactivity.

Iodine: A Double-Edged Sword

The trace mineral iodine is an essential component in the manufacture of thyroid hormone by a healthy gland. In the United States, iodine consumption varies. For at least two-thirds of the population, iodine consumption is within a good range, and for some it is even on the high side, as much as 700 mcg a day. However, iodine deficiency is not uncommon and can cause problems. As I explained in Chapter 2, too little iodine in the diet can result in goiter and an underactive thyroid. When the level of iodine in the blood and in the gland is low, it causes the thyroid cells to enlarge and proliferate as a result of stimulation by thyroid-stimulating hormone (TSH), produced by the pituitary. If you routinely engage in strenuous exercise, you may lose a considerable amount of iodine in your sweat, though this depends to a great extent on the temperature and humidity of your environment.[33] If iodine losses are not replaced, you can become depleted of iodine, which will slow down your thyroid and affect your athletic performance. Nearly 200 million people worldwide suffer from iodine deficiency and resulting goiters. In some parts of the world where fish is not a prominent food and the soil iodine content is very low, over 50 percent of the population has a goiter. Because the functioning of the thyroid gland in a developing fetus relies on the iodine supplied by the pregnant woman, women living in an iodine-deficient area may deliver babies with brain impairments. This condition is easily preventable by taking supplemental iodine.

In the United States, iodine deficiency has been rare since 1924, when table salt producers started incorporating iodine in their salt. Advice to take supplements with high amounts of iodine "to assist your thyroid" has no scientific basis and may actually be harmful for many. Because very high iodine intake can cause or precipitate autoimmune attacks on the thyroid, researchers are speculating that the increasingly high frequency of autoimmune thyroid disease being observed in the United States and Japan is somewhat related to excessive iodine intake.[34] Research has clearly established that adding iodine to the diet of people living in iodine-deficient regions has resulted in a rise in the prevalence of thyroiditis and thyroid cancer.[35]

Iodine is trapped by a large protein found in the thyroid gland, called thyroglobulin. The process of manufacturing thyroid hormone takes place in this protein. But when your intake of iodine is too high, large amounts of iodinated thyroglobulin prompt the immune system to react and cause inflammation in the thyroid, characteristic of Hashimoto's thyroiditis. Animal research has demonstrated that the severity of autoimmune thyroiditis is increased by a very high iodine intake.

Several years ago, NASA physicians consulted me because they had observed low-grade hypothyroidism in a few people participating in a ground study. The imbalance occurred within a few weeks of the subjects' beginning to consume high amounts of iodine. The amount of iodine given to these people was 4 g/L, comparable to the amount delivered to astronauts who consume recycled water with added iodine to keep it sterile in flight. In some of the ground subjects, the consequences of the high iodine intake might eventually have included an autoimmune attack on the thyroid gland. One of these people had a persistent low-grade overactive thyroid after having previously been low-grade hypothyroid. Alarmed by my warnings about the potential consequences of thyroid imbalance for both astronauts and ground subjects, NASA decided to change its sterilization system and made the study participants stop the high iodine intake.

Inadvertent intake or administration of products high in iodine can trigger a thyroid imbalance among patients with Hashimoto's thyroiditis and Graves' disease. Too much iodine can cause hypothyroidism in certain patients with Graves' disease, particularly those who had regained normal thyroid function after treatment. Clearly, consuming high amounts of iodine from taking sea kelp supplements (sea vegetables are a particularly rich source of iodine) or from using large amounts of iodized salt may represent a health hazard for thyroid patients.

Iodine excess from certain medications and contrast agents used in X-ray procedures also places thyroid patients at risk for more thyroid dysfunction. Amiodarone, a medication commonly used to correct life-threatening heart rhythm problems, contains large amounts of iodine (75 mg per tablet). Approximately 20 percent of people taking amiodarone become hypothyroid, and 2 percent develop hyperthyroidism. In parts of the world where iodine deficiency remains a problem, amiodarone causes more hyperthyroidism and less hypothyroidism than it does in the United States.

Marcie, a thirty-five-year-old housewife whose sister had been diagnosed with Hashimoto's thyroiditis and an underactive thyroid a few years ago, visited a physician because of weight gain and fatigue. Disappointed that her thyroid tests were normal, as that seemed to leave her with no explanation for her symptoms, she began reading books on nutrition, one of which recommended 2,000–3,000 mg of kelp every day as essential for a healthy thyroid. Marcie took the suggested supplements, thinking that ingesting more iodine would reduce her likelihood of having a thyroid problem like her sister's and alleviate her symptoms. As a result, however, she became afflicted by an overactive thyroid due to Graves' disease.

Among common foods, seafood contains the highest amount of iodine. These include lobsters, crabs, oysters, and other shellfish. Plant and dairy products may have some iodine if they are derived from areas that have iodine in the soil. (Soil in ocean coastal areas usually has higher iodine levels than soil in inland areas.) Other foods that contain high amounts of iodine are bread and eggs. Iodized salt, which contains 70 mcg of iodine per gram of salt, is the most common source of iodine for most Americans.

People like Marcie with a known genetic predisposition to autoimmune thyroid disease should avoid excess iodine. If any of your relatives have thyroid disease, minimize the use of iodized salt as much as possible. Although the general recommendation is that dietary consumption of iodine should not exceed 1 mg per day, I advise not consuming more than 500–600 mcg a day. The trick is to avoid both iodine deficiency and iodine excess.

Vitamin D

Vitamin D is probably best-known for its role in bone health, as vitamin D deficiency has long been known to cause rickets in children, bone loss, and even osteoporosis in adults.[36] Even if you do not have bone loss, vitamin D deficiency can make you suffer from joint and muscle pains. However, in recent years, extensive research has demonstrated that vitamin D plays a major role in the health and functioning of many organs in our bodies, and even regulates cell growth. Vitamin D deficiency is an overlooked and unrecognized epidemic. Deficiency of vitamin D has been linked to the progression of cancer, and possibly its occurrence.[37] Vitamin D also plays an important role in the brain and modulates mood. Its deficiency is thought to contribute to the occurrence of mood disorders such as seasonal affective disorder (depression that occurs during the winter months).[38] Research is also showing that vitamin D deficiency is associated with, and may be responsible for, many inflammatory and autoimmune conditions, such as multiple sclerosis, Crohn's disease, ulcerative colitis, rheumatoid arthritis, and autoimmune thyroid conditions such as Hashimoto's thyroiditis and Graves' disease. There is clearly a correlation between having an autoimmune thyroid disease and low vitamin D levels.[39] Roughly 90 percent of patients with Hashimoto's thyroiditis suffer from vitamin D deficiency, and researchers believe that vitamin D deficiency could be a trigger of this autoimmune condition. Research in Japan has also shown a correlation between low vitamin D levels and the occurrence of Graves' disease.[40] In addition to promoting autoimmunity, vitamin D deficiency can generate a state of body inflammation that can negatively affect your metabolism and cardiovascular system.

For these reasons, patients with autoimmune thyroid disease need to have their vitamin D level (25-hydroxy vitamin D) tested. For patients with low or marginal blood levels of 25-hydroxy vitamin D, I recommend vitamin D in a liquid form with or right after meals that include some fat, as vitamin D is fat-soluble. The amount of vitamin D supplemented varies from one individual to another because the GI absorption of vitamin D varies. Keeping vitamin D in an optimal range will help reduce inflammation in the body and temper immune system reactivity. It has been thought for some time that sun exposure will correct a vitamin D deficiency; however, research suggests that production of vitamin D in the skin as a result of sun exposure may be insufficient. Manufacture of vitamin D in the skin depends on several factors:

season, latitude, time of day, skin color, age, air pollution, and genes. In addition, trying to get all your vitamin D from sun exposure can put you at risk for skin cancer. For all these reasons, I highly recommend vitamin D supplementation.

Main Benefits of Vitamin D
Bone and muscle strength
Decrease in autoimmune attacks
Cancer prevention; slows down progression of thyroid cancer
Mood benefits

Exercise: When and How?

Many of my patients ask me whether they can engage in physical exercise and what type of exercise they can do, afraid that it will cause damage to their body while they are being treated for their thyroid condition. I typically do not recommend any strenuous exercise when you are still hypothyroid or hyperthyroid, because your muscles are still in a dysfunctional, sluggish mode and you risk muscle damage. However, if you have low-grade hypothyroidism, the risk of damage is much lower. Because cardiac performance depends on having perfectly well-balanced thyroid hormone levels, high-intensity exercise during hyperthyroidism (whether caused by an overactive thyroid or as a result of thyroid hormone overmedication), should be avoided as well. When thyroid hormone levels have become normal, however, I highly recommend physical exercise, not only for weight control but also because it produces psychological benefits such as improved mood and self-esteem. These are crucial for patients suffering from thyroid disease.

Regular exercise relieves tension, anger, and confusion. It alleviates depression and anxiety, and also reduces the perception of stress, which is very helpful for patients with autoimmunity. Exercise promotes good brain cell health. This beneficial effect has been suggested by animal research that has shown that exercise doubles or triples brain cell regeneration in areas of the brain that regulate mood. Exercise has the same beneficial effect on brain cells as antidepressants do.[41]

During a thyroid imbalance, before blood tests have become normal, I recommend doing only mild aerobic exercise, such as regular walking, fifteen to twenty minutes daily. This strengthens the heart and lungs and allows you to adjust to the new demands of your body as thyroid levels normalize. Avoid rigorous anaerobic, muscle-building exercise in this phase of treatment because metabolism in the muscle is either too slow or too rapid, and it may impose demands on muscles that cannot be met without damaging them.

Once your thyroid hormone levels have normalized, you need to engage in an exercise program that gradually increases your exertion. There are four main reasons a wellness program designed to provide optimal physical and mental health for thyroid patients should include exercise:

1. Exercise or regular physical activity boosts endorphin levels and alleviates low mood.
2. Exercise increases muscle mass and makes your metabolism speedier, helping you manage your weight gain problem more efficiently.
3. Exercise improves cardiovascular function and helps reduce the cardiovascular disease risk that haunts thyroid patients over time.
4. Exercise helps minimize the risk of impaired cognition associated with aging, which especially affects thyroid patients.

Assuming you are not suffering from any kind of heart condition and that you were not involved in any exercise program prior to the diagnosis and initial treatment of your thyroid condition, I recommend that you begin a three-phase program once your thyroid hormone levels have become normal and stable with treatment.

Phase one (two to four weeks): This is an initiation phase, during which you perform aerobic exercise three days a week for only thirty minutes a day. This can include walking, stair-stepping, swimming, jogging, treadmill exercise, and cycling. You should stretch for five to ten minutes prior to each session and take a cool-down period of five to ten minutes of walking or stretching after each session.

Phase two (four to six weeks): Step up to thirty to forty-five minutes of aerobic exercise five or six days a week. I recommend that you do this gradually—for example, exercise four days the first week, five days the second week, and six days the third week. Also in this phase, I recommend that you begin gentle muscle workouts of ten to fifteen minutes. A good target for muscle workouts at the end of phase two is fifteen minutes of muscle workouts three to four days a week.

Phase three: When you are ready to follow a maintenance program after the first two phases, I recommend combining aerobic exercise and muscle workouts according to the fundamentals of the 20/10 exercise program. This will help you burn fat more efficiently, even hours after you stop the exercise, as well as improve your mental and cardiovascular health.[42] (Consult my book *The Protein Boost Diet* for details of the entire exercise program.)

This exercise program will help you take control of your health once again. If you are forty or older or have any history of heart disease, consult with your physician; he or she might recommend a heart stress test prior to commencing the exercise program. Stress tests are a good idea for most people who had hypothyroidism and remained undiagnosed for a long time.

Alcohol and Nicotine: Enemies of the Thyroid

Heavy alcohol consumption and depression often go hand in hand. Depressed and alcoholic hypothyroid individuals may take their medication irregularly or stop taking it altogether, thereby precipitating another vicious cycle. Alcohol consumption also contributes to excess caloric intake and increases the risk of weight gain.

Smoking harms most of your vital organs, and the thyroid gland is no exception. Smoking can increase the risk of Graves' disease and can worsen eye disease in patients with autoimmune thyroid conditions. If you have Graves' disease and it is in remission, smoking will make you more likely to relapse.[43] The typical severity of an autoimmune attack on the thyroid is greater among pregnant women who smoked heavily prior to pregnancy. Both active and passive smoking have been proven deleterious to the fetus's thyroid. Smoking also increases the risk of having a goiter. Thiocyanate, which is a breakdown product of the cyanide in tobacco smoke, prevents the gland from utilizing iodine and will promote multinodular goiter. It also impairs thyroid hormone production and may cause hypothyroidism in a person deficient in iodine. However, the prevalence of low-grade hypothyroidism is not increased with tobacco smoking.[44]

Other factors in the environment, including mercuric chloride, silicone, anilides, vinyl chloride, toxins, and ultraviolet irradiation, can promote an autoimmune attack on the thyroid.[45] This is more likely to happen if you are genetically predisposed to having an autoimmune attack.

Medications That Can Affect Your Thyroid

In addition to avoiding excessive iodine intake, nicotine, and excessive alcohol consumption, you need to be alert to potential adverse interactions between certain medications and your thyroid system. Thyroid patients often wonder whether taking various over-the-counter medications will affect their thyroid function. Whether you are hypo- or hyperthyroid, you should not be overly concerned about taking most cold remedies and decongestants as long as your blood thyroid levels are relatively stable. Some cold remedies containing pseudoephedrine may cause a hyperthyroid person to have more symptoms of thyroid hormone excess, such as trembling, nervousness, sleep problems, and rapid heartbeat. Taking a decongestant that contains pseudoephedrine may also be a concern if you are hyperthyroid and have a heart condition. You should also avoid antihistamines that cause a drowsy effect if you have hypothyroidism and your thyroid levels are still low. Note as well that whether you have an underactive or overactive thyroid, too much caffeine may increase your anxiety symptoms and cause your heart to beat even faster.

Avoid sleeping pills and sedatives when your thyroid levels are low, as low thyroid slows the clearance of these medications from the body. Sedatives can also precipitate myxedema coma, a life-threatening condition related to very low thyroid, especially in older people.

If you are taking warfarin (Coumadin), a blood thinner used to treat phlebitis and some forms of cerebrovascular disease, you should be aware that your thyroid levels will affect the dosage needed to maintain the desired level of anticoagulant effect. If the thyroid levels rise or fall, you will need a change in the dose of warfarin.

Thyroid hormone levels also affect blood levels of many other medications. Those that need to be adjusted when you have a thyroid imbalance include beta-blockers and digitalis (which is used for congestive heart failure). Theophylline, an antiasthma drug, may also need to be adjusted. A number of medications taken for asthma may heighten the effect of thyroid hormone. Some antiasthma medications should be avoided when your thyroid levels are high.

People who develop mild hypothyroidism from taking the heart drug amiodarone should have their TSH monitored. In many patients, the hypothyroidism is transient and TSH levels will become normal over time, even when they continue to take the medication.

Hyperthyroidism from amiodarone use represents a more complex problem, since excess thyroid hormone can cause irregularities in heart rhythm and makes amiodarone less effective in controlling this problem.[46] Hyperthyroidism due to amiodarone should be promptly corrected. Two distinct types of hyperthyroidism are caused by amiodarone, however. The first type is the result of an increase in iodine uptake by the gland or an increase in the amount of thyroid hormone manufactured. The second type is due to the medication having a toxic effect on the gland, which results in damaged thyroid cells' releasing thyroid hormone into the bloodstream (similar to what happens in silent thyroiditis and subacute thyroiditis; see Chapter 6). It is important for your physician to determine which mechanism is causing the hyperthyroidism, since the treatment differs.

Interferon, a medication used to treat chronic hepatitis C, multiple sclerosis, hematological tumors, and cancer, frequently causes thyroid dysfunction. One study showed that 6.2 percent of patients taking interferon experience a thyroid dysfunction, with hypothyroidism occurring in 3.9 percent of patients and hyperthyroidism in 2.3 percent of patients.[47] Women with a preexisting autoimmune thyroid condition are at a higher risk for having a thyroid imbalance due to interferon. The most common thyroid problem is a destructive thyroiditis that causes hyperthyroidism, followed by hypothyroidism. Thyroid dysfunction is often mild and self-limited. The imbalance resolves itself in 60 percent of patients, whether you continue taking interferon or not. Thyroid gland inflammation and damage can also be caused by alemtuzumab, a medication prescribed to treat some blood conditions, and sunitinib, a medication used to treat certain cancers.

Many people with lingering depression receive a course of antidepressants (see Chapter 18), which may require an increase in the thyroid hormone dosage.[48] Patients with a known thyroid disorder who are given antidepressants must be tested more frequently and their thyroid medication dose adjusted. Otherwise, the antidepressant may be less effective in treating the depression.

Lithium can result in hypothyroidism, since it inhibits the release of thyroid hormone from the thyroid gland while causing it to retain iodine. Research has shown that lithium can promote an autoimmune attack, of the Hashimoto's thyroiditis type, on the thyroid. It can exacerbate existing Hashimoto's thyroiditis and cause more damage to the gland. A significant number of people who take lithium for mood disorders have evidence of an underactive thyroid. More rarely, lithium can induce an overactive thyroid via an autoimmune attack. Hyperthyroidism may rarely occur as a rebound phenomenon after patients discontinue lithium.

In someone with preexisting Hashimoto's thyroiditis, the addition of lithium may cause an even more profound state of hypothyroidism and may confound the mental problems associated with bipolar disorder. For this reason, manic-depressive patients treated with lithium often have thyroid testing done on a regular basis. Even if the underlying thyroid gland is normal, lithium can cause low-grade hypothyroidism, which should be treated with thyroid hormone to minimize effects on mood swings.

Important Points to Remember

- To reach and maintain overall thyroid wellness, you need to embrace a comprehensive program that includes perfecting your thyroid hormone levels, proper nutrition, addressing any sleep issues, managing stress, and taking the right supplements.
- The best diet to help thyroid patients with mood, weight control, and disease prevention is a low-glycemic-index diet high in proteins and fiber, and low in trans-fats and saturated fats.
- The right mix of vitamins and antioxidants will reduce damage to the thyroid gland and make thyroid hormone work more efficiently in the body. You also need to take omega-3 fatty acids and the right probiotics.
- You need to achieve the right balance with respect to your iodine intake: too little can make your gland underperform, and too much can be harmful to your thyroid.
- Exercise is an important component of the mind-body program. It will keep you healthy, both physically and mentally.

ACKNOWLEDGMENTS

So many people have made the writing of this book possible. First of all, my deepest gratitude goes to the patients who have taught me what books and articles did not, and to those who were kind enough to share their experiences with me for this book. These patients have made an invaluable contribution toward helping others. The hard work and dedication of researchers from around the world who have studied thyroid disease were critical in enabling me to understand and interpret the intricate interactions between the mind and the thyroid gland. A special thank-you goes to my mentors, who enhanced my passion for the thyroid: Dr. James B. Field, who was chairman of Endocrinology and Metabolism when I began my academic career at Baylor College of Medicine, and Professor Raymond Michel, who in the early 1950s was one of the researchers who discovered T3, the most active form of thyroid hormone.

There is no doubt that without the unshakable support and understanding of my wife, Noura, I would not have been able to carry out the project of writing this book. I will always be grateful to Julie Murphy Pieper, who assisted me during my academic growth and during the writing of the first edition of this book. I would like to thank Mansour Arem and Brittany Stone for their outstanding assistance and for helping me with gathering research, typing, and organizing the current edition of this book.

My gratitude to my agent, Angela Rinaldi, for her continued support. I deeply appreciate the thoroughness and talents of my editors, Leslie Meredith and Marnie Cochran, copy editor Sue Warga, and production editor Steve Messina. I also wish to thank everyone else at Ballantine who worked on this project, including Betsy Cowie, Jo Anne Metsch, Sarah Feightner, Pamela Alders, and Anna Bauer.

NOTES

PART I. **The Emerging Mind-Thyroid Connection: How a Tiny Endocrine Gland Intimately Affects Your Mood, Emotions, and Behavior**
CHAPTER 1. **Thyroid Imbalance: A Hidden Epidemic**

1. L. C. Wood, D. S. Cooper, and E. C. Ridgway, *Your Thyroid: A Home Reference,* 3rd ed. (New York: Ballantine Books, 1995), 215–19.
2. R. Arem and D. Escalante, "Subclinical Hypothyroidism: Epidemiology, Diagnosis, and Significance," *Advances in Internal Medicine* 41 (1996): 213–50.
3. S. I. Sherman, P. Nadkarni, and R. Arem, "Outcomes of a Community TSH Screening Program," abstract presented at the Seventy-ninth Annual Meeting of the Endocrine Society, Minneapolis, June 11, 1997.
4. G. J. Canaris, N. R. Manowitz, G. Mayor, and E. C. Ridgway, "The Colorado Thyroid Disease Prevalence Study," *Archives of Internal Medicine* 160, no. 4 (2000): 526–34.
5. C. Scheffer, C. Heckmann, T. Mijic, and K. H. Rudorff, "Chronic Distress Syndrome in Patients with Graves' Disease," *Medizinische Klinik* 99, no. 10 (2004): 578–84.
6. L. Wartofsky, "The Scope and Impact of Thyroid Disease," *Clinical Chemistry* 42, no. 1 (1996): 121–24.
7. R. J. Graves, "Newly Observed Affection of the Thyroid Gland in Females," *London Medical Surgical Journal* 7, part 2 (1835): 516.
8. *Collections from the Unpublished Writings of the Late C. H. Parry* (London: Underwoods, 1825).
9. W. W. Gull, "On a Cretinoid State Supervening in Adult Life in Women," *Transitional Clinical Society* (London) 7 (1873): 180–85.
10. G. Lewis and S. Wessely, "The Epidemiology of Fatigue: More Questions than Answers," *Journal of Epidemiology and Community Health* 46 (1992): 92–97.
11. R. C. Kessler, K. A. McGonagle, S. Zhao, et al., "Lifetime and Twelve-Month Prevalence of DSM-III-R Psychiatric Disorders in the United States: Results from the National Comorbidity Study," *Archives of General Psychiatry* 51 (1994): 8–19.
12. D. A. Regier, R. M. A. Hirschfeld, F. K. Goodwin, et al., "The NIMH Depression Awareness, Recognition, and Treatment Program: Structure, Aims, and Scientific Basis," *American Journal of Psychiatry* 145 (1988): 1351–57.

13. K. B. Wells, R. D. Hays, M. A. Burnam, et al., "Detection of Depressive Disorders for Patients Receiving Prepaid or Fee-for-Service Care: Results from the Medical Outcomes Study," *Journal of the American Medical Association* 262 (1989): 3298–3302.

14. W. Katon, M. Von Korff, E. Lin, et al., "Adequacy and Duration of Antidepressant Treatment in Primary Care," *Medical Care* 30 (1992): 67–76.

15. R. G. Kathol and J. W. Delahunt, "The Relationship of Anxiety and Depression to Symptoms of Hyperthyroidism Using Operational Criteria," *General Hospital Psychiatry* 8 (1986): 23–28.

16. S. Gulseren, L. Gulseren, Z. Hekimsoy, P. Cetinay, C. Ozen, and B. Tokatlioglu, "Depression, Anxiety, Health-Related Quality of Life, and Disability in Patients with Overt and Subclinical Thyroid Dysfunction," *Archives of Medical Research* 37, no. 1 (2006): 133–39.

17. B. A. Bartman and K. B. Weiss, "Women's Primary Care in the United States: A Study of Practice Variation Among Physician Specialties," *Journal of Women's Health* 2, no. 3 (1993): 261–68.

18. L. Laurence and B. Weinhouse, *Outrageous Practices: The Alarming Truth About How Medicine Mistreats Women* (New York: Random House, 1994), 259–61.

CHAPTER 2. I'm Tired of Being Tired: Could It Be My Thyroid?

1. R. Dantzer, C. J. Heijen, A. Kavelaars, et al., "The Neuroimmune Basis of Fatigue," *Trends in Neurosciences* 37, no. 1 (2014): 39–46.

2. D. W. Bates, W. Schmitt, D. Buchwald, et al., "Prevalence of Fatigue and Chronic Fatigue Syndrome in a Primary Care Practice," *Archives of Internal Medicine* 153 (1993): 2759–65.

3. K. Kroenke, D. R. Wood, A. D. Mangelsdorff, et al., "Chronic Fatigue in Primary Care: Prevalence, Patient Characteristics, and Outcome," *Journal of the American Medical Association* 260, no. 7 (1988): 929–34.

4. L. Wartofsky, "The Scope and Impact of Thyroid Disease," *Clinical Chemistry* 42, no. 1 (1996): 121–24.

5. AACE/AME Task Force on Thyroid Nodules, "American Association of Clinical Endocrinologists and Associazione Medici Endocrinologi Medical Guidelines for Clinical Practice for the Diagnosis and Management of Thyroid Nodules," *Endocrine Practice* 12, no. 1 (2006): 63–102.

6. E. Papini, R. Guglielmi, A. Bianchini, et al., "Risk of Malignancy in Nonpalpable Thyroid Nodules: Predictive Value of Ultrasound and Color-Doppler Features," *Journal of Clinical Endocrinology and Metabolism* 87, no. 5 (2002): 1941–46.

7. R. Arem and D. Escalante, "Subclinical Hypothyroidism: Epidemiology, Diagnosis, and Significance," *Advances in Internal Medicine* 41 (1996): 213–50.

8. M. Valko, D. Leibfritz, J. Moncol, et al., "Free Radicals and Antioxidants in Normal Physiological Functions and Human Disease," *International Journal of Biochemistry and Cell Biology* 39, no. 1 (2007): 44–84.

9. K. Sworczak and P. Wisniewski, "Role of Vitamins in the Prevention and Treatment of Thyroid Disorders," *Polish Journal of Endocrinology* 62, no. 4 (2011): 340–44.

10. M. J. Berry and P. R. Larsen, "Role of Selenium in Thyroid Hormone Actions," *Endocrine Reviews* 13, no. 2 (1992): 207–19.

11. F. Licastro, E. Mocchenegiani, M. Zannotti, et al., "Zinc Affects the Metabolism of Thyroid Hormones in Children with Down's Syndrome: Normalisation of Thyroid-Stimulating Hormone and of Reverse Triiodothyronine Plasmic Levels by Dietary Zinc Supplementation," *International Journal of Neuroscience* 65 (1992): 259–68.

12. J. E. Maras, O. I. Bermudez, N. Qiao, P. J. Bakun, E. L. Boody-Alter, and K. L. Tucker, "Intake of Alpha-Tocopherol Is Limited Among US Adults," *Journal of the American Dietetic Association* 104, no. 4 (2004): 567–75.

13. S. M. Getahun and F. L. Chung, "Conversion of Glucosinolates to Isothiocyanates in Humans After Ingestion of Cooked Watercress," *Cancer Epidemiology, Biomarkers and Prevention* 8, no. 5 (1999): 447–51.

14. F. Schöne, B. Rudolph, U. Kirchheim, and G. Knapp, "Counteracting the Negative Effects of Rapeseed and Rapeseed Press Cake in Pig Diets," *British Journal of Nutrition* 78, no. 6 (1997): 947–62.

15. M. C. D. S. dos Santos, C. F. L. Goncalves, M. Vaisman, et al., "Impact of Flavonoids on Thyroid Function," *Food and Chemical Toxicology* 49, no. 10 (2011): 2495–502.

16. T. Sathyapalan, A. M. Manuchehri, N. J. Thatcher, et al., "Effect of Soy Phytoestrogen Supplementation on Thyroid Status and Cardiovascular Risk Markers in Patients with Subclinical Hypothyroidism: A Randomized, Double-Blind, Crossover Study," *Journal of Clinical Endocrinology and Metabolism* 96, no. 5 (2011): 1442–49.

17. R. L. Divi, H. C. C. Chang, and D. Doerge, "Antithyroid Isoflavones from Soybean: Isolation, Characterization, and Mechanisms of Action," *Biochemical Pharmacology* 54, no. 10 (1997): 1087–96.

18. M. P. Montgomery, F. Kamel, T. M. Saldana, et al., "Incident Diabetes and Pesticide Exposure Among Licensed Pesticide Applicators: Agricultural Health Study, 1993–2003," *American Journal of Epidemiology* 167, no. 10 (2008): 1235–46.

19. G. B. Post, P. D. Cohn, and K. R. Cooper, "Perfluorooctanoic Acid (PFOA), an Emerging Drinking Water Contaminant: A Critical Review of Recent Literature," *Environmental Research* 116 (2012): 93–117.

20. T. Reinehr, "Obesity and Thyroid Function," *Molecular and Cellular Endocrinology* 316, no. 2 (2010): 165–71.

21. D. F. Zhu, Z. X. Wang, D. R. Zhang, et al., "fMRI Revealed Neural Substrate for Reversible Working Memory Dysfunction in Subclinical Hypothyroidism," *Brain* 129, no. 11 (2006): 2923–30.

22. C. Kirkegaard and J. Faber, "The Role of Thyroid Hormone in Depression," *European Journal of Endocrinology* 138 (1998): 1–9.

23. G. A. Mason, C. H. Walker, and A. J. Prange Jr., "L-Triiodothyronine: Is the Peripheral Hormone a Central Neurotransmitter?" *Neuropsychopharmacology* 8 (1993): 253–57.

24. M. Valko, D. Leibfritz, J. Moncol, et al., "Free Radicals and Antioxidants in Normal Physiological Functions and Human Disease," *International Journal of Biochemistry and Cell Biology* 39, no. 1 (2007): 44–84.

CHAPTER 3. When the Immune System Strikes the Thyroid

1. O. M. Pedersen, N. P. Aardal, T. B. Larssen, J. E. Varhaug, O. Myking, and H. Vik-Mo, "The Value of Ultrasonography in Predicting Autoimmune Thyroid Disease," *Thyroid* 10, no. 3 (2000): 251–59.

2. R. Arem and D. Escalante, "Subclinical Hypothyroidism: Epidemiology, Diagnosis, and Significance," *Advances in Internal Medicine* 41 (1996): 213–50.

3. F. Licastro, E. Mocchenegiani, M. Zannotti, et al., "Zinc Affects the Metabolism of Thyroid Hormones in Children with Down's Syndrome: Normalisation of Thyroid-Stimulating Hormone and of Reverse Triiodothyronine Plasmic Levels by Dietary Zinc Supplementation," *International Journal of Neuroscience* 65 (1992): 259–68.

4. T. G. Strieder, M. F. Prummel, J. G. Tijssen, E. Endert, and W. M. Wiersinga, "Risk

Factors for and Prevalence of Thyroid Disorders in a Cross-Sectional Study Among Healthy Female Relatives of Patients with Autoimmune Thyroid Disease," *Clinical Endocrinology* 59, no. 3 (2003): 396–401.

5. Y. Ban and Y. Tomer, "Susceptibility Genes in Thyroid Autoimmunity," *Clinical Developmental Immunology* 12, no. 1 (2005): 47–58.

6. D. A. Ringold, J. T. Nicoloff, M. Kesler, H. Davis, A. Hamilton, and T. Mack, "Further Evidence for a Strong Genetic Influence on the Development of Autoimmune Thyroid Disease: The California Twin Study," *Thyroid* 12, no. 8 (2002): 647–53.

7. J. Heward and S. C. L. Gough, "Genetic Susceptibility to the Development of Autoimmune Disease," *Clinical Science* 93 (1997): 479–91.

8. S. Wang, S. Mao, G. Zhao, and H. Wu, "Relationship Between Estrogen Receptor and Graves' Disease," *Zhonghua Wai Ke Za Zhi* 38, no. 8 (2000): 619–21.

9. V. R. Radosavljevic, S. M. Jankovic, and J. M. Marinkovic, "Stressful Life Events in the Pathogenesis of Graves' Disease," *European Journal of Endocrinology* 134 (1996): 699–701.

10. M. Maes, I. Mihaylova, and M. De Ruyter, "Lower Serum Zinc in Chronic Fatigue Syndrome (CFS): Relationships to Immune Dysfunctions and Relevance for the Oxidative Stress Status in CFS," *Journal of Affective Disorders* 90, nos. 2–3 (2006): 141–47.

11. C. Boumad and J. J. Orgiazzi, "Iodine Excess and Thyroid Autoimmunity," *Journal of Endocrinological Investigation* 26 (2003): 49–56.

12. D. A. de Luis, C. Varella, H. de la Calle, et al., "*Helicobacter pylori* Infection Is Markedly Increased in Patients with Autoimmune Atrophic Thyroiditis," *Journal of Clinical Gastroenterology* 26, no. 4 (1998): 259–63.

13. P. C. Calder and S. Kew, "The Immune System: A Target for Functional Foods?" *British Journal of Nutrition* 88, suppl. 2 (2002): S165–77.

14. M. F. Vine, L. Stein, K. Weigle, et al., "Effects on the Immune System Associated with Living Near a Pesticide Dump Site," *Environmental Health Perspectives* 108, no. 12 (2000): 1113–24.

15. H. Völzke, A. Werner, H. Wallaschofski, et al., "Occupational Exposure to Ionizing Radiation Is Associated with Autoimmune Thyroid Disease," *Journal of Clinical Endocrinology and Metabolism* 90, no. 8 (2005): 4587–92.

16. N. Takasu, T. Yamada, A. Sato, et al., "Graves' Disease Following Hypothyroidism Due to Hashimoto's Disease: Studies of Eight Cases," *Clinical Endocrinology* 33 (1990): 687–89.

17. T. Kay, R. Darwiche, W. Irawaty, M. Chong, H. Pennington, and H. Thomas, "The Role of Cytokines as Effectors of Tissue Destruction in Autoimmunity," in *Cytokines and Chemokines in Autoimmune Disease,* edited by P. Santamaria (Austin, TX: RG Landes, 2001).

18. R. Dantzer, C. J. Heijen, A. Kavelaars, et al., "The Neuroimmune Basis of Fatigue," *Trends in Neurosciences* 37, no. 1 (2014): 39–46.

19. A. J. Dunn, "Effects of Cytokines and Infections on Brain Neurochemistry," *Clinical Neuroscience Research* 6, nos. 1–2 (2006): 52–68.

20. M. G. Carta, A. Loviselli, M. C. Hardoy, et al., "The Link Between Thyroid Autoimmunity (Antithyroid Peroxidase Autoantibodies) with Anxiety and Mood Disorders in the Community: A Field of Interest for Public Health in the Future," *BMC Psychiatry* 4 (2004): 25.

21. R. Krishnadas and J. Cavanagh, "Depression: An Inflammatory Illness?" *Journal of Neurology, Neurosurgery, and Psychiatry* 83, no. 5 (2012): 495–502.

22. O. N. Pamuk and N. Cakir, "The Frequency of Thyroid Antibodies in Fibromyalgia Patients and Their Relationship with Symptoms," *Clinical Rheumatology* 26, no. 1 (2007): 55–59.

23. B. Segal, W. Thomas, X. Zhu, et al., "Oxidative Stress and Fatigue in Systemic Lupus Erythematosus," *Lupus* 21 (2012): 984–92.

24. F. Baeke, T. Takiishi, H. Korf, C. Gysemans, and C. Mathieu, "Vitamin D: Modulator of the Immune System," *Current Opinion in Pharmacology* 10, no. 4 (2010): 482–96.

25. J. A. Bravo, P. Forsythe, M. V. Chew, et al., "Ingestion of Lactobacillus Strain Regulates Emotional Behavior and Central GABA Receptor Expression in a Mouse via the Vagus Nerve," *Proceedings of the National Academy of Sciences* 108, no. 38 (2011): 16050–55.

CHAPTER 4. Stress and Thyroid Disease: Which Comes First?

1. N. Cousins, *Anatomy of an Illness as Perceived by the Patient* (New York: W. W. Norton, 1979).

2. T. M. O'Connor, D. J. O'Halloran, and F. Shanahan, "The Stress Response and the Hypothalamic-Pituitary-Adrenal Axis: From Molecule to Melancholia," *Quarterly Journal of Medicine* 93 (2000): 323–33.

3. J. K. Levey, K. E. Bell, B. L. Lachar, et al., "Psychoneuroimmunology," in *Neuroimmunology for the Clinician*, edited by Loren A. Rolak and Yadollah Harati, 35–55 (Newton, MA: Butterworth-Heinemann, 1997).

4. E. Caffro, B. Forresi, and L. S. Lievers, "Impact, Psychological Sequelae and Management of Trauma Affecting Children and Adolescents," *Current Opinions in Psychiatry* 18, no. 4 (2005): 422–28.

5. D. N. Khansari, A. J. Murgo, and R. E. Faith, "Effects of Stress on the Immune System," *Immunology Today* 11 (1990): 170–75.

6. J. K. Kiecolt-Glaser, W. B. Malarkey, and M. Chee, "Negative Behavior During Marital Conflict Is Associated with Immunological Down-Regulation," *Psychosomatic Medicine* 55 (1993): 395–409.

7. S. Cohen, A. J. Tyrell, and A. P. Smith, "Psychological Stress and Susceptibility to the Common Cold," *New England Journal of Medicine* 325 (1991): 606–12.

8. *Collections from the Writings of the Late C. H. Parry* (London: Underwoods, 1825).

9. V. R. Radosavljevic, S. M. Jankovic, and J. M. Marinkovic, "Stressful Life Events in the Pathogenesis of Graves' Disease," *European Journal of Endocrinology* 134 (1996): 699–701.

10. K. Yoshiuchi, H. Kumano, S. Nomura, et al., "Stressful Life Events and Smoking Were Associated with Graves' Disease in Women, but Not in Men," *Psychosomatic Medicine* 60 (1998): 182–85.

11. B. Harris, S. Othman, J. A. Davies, et al., "Association Between Postpartum Thyroid Dysfunction and Thyroid Antibodies and Depression," *British Medical Journal* 305, no. 6846 (1992): 152–56.

12. V. J. Pop, L. H. Maartens, G. Leusink, et al., "Are Autoimmune Thyroid Dysfunction and Depression Related?" *Journal of Clinical Endocrinology and Metabolism* 83, no. 9 (1998): 3194–97.

13. J. J. Haggerty, K. L. Evans, R. N. Golden, et al., "The Presence of Antithyroid Antibodies in Patients with Affective and Non-Affective Psychiatric Disorders," *Biological Psychiatry* 27 (1990): 51–60.

14. M. G. Carta, A. Loviselli, M. C. Hardoy, et al., "The Link Between Thyroid Autoimmunity (Antithyroid Peroxidase Autoantibodies) with Anxiety and Mood Disorders in the Community: A Field of Interest for Public Health in the Future," *BMC Psychiatry* 4 (2004): 25.

15. K. C. Hyams, F. S. Wignall, and R. Roswell, "War Syndromes and Their Evaluation: From the U.S. Civil War to the Persian Gulf War," *Annals of Internal Medicine* 125 (1996): 398–405.

16. S. Wang, "Traumatic Stress and Attachment," *Acta Physiologica Scandinavica* 161, suppl. 640 (1997): 164–69.

17. H. Brooks, "Hyperthyroidism in the Recruit," *American Journal of Medical Science* 156 (1918): 726–33.

18. R. Grelland, "Thyrotoxicosis at Ullevål Hospital in the Years 1934–44 with a Special View of Frequency of the Disease," *Acta Medica Scandinavica* 125 (1946): 108–38.

19. A. Trafford, "Me, Bush, and Graves' Disease: Many Thyroid Patients Face an Emotional Rollercoaster," *Washington Post*, May 26, 1991, p. D1.

20. S. A. Ebner, M.-C. Badonnel, L. K. Altman, et al., "Conjugal Graves' Disease," *Annals of Internal Medicine* 116 (1992): 479–81.

21. J. B. Jaspan, H. Luo, B. Ahmed, et al., "Evidence for a Retroviral Trigger in Graves' Disease," *Autoimmunity* 20 (1995): 135–42.

22. A. Fukao, M. Ito, and S. Hayashi, "The Effect of Psychological Factors on the Prognosis of Antithyroid Drug-Related Graves' Disease Patients" (abstract), *Thyroid* 5, suppl. 1 (1995): S244.

23. H. M. Voth, P. S. Holzman, J. B. Katz, et al., "Thyroid 'Hot Spots': Their Relationship to Life Stress," *Psychosomatic Medicine* 32 (1970): 561–68.

24. A. Fukao, J. Takamatsu, Y. Murakami, S. Sakane, A. Miyauchi, K. Kuma, S. Hayashi, and T. Hanafusa, "The Relationship of Psychological Factors to the Prognosis of Hyperthyroidism in Antithyroid Drug-Treated Patients with Graves' Disease," *Clinical Endocrinology* 58, no. 5 (2003): 550–55.

25. E. Moschowitz, "The Nature of Graves' Disease," *Archives of Internal Medicine* 46 (1930): 610–29.

26. D. R. Brown, Y. Wang, and A. Ward, "Chronic Psychological Effects of Exercise and Exercise Plus Cognitive Strategies," *Medicine and Science in Sports and Exercise* 27, no. 5 (1995): 765–75.

CHAPTER 5. Hypothyroidism: When the Thyroid Is Underactive

1. F. F. Cartwright, *Disease and History* (New York: Dorset Press, 1972), 105–6.

2. H. F. Stoll, "Chronic Invalidism with Marked Personality Changes Due to Myxedema," *Annals of Internal Medicine* 6 (1932): 806.

3. W. M. Easson and T. Kay, "Myxedema with Psychosis," *Archives of General Psychiatry* 14 (1966): 277–83.

4. R. Asher, "Myxedematous Madness," *British Medical Journal* 2 (1949): 555–62.

5. I. Klein and K. Ojamaa, "Thyroid Hormone and Blood Pressure Regulation," in *Hypertension: Pathophysiology, Diagnosis, and Management*, 2d ed., edited by J. H. Laragh and B. M. Brenner, 2247–62 (New York: Raven Press, 1995).

6. J. J. Series, E. M. Biggart, D. St. J. O'Reilly, et al., "Thyroid Dysfunction and Hypercholesterolaemia in the General Population of Glasgow, Scotland," *Clinica Chimica Acta* 172 (1988): 217–22.

7. M. S. Morris, A. G. Bostom, P. F. Jacques, J. Selhub, and I. H. Rosenberg, "Hyperho-

mocysteinemia and Hypercholesterolemia Associated with Hypothyroidism in the Third US National Health and Nutrition Examination Survey," *Atherosclerosis* 155, no. 1 (2001): 195–200.

8. F. Monzani, A. Dardano, and N. Caraccio, "Does Treating Subclinical Hypothyroidism Improve Markers of Cardiovascular Risk?" *Treatments in Endocrinology* 5, no. 2 (2006): 65–81.

9. E. Beghi, M. Delodovici, G. Boglium, et al., "Hypothyroidism and Polyneuropathy," *Journal of Neurology, Neurosurgery, and Psychiatry* 52 (1989): 1420–23.

10. M. A. Laylock and R. Pascuzzi, "The Neuromuscular Effects of Hypothyroidism," *Seminars in Neurology* 11, no. 3 (1991): 288–94.

11. J. Salvador, J. Iriarte, C. Silva, J. Gomez Ambrosi, A. Diez Caballero, and G. Fruhbeck, "The Obstructive Sleep Apnea Syndrome in Obesity: A Conspirator in the Shadow," *Review of the Medical University of Navarra* 48, no. 2 (2004): 55–62.

12. R. Arem and D. Escalante, "Subclinical Hypothyroidism: Epidemiology, Diagnosis, and Significance," *Advances in Internal Medicine* 41 (1996): 213–50.

13. W. M. G. Turnbridge, M. Brewis, J. M. French, et al., "Natural History of Autoimmune Thyroiditis," *British Medical Journal* 282 (1981): 258–62.

14. D. Brown and D. Hoffman, "Russian Government Continues to Hide Details of Yeltsin's Medical Problems," *Washington Post*, February 20, 1996, 3.

15. Cable News Network, "Yeltsin Didn't Look Sick," September 26, 1996.

16. Cable News Network, "Yeltsin's Health Problems Cloud Russia's Future. More than Heart Disease May Be Involved," September 21, 1996.

17. R. Arem and W. Patsch, "Lipoprotein and Apolipoprotein Levels in Subclinical Hypothyroidism," *Archives of Internal Medicine* 150 (1990): 2097–100.

18. R. Luboshitzky, A. Aviv, P. Herer, and L. Lavie, "Risk Factors for Cardiovascular Disease in Women with Subclinical Hypothyroidism," *Thyroid* 12, no. 5 (2002): 421–25.

19. J. P. Walsh, A. P. Bremner, M. K. Bulsara, et al., "Subclinical Thyroid Dysfunction as a Risk Factor for Cardiovascular Disease," *Archives of Internal Medicine* 165, no. 21 (2005): 2467–72.

20. M. M. Mya and W. S. Aronow, "Increased Prevalence of Peripheral Arterial Disease in Older Men and Women with Subclinical Hypothyroidism," *Journals of Gerontology, Series A: Biological Sciences and Medical Sciences* 58, no. 1 (2003): 68–69.

21. G. Bono, R. Fancellu, F. Blandini, G. Santoro, and M. Mauri, "Cognitive and Affective Status in Mild Hypothyroidism and Interactions with L-Thyroxine Treatment," *Acta Neurologica Scandinavica* 110, no. 1 (2004): 59–66.

22. R. Fierro-Benitez, R. Casar, J. B. Stanburly, et al., "Long-Term Effects of Correction of Iodine Deficiency on Psychomotor and Intellectual Development," in *Proceedings of the Fifth Meeting of the PAHO/WHO Technical Group on Endemic Goiter, Cretinism, and Iodine Deficiency*, edited by J. T. Dunn et al. (Washington, DC: Pan-American Health Organization, 1986).

23. E. Nyström, K. Caidahl, G. Fager, et al., "A Double-Blind Cross-over 12-Month Study of L-Thyroxine Treatment of Women with 'Subclinical' Hypothyroidism," *Clinical Endocrinology* 29 (1988): 63–76.

24. J. J. Haggerty, J. C. Garbutt, D. L. Evans, et al., "Subclinical Hypothyroidism: A Review of Neuropsychiatric Aspects," *International Journal of Psychiatry in Medicine* 20, no. 2 (1990): 193–208.

25. F. Monzani, P. Del Guerra, N. Caraccio, et al., "Subclinical Hypothyroidism: Neurobehavioral Features and Beneficial Effect of L-Thyroxine Treatment," *Clinical Investigator* 71 (1993): 367–71.

26. J. V. Felicetta, "Thyroid Changes with Aging: Significance and Management," *Geriatrics* 42 (1987): 86–92.

27. J. D. Davis, R. A. Stern, and L. A. Flashman, "Cognitive and Neuropsychiatric Aspects of Subclinical Hypothyroidism: Significance in the Elderly," *Current Psychiatry Reports* 5, no. 5 (2003): 384–90.

28. D. L. Ewins, M. N. Rossot, J. Butler, et al., "Association Between Autoimmune Thyroid Disease and Familial Alzheimer's Disease," *Clinical Endocrinology* 35 (1991): 93–96.

29. C. T. Sawin, D. Chopra, A. Azizi, et al., "The Aging Thyroid: Increased Prevalence of Elevated Serum Thyrotropin in the Elderly," *Journal of the American Medical Association* 242 (1979): 247–50.

30. F. Delange, "Neonatal Screening for Congenital Hypothyroidism: Results and Perspectives," *Hormone Research* 48 (1997): 51–61.

31. M. A. Jabbar, J. Larrea, and R. A. Shaw, "Abnormal Thyroid Function Tests in Infants with Congenital Hypothyroidism: The Influence of Soy-Based Formula," *Journal of the American College of Nutrition* 16, no. 3 (1997): 280–82.

32. H. E. Roberts, C. A. Moore, P. M. Fernhoff, et al., "Population Study of Congenital Hypothyroidism and Associated Birth Defects, Atlanta, 1979–1992," *American Journal of Medical Genetics* 71 (1997): 29–32.

33. E. Medda, A. Olivieri, M. A. Stazi, et al., "Risk Factors for Congenital Hypothyroidism: Results of a Population Case-Control Study (1997–2003)," *European Journal of Endocrinology* 153, no. 6 (2005): 765–73.

CHAPTER 6. **Hyperthyroidism: When the Thyroid Is Overactive**

1. H. F. Dunlap and F. P. Moersch, "Psychic Manifestations Associated with Hyperthyroidism," *American Journal of Psychiatry* 91 (1935): 1215–38.

2. S. Nagasaka, H. Sugimoto, T. Nakamura, et al., "Antithyroid Therapy Improves Bony Manifestations and Bone Metabolic Markers in Patients with Graves' Thyrotoxicosis," *Clinical Endocrinology* 47, no. 2 (1997): 215–21.

3. C. Erem, H. O. Ersoz, S. S. Karti, K. Ukinc, A. Hacihasanoglu, O. Deger, and M. Telatar, "Blood Coagulation and Fibrinolysis in Patients with Hyperthyroidism," *Journal of Endocrinological Investigation* 25, no. 4 (2002): 345–50.

4. P.-T. Trzepacz, I. Klein, M. Roberts, et al., "Graves' Disease: An Analysis of Thyroid Hormone Levels and Hyperthyroid Signs and Symptoms," *American Journal of Medicine* 87, no. 5 (1989): 558–61.

5. V. I. Reus, "Behavioral Aspects of Thyroid Disease in Women," *Psychiatric Clinics of North America* 12, no. 1 (1989): 153–63.

6. R. C. W. Hall, "Psychiatric Effects of Thyroid Hormone Disturbance," *Psychosomatics* 24, no. 1 (1983): 7–18.

7. B. E. Brownlie, A. M. Rae, J. W. Walshe, and J. E. Wells, "Psychoses Associated with Thyrotoxicosis—'Thyrotoxic Psychosis.' A Report of 18 Cases, with Statistical Analysis of Incidence," *European Journal of Endocrinology* 142, no. 5 (2000): 438–44.

8. P. H. Rockey and R. J. Griep, "Behavioral Dysfunction in Hyperthyroidism: Improvement with Treatment," *Archives of Internal Medicine* 140 (1980): 1194–97.

9. D. G. Folks and W. M. Petrie, "Thyrotoxicosis Presenting as Depression" (letter), *British Journal of Psychiatry* 140 (1982): 432–33.

10. P. F. Giannandrea, "The Depressed Hyperthyroid Patient," *General Hospital Psychiatry* 9 (1987): 71–74.

11. M. M. Demet, B. Ozmen, A. Deveci, S. Boyvada, H. Adiguzel, and O. Aydemir, "Depression and Anxiety in Hyperthyroidism," *Archives of Medical Research* 33, no. 6 (2002): 552–56.

12. B. Schlote, B. Nowotny, L. Schaaf, et al., "Subclinical Hyperthyroidism: Physical and Mental State of Patients," *European Archives of Psychiatry and Clinical Neuroscience* 241 (1992): 357–64.

13. B. Uzzan, J. Campos, M. Cucherat, et al., "Effects on Bone Mass of Long-Term Treatment with Thyroid Hormones: A Meta-Analysis," *Journal of Clinical Endocrinology and Metabolism* 81 (1996): 4278–89.

14. B. Biondi, S. Fazio, A. Cuocola, et al., "Impaired Cardiac Reserve and Exercise Capacity in Patients Receiving Long-Term Thyrotropin Suppressive Therapy with Levothyroxine," *Journal of Clinical Endocrinology and Metabolism* 81 (1996): 4224–28.

15. V. Fatourechi, J. P. Aniszewski, G. Z. E. Fatourechi, E. J. Atkinson, and S. J. Jacobsen, "Clinical Features and Outcome of Subacute Thyroiditis in an Incidence Cohort: Olmsted County, Minnesota, Study," *Journal of Clinical Endocrinology and Metabolism* 88, no. 5 (2003): 2100–5.

16. W. M. G. Turnbridge, D. C. Evered, R. Hall, et al., "The Spectrum of Thyroid Disease in a Community: The Whickham Survey," *Clinical Endocrinology* 7 (1977): 481–93.

17. C. Triavalle, J. Doucet, P. Chassagne, et al., "Differences in the Signs and Symptoms of Hyperthyroidism in Older and Younger Patients," *Journal of the American Geriatrics Society* 44 (1996): 50–53.

18. F. I. R. Martin and D. R. Deam, "Hyperthyroidism in Elderly Hospitalized Patients: Clinical Features and Treatment Outcomes," *Medical Journal of Australia* 164 (1996): 200–3.

CHAPTER 7. Getting the Proper Diagnosis

1. D. S. Ross, G. H. Daniels, and D. Gouveia, "The Use and Limitations of a Chemilu minescent Thyrotropin Assay as a Single Thyroid Function Test in an Outpatient Endocrine Clinic," *Journal of Clinical Endocrinology and Metabolism* 71, no. 3 (1990): 764–69.

2. K. W. Geul, I. L. L. van Sluisveld, D. E. Grobbee, et al., "The Importance of Thyroid Microsomal Antibodies in the Development of Elevated Serum TSH in Middle-Aged Women: Associations with Serum Lipids," *Clinical Endocrinology* 39 (1993): 275–80.

3. G. Michalopoulou, M. Alevizaki, G. Piperingos, et al., "High Serum Cholesterol Levels in Persons with 'High-Normal' TSH Levels: Should One Extend the Definition of Subclinical Hypothyroidism?" *European Journal of Endocrinology* 138, no. 2 (1998): 141–45.

4. I. Berlin, C. Payan, E. Corruble, and A. J. Puech, "Serum Thyroid-Stimulating-Hormone Concentration as an Index of Severity of Major Depression," *International Journal of Neuropsychopharmacology* 2, no. 2 (1999): 105–10.

5. H. J. Baskin, R. H. Cobin, D. S. Duick, et al., "American Association for Clinical Endocrinologists Medical Guidelines for Clinical Practice for the Evaluation of Treatment of Hyperthyroidism and Hypothyroidism," *Endocrine Practice* 8 (2002): 457–67.

6. M. I. Surks, G. Goswami, and G. H. Daniels, "Controversies in Clinical Endocrinology: The Thyrotropin Reference Range Should Remain Unchanged," *Journal of Clinical Endocrinology and Metabolism* 90, no. 9 (2005): 5489–96.

7. R. Arem and D. Escalante, "Subclinical Hypothyroidism: Epidemiology, Diagnosis, and Significance," *Advances in Internal Medicine* 41 (1996): 213–50.

8. J. G. Eales, "Iodine Metabolism and Thyroid-Related Functions in Organisms Lacking Thyroid Follicules: Are Thyroid Hormones Also Vitamins?" *Proceedings of the Society for Experimental Biology and Medicine* 214 (1997): 302–17.

9. G. R. B. Skinner, R. Thomas, M. Taylor, et al., "Thyroxine Should Be Tried in Clinically Hypothyroid but Biochemically Euthyroid Patients," *British Medical Journal* 314 (1997): 1764.

10. M.-F. Poirier, H. Lôo, A. Galinowski, et al., "Sensitive Assay of Thyroid-Stimulating Hormone in Depressed Patients," *Psychiatry Research* 57 (1995): 41–48.

11. R. A. Dickey and H. W. Rodbard, "American Association of Clinical Endocrinologists 'Neck Check' Promoted During Thyroid Awareness Month," *First Messenger* 5, no. 1 (1997): 1.

12. O. M. Pedersen, N. P. Aardal, T. B. Larssen, J. E. Varhaug, O. Myking, and H. Vik-Mo, "The Value of Ultrasonography in Predicting Autoimmune Thyroid Disease," *Thyroid* 10, no. 3 (2000): 251–59.

13. S. Morita, T. Arima, and M. Matsuda, "Prevalence of Nonthyroid Specific Autoantibodies in Autoimmune Thyroid Diseases," *Journal of Clinical Endocrinology and Metabolism* 80, no. 4 (1995): 1203–6.

14. B. Lindberg, U.-B. Ericsson, R. Ljung, et al., "High Prevalence of Thyroid Autoantibodies at Diagnosis of Insulin-Dependent Diabetes Mellitus in Swedish Children," *Journal of Laboratory and Clinical Medicine* 130 (1997): 585–89.

15. J. Heward and S. C. L. Gough, "Genetic Susceptibility to the Development of Autoimmune Disease," *Clinical Science* 93 (1997): 479–91.

16. E. Biro, Z. Szekanecz, L. Czirjak, et al., "Association of Systemic and Thyroid Autoimmune Diseases," *Clinical Rheumatology* 25, no. 2 (2006): 240–45.

17. M. S. Rosenthal, *The Thyroid Source Book: Everything You Need to Know*, 2d ed. (Los Angeles: Lowell House, 1996), 57.

18. J. Coll, J. Anglada, S. Tomas, et al., "High Prevalence of Subclinical Sjögren's Syndrome Features in Patients with Autoimmune Thyroid Disease," *Journal of Rheumatology* 24, no. 9 (1997): 1719–24.

19. J. S. Sloka, P. W. Phillips, M. Stefanelli, and C. Joyce, "Co-occurrence of Autoimmune Thyroid Disease in a Multiple Sclerosis Cohort," *Journal of Autoimmune Diseases* 2 (2005): 9.

20. D. P. Westerberg, J. M. Gill, B. Dave, M. J. DiPrinzio, A. Quisel, and A. Foy, "New Strategies for Diagnosis and Management of Celiac Disease," *Journal of the American Osteopathic Association* 106, no. 3 (2006): 145–51.

21. M. Hakanen, K. Luotola, J. Salmi, P. Laippala, K. Kaukinen, and P. Collin, "Clinical and Subclinical Autoimmune Thyroid Disease in Adult Celiac Disease," *Digestive Diseases and Sciences* 46, no. 12 (2001): 2631–35.

22. L. M. da Silva Kotze, R. M. Nisihara, S. R. da Rosa Utiyama, G. C. Piovezan, and L. R. Kotze, "Thyroid Disorders in Brazilian Patients with Celiac Disease," *Journal of Clinical Gastroenterology* 40, no. 1 (2006): 33–36.

23. C. L. Ch'ng, M. Biswas, A. Benton, M. K. Jones, and J. G. Kingham, "Prospective Screening for Coeliac Disease in Patients with Graves' Hyperthyroidism Using Anti-Gliadin and Tissue Transglutaminase Antibodies," *Clinical Endocrinology* 62, no. 3 (2005): 303–6.

24. E. Deressa, A. C. Wammer, J. A. Falch, and J. Jahnsen, "Bone Metabolism in Patients with Newly Diagnosed Coeliac Disease," *Tidsskrift for den Norske Laegeforening* 126, no. 9 (2006): 1201–4.

25. W. Dickey and S. A. McMillan, "Increasing Numbers at a Specialist Coeliac Clinic: Contribution of Serological Testing in Primary Care," *Digestive and Liver Disease* 37, no. 12 (2005): 928–33.

26. P. F. Peerboom, E. A. M. Hassink, R. Melkert, et al., "Thyroid Function 10–18 Years After Mantle Field Irradiation for Hodgkin's Disease," *European Journal of Cancer* 28A, no. 10 (1992): 1716–18.

27. A. Leznoff and G. L. Sussman, "Syndrome of Idiopathic Chronic Urticaria and Angioedema with Thyroid Autoimmunity: A Study of 90 Patients," *Journal of Allergy and Clinical Immunology* 84, no. 1 (1989): 66–71.

28. L. C. Hofbauer, C. Spitzweig, S. Schmauss, et al., "Graves' Disease Associated with Autoimmune Thrombocytopenic Purpura," *Archives of Internal Medicine* 157 (1997): 1033–36.

29. A. Pinchera, E. Martino, and G. Faglia, "Central Hypothyroidism," in *Werner and Ingbar's The Thyroid*, 6th ed., edited by Lewis E. Braverman and R. D. Utiger, 968–84 (Philadelphia: Lippincott, 1991).

30. M. Mori, Y. Shoda, M. Yamado, et al., "Case Report: Central Hypothyroidism Due to Isolated TRH Deficiency in a Depressive Man," *Journal of Internal Medicine* 229 (1991): 285–88.

CHAPTER 8. Thyroid Imbalance, Depression, Anxiety, and Mood Swings

1. F. Monzani, P. Del Guerra, N. Caraccio, et al., "Subclinical Hypothyroidism: Neurobehavioral Features and Beneficial Effect of L-Thyroxine Treatment," *Clinical Investigator* 71 (1993): 367–71.

2. J. Scherer, "The Prevalence of Goiter in Psychiatric Outpatients Suffering from Affective Disorders" (letter), *American Journal of Psychiatry* 151 (1994): 453.

3. M. B. Dratman and J. T. Gordon, "Thyroid Hormones as Neurotransmitters," *Thyroid* 6, no. 6 (1996): 639–47.

4. C. Kirkegaard and J. Faber, "The Role of Thyroid Hormone in Depression," *European Journal of Endocrinology* 138 (1998): 1–9.

5. G. A. Mason, C. H. Walker, and A. J. Prange Jr., "L-Triiodothyronine: Is the Peripheral Hormone a Central Neurotransmitter?" *Neuropsychopharmacology* 8 (1993): 253–57.

6. P. C. Whybrow and A. J. Prange Jr., "A Hypothesis of Thyroid-Catecholamine-Receptor Interaction: Its Relevance to Affective Illness," *Archives of General Psychiatry* 38 (1981): 106–13.

7. T. Gunnarsson, S. Sjoberg, M. Eriksson, and C. Nordin, "Depressive Symptoms in Hypothyroid Disorder with Some Observations on Biochemical Correlates," *Neuropsychobiology* 43, no. 2 (2001): 70–74.

8. J. M. Gorman, *The New Psychiatry* (New York: St. Martin's Press, 1996).

9. J. Morrison, "DSM-IV Made Easy," *The Clinician's Guide to Diagnosis* (New York: Guilford Press, 1995).

10. A. F. Thomsen, T. K. Kvist, P. K. Andersen, and L. V. Kessing, "Increased Risk of Developing Affective Disorder in Patients with Hypothyroidism: A Register-Based Study," *Thyroid* 15, no. 7 (2005): 700–7.

11. M. S. Gold, A. L. C. Pottash, and I. Extein, "'Symptomless' Autoimmune Thyroiditis in Depression," *Psychiatry Research* 6 (1982): 261–69.

12. C. B. Nemeroff, J. S. Simon, J. J. Haggerty, et al., "Antithyroid Antibodies in Depressed Patients," *American Journal of Psychiatry* 142 (1985): 840–43.

13. J. J. Haggerty, R. A. Stern, G. A. Mason, et al., "Subclinical Hypothyroidism: A Mod-

ifiable Risk Factor for Depression?" *American Journal of Psychiatry* 150, no. 3 (1993): 508–10.

14. C. Kirkegaard and J. Faber, "The Role of Thyroid Hormones in Depression," *European Journal of Endocrinology* 138 (1998): 1–9.

15. K. D. Denicoff, R. T. Joffe, M. C. Lakshmanan, et al., "Neuropsychiatric Manifestations of Altered Thyroid State," *American Journal of Psychiatry* 147, no. 1 (1990): 94–99.

16. R. H. Howland, "Thyroid Dysfunction in Refractory Depression: Implications for Pathophysiology and Treatment," *Journal of Clinical Psychiatry* 54, no. 2 (1993): 47–54.

17. R. C. Kessler, K. A. McGonagle, S. Zhao, et al., "Lifetime and 12-Month Prevalence of DSM-III-R Psychiatric Disorders in the United States. Results from the National Comorbidity Study," *Archives of General Psychiatry* 51 (1994): 8–19.

18. C. G. Lindemann, C. M. Zitrin, and D. Klein, "Thyroid Dysfunction in Phobic Patients," *Psychosomatics* 25 (1984): 603–6.

19. S. Matsubayashi, H. Tamai, Y. Matsumoto, et al., "Graves' Disease After the Onset of Panic Disorder," *Psychotherapy and Psychosomatics* 65 (1996): 277–80.

20. M. E. Lickey and B. Gordon, *Medicine and Mental Illness: The Use of Drugs in Psychiatry* (New York: Freeman, 1991).

21. J. M. Gorman, *The New Psychiatry* (New York: St. Martin's Press, 1996), 212.

22. P. Chiaroni, "Clinical Picture and Diagnosis of Bipolar Disorder," *Revue du Practicien* 55, no. 5 (2005): 493–500.

23. L. Citrome and J. F. Goldberg, "The Many Faces of Bipolar Disorder. How to Tell Them Apart," *Postgraduate Medicine* 117, no. 2 (2005): 15–16, 19–23.

24. J. F. Goldberg and C. J. Truman, "Antidepressant-Induced Mania: An Overview of Current Controversies," *Bipolar Disorder* 5, no. 6 (2003): 407–20.

25. C. Henry, D. Van den Bulke, F. Bellivier, B. Etain, F. Rouillon, and M. Leboyer, "Anxiety Disorders in 318 Bipolar Patients: Prevalence and Impact on Illness Severity and Response to Mood Stabilizer," *Journal of Clinical Psychiatry* 64, no. 3 (2003): 331–35.

26. R. W. Cowdry, T. A. Wehr, A. P. Zis, et al., "Thyroid Abnormalities Associated with Rapid-Cycling Bipolar Illness," *Archives of General Psychiatry* 40 (1983): 414–20; M. M. Kusalic, "Grade II and Grade III Hypothyroidism in Rapid-Cycling Bipolar Patients," *Neuropsychobiology* 25 (1992): 177–81.

27. Z. J. Zhang, L. Qiang, W. H. Kang, et al., "Differences in Hypothyroidism Between Lithium-Free and -Treated Patients with Bipolar Disorder," *Life Science* 78, no. 7 (2006): 771–76.

28. H. A. P. C. Oomen, A. J. M. Schipperijn, and H. A. Drexhage, "The Prevalence of Affective Disorder and in Particular of a Rapid Cycling of Bipolar Disorder in Patients with Abnormal Thyroid Function Tests," *Clinical Endocrinology* 45 (1996): 215–23.

CHAPTER 9. Medicine from the Body: Thyroid Hormone as an Antidepressant

1. G. R. Murray, "Note on Treatment of Myxoedema by Hypodermic Injections of an Extract of the Thyroid Gland of a Sheep," *British Medical Journal* 2 (1891): 796–97.

2. S. C. Kaufman, G. P. Gross, and G. L. Kennedy, "Thyroid Hormone Use: Trends in the United States from 1960 Through 1988," *Thyroid* 1, no. 4 (1991): 285–91.

3. R. T. Joffe, S. T. H. Sokolov, and W. Singer, "Thyroid Hormone Treatment of Depression," *Thyroid* 5, no. 3 (1995): 235–39.

4. A. Baumgartner, M. Eravci, G. Pinna, et al., "Thyroid Hormone Metabolism in the Rat Brain in an Animal Model of 'Behavioral Dependence' on Ethanol," *Neuroscience Letters* 227 (1997): 25–28.

5. P. Hauser, A. J. Zametkin, P. Martinez, et al., "Attention Deficit-Hyperactivity Disorder in People with Generalized Resistance to Thyroid Hormone," *New England Journal of Medicine* 328, no. 14 (1993): 997–1001.

6. B. Rozanov and M. B. Dratman, "Immunohistochemical Mapping of Brain Triiodothyronine Reveals Prominent Localization in Ventral Noradrenergic Systems," *Neuroscience* 74, no. 3 (1996): 897–915.

7. J. A. Hatterer, J. Herbert, C. Hidaka, et al., "Transthyretin in Patients with Depression," *American Journal of Psychiatry* 150 (1993): 813–15.

8. G. M. Sullivan, J. A. Hatterer, J. Herbert, X. Chen, S. P. Roose, E. Attia, J. J. Mann, L. B. Marangell, R. R. Goetz, and J. M. Gorman, "Low Levels of Transthyretin in the CFS of Depressed Patients," *American Journal of Psychiatry* 156, no. 5 (1999): 710–15.

9. J. C. Sousa, C. Grandela, J. Fernandez-Ruiz, R. de Miguel, L. de Sousa, A. I. Magalhaes, M. J. Saraiva, N. Sousa, and J. A. Palha, "Transthyretin Is Involved in Depression-Like Behavior and Exploratory Activity," *Journal of Neurochemistry* 88, no. 5 (2004): 1052–58.

10. C. Kirkegaard and J. Faber, "The Role of Thyroid Hormones in Depression," *European Journal of Endocrinology* 138 (1998): 1–9.

11. S. T. H. Sokolov, A. J. Levitt, and R. T. Joffe, "Thyroid Hormone Levels Before Unsuccessful Antidepressant Therapy Are Associated with Later Response to T3 Augmentation," *Psychiatry Research* 69 (1997): 203–6.

12. W. N. Henley and T. J. Koehnle, "Thyroid Hormones and the Treatment of Depression: An Examination of Basic Hormonal Actions in the Mature Mammalian Brain," *Synapse* 27 (1997): 36–44.

13. L. L. Altshuler, M. Bauer, M. A. Frye, M. J. Gitlin, J. Mintz, M. P. Szuba, K. L. Leight, and P. C. Whybrow, "Does Thyroid Supplementation Accelerate Tricyclic Antidepressant Response? A Review and Meta-Analysis of the Literature," *American Journal of Psychiatry* 158, no. 10 (2001): 1617–22.

14. R. T. Joffe, W. Singer, A. J. Levitt, et al., "A Placebo-Controlled Comparison of Lithium and Triiodothyronine Augmentation of Tricyclic Antidepressants in Unipolar Refractory Depression," *Archives of General Psychiatry* 50 (1993): 387–93.

15. G. Abraham, R. Milev, and J. Stuart Lawson, "T3 Augmentation of SSRI Resistant Depression," *Journal of Affective Disorders* 91, nos. 2–3 (2006): 211–15.

16. O. Agid and B. Lerer, "Algorithm-Based Treatment of Major Depression in an Outpatient Clinic: Clinical Correlates of Response to a Specific Serotonin Reuptake Inhibitor and to Triiodothyronine Augmentation," *International Journal of Neuropsychopharmacology* 6, no. 1 (2003): 41–49.

17. E. E. Feldmesser-Reiss, "The Application of Triiodothyronine in the Treatment of Mental Disorders," *Journal of Nervous and Mental Disease* 127 (1958): 540–46.

18. R. M. Post, "The Impact of Bipolar Depression," *Journal of Clinical Psychiatry* 66, suppl. 5 (2005): 5–10.

19. A. Campos-Barros, A. Musa, A. Flechner, et al., "Evidence for Circadian Variations of Thyroid Hormone Concentrations and Type II 5'-Iodothyronine Deiodinase Activity in the Rat Central Nervous System," *Journal of Neurochemistry* 68 (1997): 795–803.

20. E. Souetre, E. Salvati, T. A. Wher, et al., "Twenty-Four-Hour Profiles of Body Temperature and Plasma TSH in Bipolar Patients During Depression and During Remission and in Normal Control Subjects," *American Journal of Psychiatry* 145, no. 9 (1988): 1133–37.

21. R. E. Noble, "Depression in Women," *Metabolism* 54, suppl. 1 (2005): 49–52.

22. N. Konno and K. Morikawa, "Seasonal Variation of Serum Thyrotropin Concentration and Thyrotropin Response to Thyrotropin-Releasing Hormone in Patients with Primary Hypothyroidism on Constant Replacement Dosage of Thyroxine," *Journal of Clinical Endocrinology and Metabolism* 54 (1982): 1118–24.

23. M. S. Bauer and P. C. Whybrow, "Rapid-Cycling Bipolar Affective Disorder," part 2, "Treatment of Refractory Rapid Cycling with High-Dose Levothyroxine: A Preliminary Study," *Archives of General Psychiatry* 47 (1990): 435–40.

24. J. S. Manning, R. F. Haykal, P. D. Connor, P. D. Cunningham, W. C. Jackson, and S. Long, "Sustained Remission with Lamotrigine Augmentation or Monotherapy in Female Resistant Depressives with Mixed Cyclothymic-Dysthymic Temperament," *Journal of Affective Disorders* 84, nos. 2–3 (2005): 259–66.

25. O. Brawman-Mintzer, R. G. Knapp, and P. J. Nietert, "Adjunctive Risperidone in Generalized Anxiety Disorder: A Double-Blind, Placebo-Controlled Study," *Journal of Clinical Psychiatry* 66, no. 10 (2005): 1321–25.

26. M. Bauer, E. D. London, N. Rasgon, et al., "Supraphysiological Doses of Levothyroxine Alter Regional Cerebral Metabolism and Improve Mood in Bipolar Depression," *Molecular Psychiatry* 10, no. 5 (2005): 456–69.

27. L. Gyulai, J. Jaggi, M. S. Bauer, et al., "Bone Mineral Density and L-Thyroxine Treatment in Rapidly Cycling Bipolar Disorder," *Biological Psychiatry* 47 (1990): 503–6.

28. M. Bauer, H. Baur, A. Berghofer, A. Strohle, R. Hellweg, B. Muller-Oerlinghausen, and A. Baumgartner, "Effects of Supraphysiological Thyroxine Administration in Healthy Controls and Patients with Depressive Disorders," *Journal of Affective Disorders* 68, nos. 2–3 (2002): 285–94.

PART II. No, You Are Not Making It Up: Common Emotional and Physical Interactions
CHAPTER 10. The Struggle with Weight Gain and Sluggish Metabolism

1. R. J. Kuczmarski, K. M. Flegal, S. M. Campbell, et al., "Increasing Prevalence of Overweight Among U.S. Adults: The National Health and Nutrition Examination Surveys, 1960–1991," *Journal of the American Medical Association* 272, no. 3 (1994): 205–11.

2. M. A. Michalaki, A. G. Vagenakis, A. S. Leonardou, et al., "Thyroid Function in Humans with Morbid Obesity," *Thyroid* 16, no. 1 (2006): 73–78.

3. M. J. Muller, "Thyroid Hormones and Energy and Fat Balance," *European Journal of Endocrinology* 136 (1997): 267–68.

4. J. Y. Lee, N. Takahashi, M. Yasubuchi, et al., "Triiodothyronine Induces UCP1 Expression and Mitochondrial Biogenesis in Human Adipocytes," *American Journal of Physiology: Cell Physiology* 302, no. 2 (2012): C463–72.

5. U. Feldt-Rasmussen, "Thyroid and Leptin," *Thyroid* 17, no. 5 (2007): 413–20.

6. G. Brenta, "Why Can Insulin Resistance Be a Natural Consequence of Thyroid Dysfunction," *Journal of Thyroid Research* 2011, article ID 152850 (2011), doi:10.4061/2011/152850.

7. A. M. Wren, C. J. Small, H. L. Ward, et al., "The Novel Hypothalamic Peptide Ghrelin Stimulates Food Intake and Growth Hormone Secretion," *Neuroendocrinology* 141, no. 11 (2000): 4325–28.

8. D. S. Weigle, D. E. Cummings, et al., "Roles of Leptin and Ghrelin in the Loss of Body Weight Caused by a Low Fat, High Carbohydrate Diet," *Journal of Clinical Endocrinology and Metabolism* 88, no. 4 (2003): 1577–86.

9. K. W. Nowak, P. Kaczmarek, P. Mackowiak, et al., "Rat Thyroid Gland Expresses the Long Form of Leptin Receptors, and Leptin Stimulates the Fuction of the Gland in Euthyroid Non-Fasted Animals," *International Journal of Molecular Medicine* 9, no. 1 (2002): 31–34.

10. T. Reinehr, "Obesity and Thyroid Function," *Molecular and Cellular Endocrinology* 316, no. 2 (2010): 165–71.

11. O. J. Marston, A. S. Garfield, and L. K. Heisler, "Role of Central Serotonin and Melanocortin Systems in the Control of Energy Balance," *European Journal of Pharmacology* 660, no. 1 (2011): 70–79.

12. L. Lu, B. Wang, Z. Shan, et al., "The Correlation Between Thyrotropin and Dyslipidemia in a Population-Based Study," *Journal of Korean Medical Science* 26, no. 2 (2011): 243–49.

13. J. Y. Lee, N. Takahashi, M. Yasubuchi, et al., "Triiodothyronine Induces UCP1 Expression and Mitochondrial Biogenesis in Human Adipocytes," *American Journal of Physiology: Cell Physiology* 302, no. 2 (2012): C463–72.

14. J. Daykin Dale, R. Holder, M. C. Sheppard, and J. A. Franklyn, "Weight Gain Following Treatment of Hyperthyroidism," *Clinical Endocrinology* 55, no. 2 (2001): 233–39.

15. F. Celsing, S. H. Westing, U. Adamson, et al., "Muscle Strength in Hyperthyroid Patients Before and After Medical Treatment," *Clinical Physiology* 10 (1990): 545–50.

16. A. F. Attanasio, D. Mo, E. M. Erfurth, et al., "Prevalence of Metabolic Syndrome in Adult Hypopituitary Growth Hormone (GH)–Deficient Patients Before and After GH Replacement," *Journal of Clinical Endocrinology and Metabolism* 95, no. 1 (2010): 74–81.

17. Food Allergy Research and Education, "Food Allergy Facts and Statistics for the U.S.," http://www.foodallergy.org/file/facts-stats.pdf, accessed December 2, 2016.

18. B. Halliwell, "Oxygen Radicals: A Common Sense Look at Their Nature and Medical Importance," *Medical Biology* 62, no. 2 (1984): 71–77.

19. B. Dziedzic, J. Szemraj, J. Bartkowiak, and A. Walczewska, "Various Dietary Fats Differentially Change the Gene Expression of Neuropeptides Involved in Body Weight Regulation in Rats," *Journal of Neuroendocrinology* 19, no. 5 (2007): 364–73.

20. D. A. Zellner, S. Loaiza, Z. Gonzalez, et al., "Food Selection Changes Under Stress," *Physiology and Behavior* 87, no. 4 (2006): 789–93.

21. E. Van Cauter and K. L. Knutson, "Sleep and the Epidemic of Obesity in Children and Adults," *European Journal of Endocrinology* 159, no. 1 (2008): S59–66.

22. D. Kunz, R. Mahlberg, C. Muller, et al., "Melatonin in Patients with Reduced REM Sleep Duration: Two Randomized Controlled Trials," *Journal of Clinical Endocrinology and Metabolism* 89, no. 1 (2004): 128–34.

23. S. C. Chu, Y. C. Chou, J. Y. Liu, et al., "Fluctuation of Serum Leptin Level in Rats After Ovariectomy and the Influence of Estrogen Supplement," *Life Sciences* 64, no. 24 (1999): 2299–306.

24. R. Arem and D. Escalante, "Subclinical Hypothyroidism: Epidemiology, Diagnosis, and Significance," *Advances in Internal Medicine* 41 (1996): 213–50.

25. O. E. Janssen, N. Mehlmauer, S. Hahn, A. H. Offner, and R. Gartner, "High Prevalence of Autoimmune Thyroiditis in Patients with Polycystic Ovary Syndrome," *European Journal of Endocrinology* 150, no. 3 (2004): 363–69.

26. L. Starka, M. Duskova, I. Cermakova, J. Vrbikova, and M. Hill, "Premature Andro-

genic Alopecia and Insulin Resistance. Male Equivalent of Polycystic Ovary Syndrome?" *Endocrine Regulations* 39, no. 4 (2005): 127–31.

27. D. A. Ehrmann, "Polycystic Ovary Syndrome," *New England Journal of Medicine* 352, no. 12 (2005): 1223–36.

28. M. A. Birdsall and C. M. Farquhar, "Polycystic Ovaries in Pre- and Post-Menopausal Women," *Clinical Endocrinology* 44, no. 3 (1996): 269–76.

29. D. A. Ehrmann, R. B. Barnes, R. L. Rosenfield, M. K. Cavaghan, and J. Imperial, "Prevalence of Impaired Glucose Tolerance and Diabetes in Women with Polycystic Ovary Syndrome," *Diabetes Care* 22, no. 1 (1999): 141–46.

30. R. S. Legro, D. Driscoll, J. F. Strauss III, J. Fox, and A. Dunaif, "Evidence for a Genetic Basis for Hyperandrogenemia in Polycystic Ovary Syndrome," *Proceedings of the National Academy of Sciences* 95, no. 25 (1998): 14956–60.

31. K. G. Klipstein and J. F. Goldberg, "Screening for Bipolar Disorder in Women with Polycystic Ovary Syndrome: A Pilot Study," *Journal of Affective Disorders* 91, nos. 2–3 (2006): 205–9.

32. H. Kahal, S. L. Atkin, and T. Sathyapalan, "Pharmacological Treatment of Obesity in Patients with Polycystic Ovary Syndrome," *Journal of Obesity*, article ID 402052 (2011), doi:10.1155/2011/402052.

CHAPTER 11. Hormones of Desire: The Thyroid and Your Sex Life

1. R. W. Lewis, K. S. Fugl-Meyer, R. Bosch, A. R. Fugl-Meyer, E. O. Laumann, E. Lizza, and A. Martin-Morales, "Epidemiology/Risk Factors of Sexual Dysfunction," *Journal of Sexual Medicine* 1, no. 1 (2004): 35–39.

2. E. Lambreva, R. Klaghofer, and C. Buddeberg, "Psychosocial Aspects of Patients with Sexual Dysfunction," *Schweiz Rundschau für Medizin Praxis* 95, no. 7 (2006): 226–31.

3. R. N. Pauls, S. D. Kleeman, and M. M. Karram, "Female Sexual Dysfunction: Principles of Diagnosis and Therapy," *Obstetrical and Gynecological Survey* 60, no. 3 (2005): 196–205.

4. G. Corona, L. Petrone, E. Mannucci, V. Ricca, G. Balercia, R. Giommi, G. Forti, and M. Maggi, "The Impotent Couple: Low Desire," *International Journal of Andrology* 28, suppl. 2 (2005): 46–52.

5. C. Araki, "Sexuality of Aging Couples—From Women's Point of View," *Hinyokika Kiyo* 51, no. 9 (2005): 591–94.

6. P. Kadioglu, A. S. Yalin, O. Tiryakioglu, N. Gazioglu, G. Oral, O. Sanli, K. Onem, and A. Kadioglu, "Sexual Dysfunction in Women with Hyperprolactinemia: A Pilot Study Report," *Journal of Urology* 174, no. 5 (2005): 1921–25.

7. C. Longcope, "The Male and Female Reproductive Systems in Hypothyroidism," in *Werner and Ingbar's The Thyroid*, 6th ed., edited by L. D. Braverman and R. D. Utiger, 1052–55 (Philadelphia: Lippincott, 1991).

8. S. R. Davis, A. T Guay, J. L. Shifren, and N. A. Mazer, "Endocrine Aspects of Female Sexual Dysfunction," *Journal of Sexual Medicine* 1, no. 1 (2004): 82–86.

9. C. Longcope, "The Male and Female Reproductive Systems in Thyrotoxicosis," in *Werner and Ingbar's The Thyroid*, 6th ed., edited by L. D. Braverman and R. D. Utiger, 828–35 (Philadelphia: Lippincott, 1991).

10. W. F. Bergfeld, "Androgenic Alopecia: An Overview," *Seventh Symposium on Alopecia, in Dermatology: Capsule and Comment*, edited by H. P. Badin, 1–10 (New York: HP Publishing, 1988).

11. B. J. Kumar, M. L. Khurana, A. C. Ammini, et al., "Reproductive Endocrine Func-

tions in Men with Primary Hypothyroidism: Effect of Thyroxine Replacement," *Hormone Research* 34 (1990): 215–18.

12. R. W. Hudson and A. L. Edwards, "Testicular Function in Hyperthyroidism," *Journal of Andrology* 13 (1992): 117–24.

13. J. Lever and P. Schwartz, "When Sex Hurts: Finding the Causes of Your Pain During Intercourse," *Sexual Health* 1 (1997): 64–66.

14. A. J. Wright, "Lichen Sclerosus and Thyroid Disease" (letter), *Journal of Reproductive Medicine* 43 (1998): 240.

15. C. Penner and J. Penner, *The Gift of Sex: A Guide to Sexual Fulfillment* (Waco, TX: Word Publishing, 1981).

16. M. J. Taylor, L. Rudkin, and K. Hawton, "Strategies for Managing Antidepressant-Induced Sexual Dysfunction: Systematic Review of Randomised Controlled Trials," *Journal of Affective Disorders* 88, no. 3 (2005): 241–54.

17. A. H. Clayton, J. K. Warnock, S. G. Kornstein, R. Pinkerton, A. Sheldon-Keller, and E. L. McGarvey, "A Placebo-Controlled Trial of Bupropion SR as an Antidote for Selective Serotonin Reuptake Inhibitor-Induced Sexual Dysfunction," *Journal of Clinical Psychiatry* 65, no. 1 (2004): 62–67.

18. B. B. Sherwin, "Affective Changes with Estrogen and Androgen Replacement Therapy in Surgically Menopausal Women," *Journal of Affective Disorders* 14 (1988): 177–87.

19. J. Suckling, A. Lethaby, and R. Kennedy, "Local Oestrogen for Vaginal Atrophy in Postmenopausal Women," *Cochrane Database System Review* 4 (2003): CD001500.

CHAPTER 12. "You've Changed": When the Thyroid and Relationships Collide

1. J. Gray, *Men Are from Mars, Women Are from Venus* (New York: HarperCollins, 1992).

2. P. H. Rockey and R. J. Griep, "Behavioral Dysfunction in Hyperthyroidism," *Archives of Internal Medicine* 140 (1980): 1194–97.

CHAPTER 13. Overlapping Symptoms: Adrenal Fatigue, Fibromyalgia, Hypoglycemia, and Chronic Fatigue Syndrome

1. G. Lewis and S. Wessely, "The Epidemiology of Fatigue: More Questions than Answers," *Journal of Epidemiology and Community Health* 46 (1992): 92–97.

2. K. Kroenke, D. R. Wood, A. D. Mangelsdorff, et al., "Chronic Fatigue in Primary Care: Prevalence, Patient Characteristics, and Outcome," *Journal of the American Medical Association* 260 (1988): 929–34.

3. M. G. Carta, M. C. Hardoy, M. F. Boi, S. Mariotti, B. Carpiniello, and P. Usai, "Association Between Panic Disorder, Major Depressive Disorder and Celiac Disease: A Possible Role of Thyroid Autoimmunity," *Journal of Psychosomatic Research* 53, no. 3 (2002): 789–93.

4. A. M. Sawka, V. Fatourechi, B. F. Boeve, and B. Mokri, "Rarity of Encephalopathy Associated with Autoimmune Thyroiditis: A Case Series from Mayo Clinic from 1950 to 1996," *Thyroid* 12, no. 5 (2002): 393–98.

5. L. B. Krupp and D. Pollina, "Neuroimmune and Neuropsychiatric Aspects of Chronic Fatigue Syndrome," *Advances in Neuroimmunology* 6 (1996): 155–67.

6. W. K. Cho and G. H. Stollerman, "Chronic Fatigue Syndrome," *Hospital Practice* 27 (1992): 221–45.

7. J. R. Greenfield and K. Samaras, "Evaluation of Pituitary Function in the Fatigued

Patient: A Review of 59 Cases," *European Journal of Endocrinology* 154, no. 1 (2006): 147–57.

8. J. C. Smith, "Hormone Replacement Therapy in Hypopituitarism," *Expert Opinion in Pharmacotherapy* 5, no. 5 (2004): 1023–31.

9. A. De Bellis, A. Bizzarro, M. Conte, S. Perrino, C. Coronella, S. Solimeno, A. M. Sinisi, L. A. Stile, G. Pisano, and A. Bellastella, "Antipituitary Antibodies in Adults with Apparently Idiopathic Growth Hormone Deficiency and in Adults with Autoimmune Endocrine Diseases," *Journal of Clinical Endocrinology and Metabolism* 88, no. 2 (2003): 650–54.

10. M. Nishino, S. Yabe, M. Murakami, T. Kanda, and I. Kobayashi, "Detection of Antipituitary Antibodies in Patients with Autoimmune Thyroid Disease," *Endocrine Journal* 48, no. 2 (2001): 185–91.

11. A. A. Kasperlik-Zaluska, B. Czarnocka, W. Czech, J. Walecki, A. M. Makowska, J. Brzezinski, and J. Aniszewski, "Secondary Adrenal Insufficiency Associated with Autoimmune Disorders: A Report of Twenty-Five Cases," *Clinical Endocrinology* 49, no. 6 (1998): 779–83.

12. G. Aimaretti and E. Ghigo, "Traumatic Brain Injury and Hypopituitarism," *Scientific World Journal* 15, no. 5 (2005): 777–81.

13. D. H. Su, Y. C. Chang, and C. C. Chang, "Post-Traumatic Anterior and Posterior Pituitary Dysfunction," *Journal of the Formosan Medical Association* 104, no. 7 (2005): 463–67.

14. V. Popovic, "GH Deficiency as the Most Common Pituitary Defect After TBI: Clinical Implications," *Pituitary* 8, nos. 3–4 (2005): 239–43.

15. L. De Marinis, S. Bonadonna, A. Bianchi, G. Maira, and A. Giustina, "Extensive Clinical Experience: Primary Empty Sella," *Journal of Clinical Endocrinology and Metabolism* 90, no. 9 (2005): 5471–77.

16. R. C. Cuneo, F. Salomon, G. A. McGauley, et al., "The Growth Hormone Deficiency Syndrome in Adults," *Clinical Endocrinology* 37 (1992): 387–97.

17. T. Mahajan, A. Crown, S. Checkley, A. Farmer, and S. Lightman, "Atypical Depression in Growth Hormone Deficient Adults, and the Beneficial Effects of Growth Hormone Treatment on Depression and Quality of Life," *European Journal of Endocrinology* 151, no. 3 (2004): 325–32.

18. R. M. Bennett, "Adult Growth Hormone Deficiency in Patients with Fibromyalgia," *Current Rheumatology Reports* 4, no. 4 (2002): 306–12.

19. F. Wolfe, H. A. Smythe, M. B. Yunus, et al., "The American College of Rheumatology 1990 Criteria for the Classification of Fibromyalgia: Report of the Multicenter Criteria Committee," *Arthritis and Rheumatism* 33 (1990): 160–72.

20. S. Ozgocmen, H. Ozyurt, S. Sogut, and O. Akyol, "Current Concepts in the Pathophysiology of Fibromyalgia: The Potential Role of Oxidative Stress and Nitric Oxide," *Rheumatology International* 26, no. 7 (2006): 585–97.

21. S. Bagis, L. Tamer, G. Sahin, R. Bilgin, H. Guler, B. Ercan, and C. Erdogan, "Free Radicals and Antioxidants in Primary Fibromyalgia: An Oxidative Stress Disorder?" *Rheumatology International* 25, no. 3 (2005): 188–90.

22. D. Berg, L. H. Berg, J. Couvaras, and H. Harrison, "Chronic Fatigue Syndrome (CFS) and/or Fibromyalgia (FM) as a Variation of Antiphospholipid Antibody Syndrome (APS): An Explanatory Model and Approach to Laboratory Diagnosis," *Blood Coagulation and Fibrinolysis* 10 (1999): 1–4.

23. R. L. Garrison and P. C. Breeding, "A Metabolic Basis for Fibromyalgia and Its Related Disorders: The Possible Role of Resistance to Thyroid Hormone," *Medical Hypotheses* 61, no. 2 (2003): 182–89.

24. J. C. Lowe, R. L. Garrison, A. Reichman, et al., "Triiodothyronine (T3) Treatment of Euthyroid Fibromyalgia: A Small-N Replication of a Double-Blind Placebo-Controlled Crossover Study," *Clinical Bulletin of Myofascial Therapy* 2, no. 4 (1997): 71–88.

25. J. C. Lowe, "Results of an Open Trial of T3 Therapy with 77 Euthyroid Female Fibromyalgia Patients," *Clinical Bulletin of Myofascial Therapy* 2, no. 1 (1997): 35–37.

26. O. N. Pamuk and N. Cakir, "The Frequency of Thyroid Antibodies in Fibromyalgia Patients and Their Relationship with Symptoms," *Clinical Rheumatology* 26, no. 1 (2007): 55–59.

27. L. S. Ribiero and F. A. Proietti, "Interrelations Between Fibromyalgia, Thyroid Auto-antibodies, and Depression," *Journal of Rheumatology* 31, no. 10 (2004): 2036–40.

28. J. B. Shiroky, M. Cohen, M. L. Ballachey, et al., "Thyroid Dysfunction in Rheumatoid Arthritis: A Controlled Prospective Survey," *Annals of Rheumatic Diseases* 52 (1993): 454–56.

29. H. J. Lucas, C. M. Brauch, L. Settas, and T. C. Theoharides, "Fibromyalgia—New Concepts of Pathogenesis and Treatment," *International Journal of Immunopathology and Pharmacology* 19, no. 1 (2006): 5–10.

30. M. L. Shuer, "Fibromyalgia: Symptom Constellation and Potential Therapeutic Options," *Endocrine* 22, no. 1 (2003): 67–76.

31. O. N. Pamuk and N. Cakir, "The Variation in Chronic Widespread Pain and Other Symptoms in Fibromyalgia Patients. The Effects of Menses and Menopause," *Clinical and Experimental Rheumatology* 23, no. 6 (2005): 778–82.

32. G. O. Littlejohn and E. K. Guymer, "Fibromyalgia Syndrome: Which Antidepressant Drug Should We Choose," *Current Pharmaceutical Design* 12, no. 1 (2006): 3–9.

33. L. J. Crofford, M. C. Rowbotham, and P. J. Mease, et al., "Pregabalin for the Treatment of Fibromyalgia Syndrome: Results of a Randomized, Double-Blind, Placebo-Controlled Trial," *Arthritis and Rheumatology* 52, no. 4 (2005): 1264–73.

34. K. Kaartinen, K. Lammi, M. Hypen, M. Nenonen, O. Hanninen, and A. L. Rauma, "Vegan Diet Alleviates Fibromyalgia Symptoms," *Scandinavian Journal of Rheumatology* 29, no. 5 (2000): 308–13.

35. H. M. Taggart, C. L. Arslanian, S. Bae, and K. Singh, "Effects of Tai Chi Exercise on Fibromyalgia Symptoms and Health-Related Quality of Life," *Orthopedic Nursing* 22, no. 5 (2003): 353–60.

36. R. Bonadonna, "Meditation's Impact on Chronic Illness," *Holistic Nursing Practice* 17, no. 6 (2003): 309–19.

37. B. B. Singh, W. S. Wu, S. H. Hwang, R. Khorsan, C. Der-Martirosian, S. P. Vinjamury, C. N. Wang, and S. Y. Lin, "Effectiveness of Acupuncture in the Treatment of Fibromyalgia," *Alternative Therapies in Health and Medicine* 12, no. 2 (2006): 34–41.

38. R. M. Bennett, S. C. Clark, and J. Walczyk, "A Randomized, Double-Blind, Placebo-Controlled Study of Growth Hormone in the Treatment of Fibromyalgia," *American Journal of Medicine* 104 (1998): 227–31.

39. A. Schluderberg, S. E. Strauss, P. Peterson, et al., "NIH Conference on Chronic Fatigue Syndrome Research: Definition and Medical Outcome Assessment," *Annals of Internal Medicine* 117 (1992): 325–31.

40. D. W. Bates, W. Schmitt, D. Buchwald, et al., "Prevalence of Fatigue and Chronic Fatigue Syndrome in a Primary Care Practice," *Archives of Internal Medicine* 153 (1993): 2759–65.

41. A. C. Logan, A. Venket Rao, and D. Irani, "Chronic Fatigue Syndrome: Lactic Acid Bacteria May Be of Therapeutic Value," *Medical Hypotheses* 60, no. 6 (2003): 915–23.

42. M. Maes, I. Mihaylova, and M. De Ruyter, "Lower Serum Zinc in Chronic Fatigue

Syndrome (CFS): Relationships to Immune Dysfunctions and Relevance for the Ox-idative Stress Status in CFS," *Journal of Affective Disorders* 90, nos. 2–3 (2006): 141–47.

43. M. R. Werbach, "Nutritional Strategies for Treating Chronic Fatigue Syndrome," *Alternative Medicine Review* 5, no. 2 (2000): 93–108.

44. D. Racciatti, M. T. Guagnano, J. Vecchiet, P. L. De Remigis, E. Pizzigallo, R. Della Vecchia, T. Di Sciascio, D. Merlitti, and S. Sensi, "Chronic Fatigue Syndrome: Circa-dian Rhythm and Hypothalamic-Pituitary-Adrenal Axis Impairment," *International Journal of Immunopathology and Pharmacology* 14, no. 1 (2001): 11–15.

45. B. L. Farris, "Prevalence of Post-Glucose-Load Glycosuria and Hypoglycemia in a Group of Healthy Young Men," *Diabetes* 23 (1974): 189.

46. J. Yager and R. T. Young, "Nonhypoglycemia Is an Epidemic Condition," *New England Journal of Medicine* 291 (1974): 907.

47. S. E. Langer and J. F. Scheer, *Solved: The Riddle of Illness* (New Canaan, CT: Keats Publishing, 1984).

PART III. Women's Thyroid Problems: Your Symptoms Are Not All in Your Head
CHAPTER 14. Premenstrual Syndrome and Menopause: Tuning the Cycles

1. G. E. Krassas, "Thyroid Disease and Female Reproduction," *Fertility and Sterility* 74, no. 6 (2000); 1063–70.

2. R. Arem and D. Escalante, "Subclinical Hypothyroidism: Epidemiology, Diagnosis, and Significance," *Advances in Internal Medicine* 41 (1996): 213–50.

3. D. I. W. Phillips, J. H. Lazarus, and B. R. Butlano, "The Influence of Pregnancy and Reproductive Span on the Occurrence of Autoimmune Thyroiditis," *Clinical Endo-crinology* 32 (1990): 301–6.

4. American Psychiatric Association, *Diagnostic and Statistical Manual of Mental Disor-ders*, 5th ed. (Washington, DC: American Psychiatric Association, 2013).

5. X. Gonda and G. Bagdy, "Neurochemical Background of the Premenstrual Syn-drome: The Role of the Serotoninergic System," *Neuropsychopharmacologia Hungar-ica* 6, no. 3 (2004): 153–62.

6. T. Backstrom, L. Andreen, V. Birzniece, et al., "The Role of Hormones and Hor-monal Treatments in Premenstrual Syndrome," *CNS Drugs* 17, no. 5 (2003): 325–42.

7. N. Anim-Nyame, C. Domoney, N. Panay, J. Jones, J. Alaghband-Zadeh, and J. W. Studd, "Plasma Leptin Concentrations Are Increased in Women with Premenstrual Syndrome," *Human Reproduction* 15, no. 11 (2000): 2329–32.

8. S. W. Masho, T. Adera, and J. South-Paul, "Obesity as a Risk Factor for Premen-strual Syndrome," *Journal of Psychosomatic Obstetrics and Gynaecology* 26, no. 1 (2005): 33–39.

9. B. L. Perry, D. Miles, K. Burruss, and D. S. Svikis, "Premenstrual Symptomatology and Alcohol Consumption in College Women," *Journal of Studies on Alcohol* 65, no. 4 (2004): 464–68.

10. M. W. Ward and T. D. Holimon, "Calcium Treatment for Premenstrual Syndrome," *Annals of Pharmacotherapy* 33, no. 12 (1999): 1356–58.

11. U. Halbreich, J. Borenstein, T. Pearlstein, and L. S. Kahn, "The Prevalence, Impair-ment, Impact, and Burden of Premenstrual Dysphoric Disorder (PMS/PMDD)," *Psychoneuroendocrinology* 28, suppl. 3 (2003): 1–23.

12. I. Hassan, K. M. Ismail, and S. O'Brien, "PMS in the Perimenopause," *Journal of the British Menopause Society* 10, no. 4 (2004): 151–56.

13. M. Richards, D. R. Rubinow, R. C. Daly, and P. J. Schmidt, "Premenstrual Symptoms and Perimenopausal Depression," *American Journal of Psychiatry* 163, no. 1 (2006): 133–37.

14. M. C. Hsiao, C. C. Hsiao, and C. Y. Liu, "Premenstrual Symptoms and Premenstrual Exacerbation in Patients with Psychiatric Disorders," *Psychiatry and Clinical Neurosciences* 58, no. 2 (2004): 186–90.

15. P. J. Schmidt, G. N. Grover, P. P. Roy-Byrne, et al., "Thyroid Function in Women with Premenstrual Syndrome," *Journal of Clinical Endocrinology and Metabolism* 76 (1993): 671–74.

16. N. D. Brayshaw and D. D. Brayshaw, "Thyroid Hypofunction in Premenstrual Syndrome," *New England Journal of Medicine* 315 (1986): 1486–87.

17. A. Rapkin, "A Review of Treatment of Premenstrual Syndrome and Premenstrual Dysphoric Disorder," *Psychoneuroendocrinology* 28, suppl. 3 (2003): 39–53.

18. E. W. Freeman, "Luteal Phase Administration of Agents for the Treatment of Premenstrual Dysphoric Disorder," *CNS Drugs* 18, no. 7 (2004): 453–68.

19. M. Steiner, T. Pearlstein, L. S. Cohen, J. Endicott, S. G. Kornstein, C. Roberts, D. L. Roberts, and K. Yonkers, "Expert Guidelines for the Treatment of Severe PMS, PMDD, and Comorbidities: The Role of SSRIs," *Journal of Women's Health* 15, no. 1 (2006): 57–69.

20. M. Bryant, A. Cassidy, C. Hill, J. Powell, D. Talbot, and L. Dye, "Effect of Consumption of Soy Isoflavones on Behavioural, Somatic and Affective Symptoms in Women with Premenstrual Syndrome," *British Journal of Nutrition* 93, no. 5 (2005): 731–39.

21. E. R. Bertone-Johnson, S. E. Hankinson, A. Bendich, S. R. Johnson, W. C. Willett, and J. E. Manson, "Calcium and Vitamin D Intake and Risk of Incident Premenstrual Syndrome," *Archives of Internal Medicine* 165, no. 11 (2005): 1246–52.

22. R. J. Shamberger, "Calcium, Magnesium, and Other Elements in the Red Blood Cells and Hair of Normals and Patients with Premenstrual Syndrome," *Biological Trace Element Research* 94, no. 2 (2003): 123–29.

23. A. M. Levin, "Pre-menstrual Syndrome: A New Concept in Its Pathogenesis and Treatment," *Medical Hypotheses* 62, no. 1 (2004): 130–32.

24. G. Altman, K. C. Cain, S. Motzer, M. Jarrett, R. Burr, and M. Heitkemper, "Increased Symptoms in Female IBS Patients with Dysmenorrhea and PMS," *Gastroenterology Nursing* 29, no. 1 (2006): 4–11.

25. M. C. De Souza, A. F. Walker, P. A. Robinson, and K. Bolland, "A Synergistic Effect of a Daily Supplement for 1 Month of 200 mg Magnesium Plus 50 mg Vitamin B_6 for the Relief of Anxiety-Related Premenstrual Symptoms: A Randomized, Double-Blind, Crossover Study," *Journal of Women's Health and Gender-Based Medicine* 9, no. 2 (2000): 131–39.

26. M. J. Walsh and B. I. Polus, "A Randomized, Placebo-Controlled Clinical Trial on the Efficacy of Chiropractic Therapy on Premenstrual Syndrome," *Journal of Manipulative Physiological Therapeutics* 22, no. 9 (1999): 582–85.

27. D. Habek, J. C. Habek, and A. Barbir, "Using Acupuncture to Treat Premenstrual Syndrome," *Archives of Gynecology and Obstetrics* 267, no. 1 (2002): 23–26.

28. A. E. Schindler, "Thyroid Function and Postmenopause," *Gynecological Endocrinology* 17, no. 1 (2003): 79–85.

29. P. A. Kaufert, P. Gilbert, and R. Tate, "The Manitoba Project: A Reexamination of the Link Between Menopause and Depression," *Maturitas* 14, no. 2 (1992): 143–56.

30. N. E. Avis, P. A. Kaufert, M. Lock, et al., "The Evolution of Menopausal Symptoms," *Balliere's Clinical Endocrinology and Metabolism* 7 (1993): 17–32.

31. D. J. Cooke and J. G. Green, "Types of Life Events in Relation to Symptoms at the Climacterium," *Journal of Psychosomatic Research* 25 (1981): 5–11.
32. A. Holte and A. Mikkelson, "Psychosocial Determinants of Menopausal Complaints," *Maturitas* 13 (1991): 193–203.
33. C. Northrup, *Women's Bodies, Women's Wisdom: Creating Physical and Emotional Health and Healing* (New York: Bantam Books, 2010).
34. J. E. Rossouw, G. L. Anderson, R. L. Prentice, et al., "Risks and Benefits of Estrogen Plus Progestin in Healthy Postmenopausal Women: Principal Results from the Women's Health Initiative Randomized Controlled Trial," *Journal of the American Medical Association* 288, no. 3 (2002): 321–33.
35. R. A. Medina, E. Aranda, C. Verdugo, S. Kato, and G. I. Owen, "The Action of Ovarian Hormones in Cardiovascular Disease," *Biological Research* 36, nos. 3–4 (2003): 325–41.
36. E. L. Klaiber, W. Vogel, and S. Rako, "A Critique of the Women's Health Initiative Hormone Therapy Study," *Fertility and Sterility* 84, no. 6 (2005): 1589–601.
37. R. A. Medina, E. Aranda, C. Verdugo, S. Kato, and G. I. Owen, "The Action of Ovarian Hormones in Cardiovascular Disease," *Biological Research* 36, nos. 3–4 (2003): 325–41.
38. J. A. Raza, R. A. Reinhart, and A. Movahed, "Ischemic Heart Disease in Women and the Role of Hormone Therapy," *International Journal of Cardiology* 96, no. 1 (2004): 7–19.
39. A. H. MacLennan, A. W. Taylor, and D. H. Wilson, "Hormone Therapy Use After the Women's Health Initiative," *Climacteric* 7, no. 2 (2004): 138–42.
40. R. A. Lobo, "Appropriate Use of Hormones Should Alleviate Concerns of Cardiovascular and Breast Cancer Risk," *Maturitas* 51, no. 1 (2005): 98–109.
41. P. This, "Hormonal Replacement Therapy and Breast Cancer," *Revue du Practicien* 55, no. 4 (2005): 377–82.
42. J. L. Kuijpens, I. Nyklictek, M. W. Louwman, T. A. Weetman, V. J. Pop, and J. W. CoeBergh, "Hypothyroidism Might Be Related to Breast Cancer in Post-Menopausal Women," *Thyroid* 15, no. 11 (2005): 1253–59.
43. M. Holzbauer and M. B. Youdim, "The Oestrous Cycle and Monoamine Oxidase Activity," *British Journal of Pharmacology* 48 (1973): 600–8.
44. A. Cagnacci, S. Arangino, F. Baldassari, C. Alessandrini, S. Landi, and A. Volpe, "A Combination of the Central Effects of Different Progestins Used in Hormone Replacement Therapy," *Maturitas* 48, no. 4 (2004): 456–62.
45. P. G. Sator, J. B. Schmidt, T. Rabe, and C. C. Zouboulis, "Skin Aging and Sex Hormones in Women—Clinical Perspectives for Intervention by Hormone Replacement Therapy," *Experimental Dermatology* 13, suppl. 4 (2004): 36–40.
46. U. Gaspard and F. Van den Brule, "Medication of the Month. Angeliq: New Hormonal Therapy of Menopause, with Antialdosterone and Antiandrogenic Properties," *Revue Médicale de Liège* 59, no. 3 (2004): 162–66.
47. A. S. Dobs, T. Nguyen, C. Pace, and C. P. Roberts, "Differential Effects of Oral Estrogen Versus Oral Estrogen-Androgen Replacement Therapy on Body Composition in Postmenopausal Women," *Journal of Clinical Endocrinology and Metabolism* 87, no. 4 (2002): 1509–16.
48. A. D. Genazzani, M. Stomati, F. Bernardi, M. Pieri, L. Rovati, and A. R. Genazzani, "Long-Term Low-Dose Dehydroepiandrosterone Oral Supplementation in Early and Late Postmenopausal Women Modulates Endocrine Parameters and Synthesis of Neuroactive Steroids," *Fertility and Sterility* 80, no. 6 (2003): 1495–501.

49. H. D. Nelson, K. K. Vesco, E. Haney, R. Fu, A. Nedrow, J. Miller, C. Nicolaidis, M. Walker, and L. Humphrey, "Nonhormonal Therapies for Menopausal Hot Flashes: Systematic Review and Meta-Analysis," *Journal of the American Medical Association* 295, no. 17 (2006): 2057–71.

50. E. Petri Nahas, J. Nahas Neto, L. De Luca, P. Traiman, A. Pontes, and I. Dalben, "Benefits of Soy Germ Isoflavones in Postmenopausal Women with Contraindication for Conventional Hormone Replacement Therapy," *Maturitas* 48, no. 4 (2004): 372–80.

51. T. Low Dog, "Menopause: A Review of Botanical Dietary Supplements," *American Journal of Medicine* 118, suppl. 2 (2005): 98–108.

52. K. Winther, E. Rein, and C. Hedman, "Femal, a Herbal Remedy Made from Pollen Extracts, Reduces Hot Flushes and Improves Quality of Life in Menopausal Women: A Randomized, Placebo-Controlled, Parallel Study," *Climacteric* 8, no. 2 (2005): 162–70.

53. J. J. Curcio, L. S. Kim, D. Wollner, and B. A. Pockaj, "The Potential of 5-Hydroxytryptophan for Hot Flash Reduction: A Hypothesis," *Alternative Medicine Review* 10, no. 3 (2005): 216–21.

CHAPTER 15. Thyroid Balance for Healthy Pregnancy

1. L. P. Salzer, *Surviving Infertility* (New York: Harper Perennial, 1991).

2. E. Erikson, *Childhood and Society* (New York: Norton, 1950).

3. I. Gerhard, T. Becker, W. Eggert-Kruse, et al., "Thyroid and Ovarian Function in Infertile Women," *Human Reproduction* 6 (1991): 338–45.

4. K. Poppe, D. Glinoer, A. Van Steirteghem, H. Tournaye, P. Devroey, J. Schiettecatte, and B. Velkeniers, "Thyroid Dysfunction and Autoimmunity in Infertile Women," *Thyroid* 12, no. 11 (2002): 997–1001.

5. I. Gerhard, W. Eggert-Kruse, K. Merzoug, et al., "Thyrotropin-Releasing Hormone (TRH) and Metoclopramide Testing in Infertile Women," *Gynecological Endocrinology* 5, no. 1 (1991): 15–32.

6. T. Maruo, K. Katayama, H. Matuso, et al., "Maintaining Early Pregnancy in Threatened Abortion," *Acta Endocrinologica* 127 (1992): 118–22.

7. A. Singh, Z. N. Dantas, S. C. Stone, et al., "Presence of Thyroid Antibodies in Early Reproductive Failure: Biochemical Versus Clinical Pregnancies," *Fertility and Sterility* 63, no. 2 (1995): 277–81.

8. J. E. Haddow, G. E. Palomaki, W. C. Allan, J. R. Williams, G. J. Knight, J. Gagnon, et al., "Maternal Thyroid Deficiency During Pregnancy and Subsequent Neuropsychological Development of the Child," *New England Journal of Medicine* 341 (1999): 549–55.

9. J. F. Rovet, "Neurodevelopmental Consequences of Maternal Hypothyroidism During Pregnancy," *Thyroid* 14 (2004): 710.

10. D. Glinoer, "The Regulation of Thyroid Function in Pregnancy: Pathways of Endocrine Adaptation from Physiology to Pathology," *Endocrine Reviews* 18, no. 3 (1997): 404–33.

11. A. S. Leung, L. K. Millar, P. P. Koonings, et al., "Perinatal Outcome in Hypothyroid Pregnancies," *Obstetrics and Gynecology* 81, no. 3 (1993): 349–53.

12. M. B. Zimmermann, H. Burgi, and R. F. Hurrell, "Iron Deficiency Predicts Poor Maternal Thyroid Status During Pregnancy," *Journal of Clinical Endocrinology and Metabolism* 92 (2007): 3436–40.

13. F. Vermiglio, V. P. Lo Presti, M. Moleti, M. Sidoti, G. Tortorella, G. Scaffidi, et al., "Attention Deficit and Hyperactivity Disorders in the Offspring of Mothers Exposed to Mild-Moderate Iodine Deficiency: A Possible Novel Iodine Deficiency Disorder in Developed Countries," *Journal of Clinical Endocrinology and Metabolism* 89 (2004): 6054–60.

CHAPTER 16. Postpartum Depression: The Hormonal Link

1. Columbia University College of Physicians and Surgeons, *Complete Home Guide to Mental Health*, edited by F. I. Kass, et al. (New York: Henry Holt, 1995).
2. G. P. Redmond, "Thyroid Dysfunction and Women's Reproductive Health," *Thyroid* 14, suppl. 1 (2004): S5–15.
3. J.-E.-D. Esquirol, *Des maladies mentales considerées sous les rapports médical, hygiénique et médico-légal*, vol. 1 (Paris: J. B. Baillière, 1838).
4. I. F. Brockington and R. Kumar, eds., *Motherhood and Mental Illness* (London: Academic Press, 1982).
5. T. H. Chen, T. H. Lan, C. Y. Yang, and K. D. Juang, "Postpartum Mood Disorders May Be Related to a Decreased Insulin Level After Delivery," *Medical Hypotheses* 66, no. 4 (2006): 820–23.
6. N. I. Gavin, B. N. Gaynes, K. N. Lohr, S. Meltzer-Brody, G. Gartlehner, and T. Swinson, "Perinatal Depression: A Systematic Review of Prevalence and Incidence," *Obstetrics and Gynecology* 106 (2005): 1071–83.
7. D. F. Hay, S. Pawlby, A. Angold, G. T. Harold, and D. Sharp, "Pathways to Violence in the Children of Mothers Who Were Depressed Postpartum," *Developmental Psychology* 39, no. 6 (2003): 1083–94.
8. A. Rahman, Z. Iqbal, J. Bunn, H. Lovel, and R. Harrington, "Impact of Maternal Depression on Infant Nutritional Status and Illness: A Cohort Study," *Archives of General Psychiatry* 61, no. 9 (2004): 946–52.
9. J. A. Hamilton and P. N. Harberger, eds., *Postpartum Psychiatric Illness: A Picture Puzzle* (Philadelphia: University of Pennsylvania Press, 1992).
10. M. Bloch, N. Rotenberg, D. Koren, and E. Klein, "Risk Factors for Early Postpartum Depressive Symptoms," *General Hospital Psychiatry* 28, no. 1 (2006): 3–8.
11. J. W. Rich-Edwards, K. Kleinman, A. Abrams, et al., "Sociodemographic Predictors of Antenatal and Postpartum Depressive Symptoms Among Women in a Medical Group Practice," *Journal of Epidemiology and Community Health* 60, no. 3 (2006): 221–27.
12. E. J. Corwin, J. Brownstead, N. Barton, S. Heckard, and K. Morin, "The Impact of Fatigue on the Development of Postpartum Depression," *Journal of Obstetrics, Gynecology, and Neonatal Nursing* 34, no. 5 (2005): 577–86.
13. J. Heron, N. Craddock, and I. Jones, "Postnatal Euphoria: Are 'the Highs' an Indicator of Bipolarity?" *Bipolar Disorder* 7, no. 2 (2005): 103–10.
14. A. Wenzel, E. N. Haugen, L. C. Jackson, and K. Robinson, "Prevalence of Generalized Anxiety at Eight Weeks Postpartum," *Archives of Women's Mental Health* 6, no. 1 (2003): 43–49.
15. W. M. Ord, "Report of a Committee of the Clinical Society of London, Nominated December 14, 1883, to Investigate the Subject of Myxoedema," *Transactions of the Clinical Society of London* (suppl.) 21, no. 18 (1888).
16. B. Harris, S. Othman, J. A. Davies, et al., "Association Between Postpartum Thyroid Dysfunction and Thyroid Antibodies and Depression," *British Medical Journal* 305, no. 6846 (1992): 152–56.

17. F. Monaco, "Classification of Thyroid Diseases: Suggestions for a Revision," *Journal of Clinical Endocrinology and Metabolism* 88, no. 4 (2003): 1428–32.

18. J. H. Lazarus, "Thyroid Dysfunction: Reproduction and Postpartum Thyroiditis," *Seminars in Reproductive Medicine* 20, no. 4 (2002): 381–88.

19. T. F. Nikolai, S. L. Turney, and R. C. Roberts, "Postpartum Lymphocytic Thyroiditis: Prevalence, Clinical Course, and Long-Term Follow-Up," *Archives of Internal Medicine* 147 (1987): 221–24.

20. D. Benhaim Rochester and T. F. Davies, "Increased Risk of Graves' Disease After Pregnancy," *Thyroid* 15, no. 11 (2005): 1287–90.

21. Y. Hidaka, T. Hada, and N. Amino, "Postpartum Autoimmune Thyroid Syndrome," *Nippon Rinsho* 57, no. 8 (1999): 1775–78.

22. J. L. Kuijpens, H. L. Vader, H. A. Drexhage, W. M. Wiersinga, M. J. van Son, and V. J. Pop, "Thyroid Peroxidase Antibodies During Gestation Are a Marker for Subsequent Depression Postpartum," *European Journal of Endocrinology* 145, no. 5 (2001): 579–84.

23. H. Guan, C. Li, Y. Li, C. Fan, Y. Teng, Z. Shan, and W. Teng, "High Iodine Intake Is a Risk Factor of Post-Partum Thyroiditis: Result of a Survey from Shenyang, China," *Journal of Endocrinological Investigation* 28, no. 10 (2005): 876–81.

24. S. Othman, D. I. W. Phillips, A. B. Parkes, et al., "A Long-Term Follow-up of Postpartum Thyroiditis," *Clinical Endocrinology* 32 (1990): 559–64.

25. C. C. Hayslip, H. G. Fein, V. M. O'Donnell, et al., "The Value of Serum Antimicrosomal Antibody Testing in Screening for Symptomatic Postpartum Thyroid Dysfunction," *American Journal of Obstetrics and Gynecology* 159 (1988): 203–9.

26. D. E. Stewart, A. M. Addison, G. E. Robinson, et al., "Thyroid Function in Psychosis Following Childbirth," *American Journal of Psychiatry* 145, no. 12 (1988): 1579–81.

27. S. Misri and X. Kostaras, "Benefits and Risks to Mother and Infant of Drug Treatment for Postnatal Depression," *Drug Safety* 25, no. 13 (2002): 903–11.

28. M. P. Freeman, J. R. Hibbeln, K. L. Wisner, B. H. Brumbach, M. Watchman, and A. J. Gelenberg, "Randomized Dose-Ranging Pilot Trial of Omega-3 Fatty Acids for Postpartum Depression," *Acta Psychiatrica Scandinavica* 113, no. 1 (2006): 31–35.

29. T. H. Chen, T. H. Lan, C. Y. Yang, and K. D. Juang, "Postpartum Mood Disorders May Be Related to a Decreased Insulin Level After Delivery," *Medical Hypotheses* 66, no. 4 (2006): 820–23.

PART IV. Overcoming Thyroid Disease: The Journey to Wellness
CHAPTER 17. Treating the Imbalance

1. U. M. Kabadi and M. M. Kabadi, "Serum Thyrotropin in Primary Hypothyroidism: A Reliable and Accurate Predictor of Optimal Daily Levothyroxine Dose," *Endocrine Practitioner* 7, no. 1 (2001): 16–18.

2. M. I. Surks, "Treatment of Hypothyroidism," in *Werner and Ingbar's The Thyroid*, 6th ed., edited by Lewis E. Braverman and R. D. Utiger, 1099–103 (Philadelphia: Lippincott, 1991).

3. E. Roti, R. Minelli, and E. Gardini, "The Use and Misuse of Thyroid Hormone," *Endocrine Reviews* 14, no. 4 (1993): 401–23.

4. *Approved Drug Products with Therapeutic Equivalence Evaluations*, 24th edition, Cumulative Supplement 6, Prepared by Office of Pharmaceutical Science, Office of Generic Drugs, Center for Drug Evaluation and Research, FDA, June 2004.

5. V. Blakesley, W. Awni, C. Locke, T. Ludden, G. R. Granneman, and L. E. Braverman,

"Are Bioequivalence Studies of Levothyroxine Sodium Formulations in Euthyroid Volunteers Reliable?" *Thyroid* 14 (2004): 191–200.

6. P. C. Whybrow, "Behavioral and Psychiatric Aspects of Hypothyroidism," in *Werner and Ingbar's The Thyroid*, 6th ed., edited by Lewis E. Braverman and R. D. Utiger, 1078–83 (Philadelphia: Lippincott, 1991).

7. D. S. Ross, G. H. Daniels, and D. Gouvela, "The Use and Limitations of a Chemiluminescent Thyrotropin Assay as a Single Thyroid Function Test in an Outpatient Endocrine Clinic," *Journal of Clinical Endocrinology and Metabolism* 71, no. 3 (1990): 764–69.

8. B. Biondi, S. Fazio, A. Cuocolo, et al., "Impaired Cardiac Reserve and Exercise Capacity in Patients Receiving Long-Term Thyrotropin Suppressive Therapy with Levothyroxine," *Journal of Clinical Endocrinology and Metabolism* 81 (1996): 4224–28.

9. B. Uzzan, J. Campos, M. Cucherat, et al., "Effects on Bone Mass of Long-Term Treatment with Thyroid Hormones: A Meta-Analysis," *Journal of Clinical Endocrinology and Metabolism* 81 (1996): 4278–89.

10. B. Scholte, B. Nowotny, L. Schaaf, et al., "Subclinical Hyperthyroidism: Physical and Mental State of Patients," *European Archives of Psychiatry and Clinical Neuroscience* 241 (1992): 357–64.

11. M. T. McDermott, B. R. Haugen, D. C. Lezotte, S. Seggelke, and E. C. Ridgway, "Management Practices Among Primary Care Physicians and Thyroid Specialists in the Care of Hypothyroid Patients," *Thyroid* 11, no. 8 (2001): 757–64.

12. B. M. Arafah, "Increased Need for Thyroxine in Women with Hypothyroidism During Estrogen Therapy," *New England Journal of Medicine* 344, no. 23 (2001): 1743–49.

13. G. B. Anker, P. E. Lønning, A. Aakvaag, et al., "Thyroid Function in Postmenopausal Breast Cancer Patients Treated with Tamoxifen," *Scandinavian Journal of Clinical Laboratory Investigation* 58 (1998): 103–7.

14. E. Lesho and R. E. Jones, "Hypothyroid Graves' Disease," *Southern Medical Journal* 90, no. 12 (1997): 1201–3.

15. N. Takasu, T. Yamada, A. Sato, et al., "Graves' Disease Following Hypothyroidism Due to Hashimoto's Disease: Studies of Eight Cases," *Clinical Endocrinology* 33 (1990): 687–89.

16. R. Comtois, L. Faucher, and L. Lafleche, "Outcome of Hypothyroidism Caused by Hashimoto's Thyroiditis," *Archives of Internal Medicine* 155 (1995): 1404–8.

17. A. H. Saliby, C. Larosa, R. Rachid, et al., "Changes in Levothyroxine Dose Requirements in the Follow-up of Patients with Primary Hypothyroidism," abstract presented at the Sixty-ninth Annual Meeting of the American Thyroid Association, November 13, 1996.

18. H. T. Stelfox, S. B. Ahmed, J. Fiskio, and D. W. Bates, "An Evaluation of the Adequacy of Outpatient Monitoring of Thyroid Replacement Therapy," *Journal of Evaluation in Clinical Practice* 10, no. 4 (2004): 525–30.

19. G. S. Kurland, M. W. Hamolsky, and A. S. Freedberg, "Studies in Non-Myxedematous Hypometabolism," *Journal of Clinical Endocrinology* 15 (1955): 1354–66.

20. B. O. Barnes and L. Galton, *Hypothyroidism: The Unsuspected Illness* (New York: Harper and Row, 1976).

21. B. Barnes, "Basal Temperature Versus Basal Metabolism," *Journal of the American Medical Association* 119 (1942): 1072–74.

22. E. D. Wilson, *Wilson's Syndrome: The Miracle of Feeling Well* (Orlando, FL: Cornerstone Publishing, 1991).

23. R. Arem, "When to Choose Radioactive Iodine, Drugs, or Surgery," *Consultant* 28, no. 9 (1989): 21–35.

24. A. P. Johnstone, J. C. Cridland, C. R. Da Costa, S. S. Nussey, and P. S. Shepherd, "A Functional Site on the Human TSH Receptor: A Potential Therapeutic Target in Graves' Disease," *Clinical Endocrinology* 59, no. 4 (2003): 437–41.

25. J. A. Franklyn, "The Management of Hyperthyroidism," *New England Journal of Medicine* 330, no. 24 (1994): 1731–38.

26. T. Misaki, Y. Iida, K. Kasagi, and J. Konishi, "Seasonal Variation in Relapse Rate of Graves' Disease After Thionamide Drug Treatment," *Endocrine Journal* 50, no. 6 (2003): 669–72.

27. J. Tajiri and S. Noguchi, "Antithyroid Drug-Induced Agranulocytosis: How Has Granulocyte Colony-Stimulating Factor Changed Therapy?" *Thyroid* 15, no. 3 (2005): 292–97.

28. T. Kashiwai, Y. Hidaka, T. Takano, et al., "Practical Treatment with Minimum Maintenance Dose of Anti-Thyroid Drugs for Prediction of Remission in Graves' Disease," *Endocrine Journal* 50, no. 1 (2003): 45–49.

29. J. M. H. Deklerk, J. W. Van Isselt, A. Van Dijk, et al., "Iodine-131 Therapy in Sporadic Nontoxic Goiter," *Journal of Nuclear Medicine* 38, no. 3 (1997): 372–76.

30. S. J. Bonnema, F. N. Bennedbaek, A. Veje, J. Marving, and L. Hegedus, "Propylthiouracil Before (131)I Therapy of Hyperthyroid Diseases: Effect on Cure Rate Evaluated by a Randomized Clinical Trial," *Journal of Clinical Endocrinology and Metabolism* 89, no. 9 (2004): 4439–44.

31. V. A. Andrade, J. L. Gross, and A. L. Maia, "The Effect of Methimazole Pretreatment on the Efficacy of Radioactive Iodine Therapy in Graves' Hyperthyroidism: One-Year Follow-up of a Prospective, Randomized Study," *Journal of Clinical Endocrinology and Metabolism* 86, no. 8 (2001): 3488–93.

32. A. M. Ahmad, M. Ahmad, and E. T. Young, "Objective Estimates of the Probability of Developing Hypothyroidism Following Radioactive Iodine Treatment of Thyrotoxicosis," *European Journal of Endocrinology* 146, no. 6 (2002): 767–75.

33. E. K. Alexander and P. R. Larsen, "High Dose of (131)I Therapy for the Treatment of Hyperthyroidism Caused by Graves' Disease," *Journal of Clinical Endocrinology and Metabolism* 87, no. 3 (2002): 1073–77.

34. L. E. Holm, P. Hall, K. Wicklund, et al., "Cancer Risk After Iodine-131 Therapy for Hyperthyroidism," *Journal of the National Cancer Institute* 83 (1991): 1072–77.

35. H. Jonsson and S. Mattsson, "Excess Radiation Absorbed Doses from Non-Optimized Radioiodine Treatment of Hyperthyroidism," *Radiation Protection Dosimetry* 108, no. 2 (2004): 107–14.

36. S. T. Tietgens and M. C. Leinung, "Thyroid Storm," *Medical Clinics of North America* 79, no. 1 (1995): 169–84.

37. C. C. Wang, J. Chen, Y. Z. Hu, D. B. Wu, and Y. H. Xu, "Endoscopic Thyroidectomy with 150 Cases" [Chinese], *Zhonghua Wai Ke Za Zhi* 42, no. 11 (2004): 675–77.

38. H. Xiao, W. Zhuang, S. Wang, B. Yu, G. Chen, M. Zhou, and N. C. Wong, "Arterial Embolization: A Novel Approach to Thyroid Ablative Therapy for Graves' Disease," *Journal of Clinical Endocrinology and Metabolism* 87, no. 8 (2002): 3583–89.

39. W. B. Kim, S. M. Han, T. Y. Kim, et al., "Ultrasonographic Screening for Detection of Thyroid Cancer in Patients with Graves' Disease," *Clinical Endocrinology* 60, no. 6 (2004): 719–25.

40. G. Pellegriti, A. Belfiore, D. Giuffrida, L. Lupo, and R. Vigneri, "Outcome of Differentiated Thyroid Cancer in Graves' Patients," *Journal of Clinical Endocrinology and Metabolism* 83, no. 8 (1998): 2805–9.

41. M. A. Emanuele, M. H. Brooks, D. L. Gordon, et al., "Agoraphobia and Hyperthyroidism," *American Journal of Medicine* 86 (1989): 484–86.

42. J. H. Lazarus, "Antithyroid Drug Treatment," *Clinical Endocrinology* 45 (1996): 517–18.

43. A. Toft, "Transient Hypothyroidism," *Clinical Endocrinology* 46 (1997): 7–8.

44. T. Maruo, K. Katayama, H. Matsuo, et al., "Maintaining Early Pregnancy in Threatened Abortion," *Acta Endocrinologica* 127 (1992): 118–22.

45. E. Roti, S. Minelli, and M. Salvi, "Management of Hyperthyroidism and Hypothyroidism in Pregnant Women," *Journal of Clinical Endocrinology and Metabolism* 81, no. 5 (1996): 1679–82.

46. Y. Nakagawa, K. Mori, S. Hoshikawa, M. Yamamoto, S. Ito, and K. Yoshida, "Postpartum Recurrence of Graves' Hyperthyroidism Can Be Prevented by the Continuation of Antithyroid Drugs During Pregnancy," *Clinical Endocrinology* 57, no. 4 (2002): 467–71.

CHAPTER 18. Curing the Lingering Effects of Thyroid Imbalance

1. H. Leigh, "Cerebral Effects of Endocrine Disease," in *Principles and Practice of Endocrinology and Metabolism*, 2d ed., edited by K. L. Becker et al. (Philadelphia: Lippincott, 1995), 1695.

2. P. C. Whybrow, "Behavioral and Psychiatric Aspects of Hypothyroidism," in *Werner and Ingbar's The Thyroid*, 6th ed., edited by Lewis E. Braverman and R. D. Utiger, 1078–83 (Philadelphia: Lippincott, 1991).

3. R. A. Stern, B. Robinson, A. R. Thorner, et al., "A Survey Study of Neuropsychiatric Complaints in Patients with Graves' Disease," *Journal of Neuropsychiatry and Clinical Neurosciences* 8 (1996): 181–85.

4. M. Abraham-Nordling, O. Torring, B. Hamberger, G. Lundell, L. Tallstedt, J. Calissendorff, and G. Wallin, "Graves' Disease: A Long-Term Quality-of-Life Follow-up of Patients Randomized to Treatment with Antithyroid Drugs, Radioiodine, or Surgery," *Thyroid* 15, no. 11 (2005): 1279–86.

5. C. Scheffer, C. Heckmann, T. Mijic, and K. H. Rudorff, "Chronic Distress Syndrome in Patients with Graves' Disease" [German], *Medizinische Klinik* 99, no. 10 (2004): 578–84.

6. P. Thygesen, K. Hermann, and R. Willanger, "Concentration Camp in Denmark: Persecution, Disease, Disability, Compensation. A 23-Year Follow-up. A Survey of the Long-Term Effect of Severe Environmental Stress," *Danish Medical Bulletin* 17 (1970): 65–108.

7. J. Kabat-Zinn, *Full Catastrophe Living: Using the Wisdom of Your Body and Mind to Face Stress, Pain, and Illness* (New York: Bantam, 2013).

8. J. A. Astin, S. L. Shapiro, D. M. Eisenberg, and K. L. Forys, "Mind-Body Medicine: State of the Science, Implications for Practice," *Journal of the American Board of Family Practice* 16 (2003): 131–47.

9. J. A. Dusek, B. H. Chang, J. Zaki, et al., "Association Between Oxygen Consumption and Nitric Oxide Production During the Relaxation Response," *Medical Science Monitor* 12, no. 1 (2006): CR1–10.

10. D. R. Brown, Y. Wang, A. Ward, et al., "Chronic Psychological Effects of Exercise and Exercise Plus Cognitive Strategies," *Medicine and Science in Sports and Exercise* 27, no. 5 (1995): 765–75.

11. R. E. Taylor-Piliae, W. L. Haskell, C. M. Waters, and E. S. Froelicher, "Change in

Perceived Psychosocial Status Following a 12-Week Tai Chi Exercise Programme," *Journal of Advanced Nursing* 54, no. 3 (2006): 313–29.

12. R. Bonadonna, "Meditation's Impact on Chronic Illness," *Holistic Nursing Practice* 17, no. 6 (2003): 309–19.

13. J. A. Astin, B. M. Berman, B. Bausell, W. L. Lee, M. Hochberg, and K. L. Forys, "The Efficacy of Mindfulness Meditation Plus Qigong Movement Therapy in the Treatment of Fibromyalgia: A Randomized Controlled Trial," *Journal of Rheumatology* 30, no. 10 (2003): 2557–62.

14. S. A. Green, "Office Psychotherapy for Depression in the Primary Care Setting," *American Journal of Medicine* 101, no. 6A, suppl. (1996): 37–44.

15. I. Elkin, M. Shea, J. Warkins, et al., "National Institute of Mental Health Treatment of Depression: Collaborative Research Program: General Effectiveness of Treatments," *Archives of General Psychiatry* 46 (1989): 971–83.

16. S. H. Kennedy, H. F. Andersen, and R. W. Lam, "Efficacy of Escitalopram in the Treatment of Major Depressive Disorder Compared with Conventional Selective Serotonin Reuptake Inhibitors and Venlafaxine XR: A Meta-Analysis," *Journal of Psychiatry and Neuroscience* 31, no. 2 (2006): 122–31.

17. S. Kasper, C. Spadone, P. Verpillat, and J. Angst, "Onset of Action of Escitalopram Compared with Other Antidepressants: Results of a Pooled Analysis," *International Clinical Psychopharmacology* 21, no. 2 (2006): 105–10.

18. A. K. Ashton, A. Mahmood, and F. Iqbal, "Improvements in SSRI/SNRI-Induced Sexual Dysfunction by Switching to Escitalopram," *Journal of Sex and Marital Therapy* 31, no. 3 (2005): 257–62.

19. S. M. Stahl, M. M. Grady, C. Moret, and M. Briley, "SNRIs: Their Pharmacology, Clinical Efficacy, and Tolerability in Comparison with Other Classes of Antidepressants," *CNS Spectrums* 10, no. 9 (2005): 732–47.

20. J. I. Hudson, M. M. Wohlreich, D. K. Kajdasz, C. H. Mallinckrodt, J. G. Watkin, and O. V. Martynov, "Safety and Tolerability of Duloxetine in the Treatment of Major Depressive Disorder: Analysis of Pooled Data from Eight Placebo-Controlled Clinical Trials," *Human Psychopharmacology* 20, no. 5 (2005): 327–41.

21. M. Fava, A. J. Rush, M. E. Thase, A. Clayton, S. M. Stahl, J. F. Pradko, and J. A. Johnston, "15 Years of Clinical Experience with Bupropion HCl: From Bupropion to Bupropion SR to Bupropion XL," *Primary Care Companion Journal of Clinical Psychiatry* 7, no. 3 (2005): 106–13.

22. J. G. Waxmonsky, "Nonstimulant Therapies for Attention-Deficit Hyperactivity Disorder (ADHD) in Children and Adults," *Essential Psychopharmacology* 6, no. 5 (2005): 262–76.

23. G. Rubio, L. San, F. Lopez-Munoz, and C. Alamo, "Reboxetine Adjunct for Partial or Nonresponders to Antidepressant Treatment," *Journal of Affective Disorders* 81, no. 1 (2004): 67–72.

24. L. L. Altshuler, L. S. Cohen, M. L. Moline, D. A. Khan, D. Carpenter, J. P. Docherty, and R. W. Ross, "Treatment of Depression in Women: A Summary of the Expert Consensus Guidelines," *Journal of Psychiatric Practice* 7, no. 3 (2001): 185–208.

25. B. C. Prator, "Serotonin Syndrome," *Journal of Neuroscience Nursing* 38, no. 2 (2006): 102–5.

26. O. Tajima, "Recent Trends in Pharmacotherapy for Anxiety Disorders," *Nihon Shinkei Seishin Yakurigaku Zasshi* 24, no. 3 (2004): 133–36.

27. S. Pridmore and Y. Turnier-Shea, "Medication Options in the Treatment of

Treatment-Resistant Depression," *Australian and New Zealand Journal of Psychiatry* 38, no. 4 (2004): 219–25.

28. H. Marin and M. A. Menza, "The Management of Fatigue in Depressed Patients," *Essential Psychopharmacology* 6, no. 4 (2005): 185–92.

29. S. E. Murphy, C. Longhitano, R. E. Ayres, P. J. Cowen, and C. J. Harmer, "Tryptophan Supplementation Induces a Positive Bias in the Processing of Emotional Material in Healthy Female Volunteers," *Psychopharmacology* 187, no. 1 (2006): 121–30.

30. C. Hudson, S. P. Hudson, T. Hecht, and J. MacKenzie, "Protein Source Tryptophan Versus Pharmaceutical Grade Tryptophan as an Efficacious Treatment for Chronic Insomnia," *Nutritional Neuroscience* 8, no. 2 (2005): 121–27.

31. Y. T. Das, M. Bagchi, D. Bagchi, and H. G. Preuss, "Safety of 5-hydroxy-L-tryptophan," *Toxicology Letters* 150, no. 1 (2004): 111–22.

32. B. M. Cortese and K. L. Phan, "The Role of Glutamate in Anxiety and Related Disorders," *CNS Spectrums* 10, no. 10 (2005): 820–30.

33. H. J. Heo and C. Y. Lee, "Protective Effects of Quercetin and Vitamin C Against Oxidative Stress-Induced Neurodegeneration," *Journal of Agricultural and Food Chemistry* 52, no. 25 (2004): 7514–17.

34. G. S. Kelly, "Rhodiola Rosea: A Possible Plant Adaptogen," *Alternative Medicine Review* 6, no. 3 (2001): 293–302.

35. A. Panossian and H. Wagner, "Stimulating Effect of Adaptogens: An Overview with Particular Reference to Their Efficacy Following Single Dose Administration," *Phytotherapy Research* 19, no. 10 (2005): 819–38.

36. G. Chamorro, M. Salazar, K. G. Araujo, C. P. dos Santos, G. Ceballos, and L. F. Castillo, "Update on the Pharmacology of Spirulina, an Unconventional Food" [Spanish], *Archivos Latinoamericanos de Nutrición* 52, no. 3 (2002): 232–40.

37. M. D. Edden and M. S. Torre, "Physician's Guide to Herbs," *Practical Diabetology* 16, no. 1 (1997): 10–20.

38. M. Auf'mkolk, J. C. Ingbar, K. Kubota, et al., "Extracts and Auto-Oxidized Constituents of Certain Plants Inhibit the Receptor-Binding and the Biological Activity of Graves' Immunoglobulins," *Endocrinology* 116, no. 5 (1985): 1687–93.

39. M. Mennemeier, R. D. Garner, and K. M. Heilman, "Memory, Mood and Measurement in Hypothyroidism," *Journal of Clinical and Experimental Neuropsychology* 15, no. 5 (1993): 822–31.

40. H. Perrild, J. M. Hansen, K. Arnung, et al., "Intellectual Impairment After Hyperthyroidism," *Acta Endocrinologica* 112 (1986): 185–91.

41. M. Bommer, T. Eversmann, R. Pickhardt, et al., "Psychopathological and Neuropsychological Symptoms in Patients with Subclinical and Remitted Hyperthyroidism," *Klinische Wochenschrift* 68 (1990): 552–58.

42. L. S. Chia, J. E. Thompson, and M. A. Moscarello, "Changes in Lipid Phase Behavior in Human Myelin During Maturation and Aging" (letter), *Federation of European Biochemical Societies* 157 (1983): 155–58.

43. A. McCaddon, B. Regland, P. Hudson, and G. Davies, "Functional Vitamin B_{12} Deficiency and Alzheimer Disease," *Neurology* 58, no. 9 (2002): 1395–99.

44. J. M. Pasquini and A. M. Adamo, "Thyroid Hormones and the Central Nervous System," *Developmental Neuroscience* 16 (1994): 1–8.

45. J. Bernal and J. Nunez, "Thyroid Hormones and Brain Development," *European Journal of Endocrinology* 133 (1995): 390–98.

46. B. L. Jorissen, F. Brouns, M. P. Van Boxtel, and W. J. Riedel, "Safety of Soy-Derived Phosphatidylserine in Elderly People," *Nutritional Neuroscience* 5, no. 5 (2002): 337–43.

47. I. Skoog, L. Nilsson, B. Palmertz, et al., "A Population-Based Study of Dementia in 85-Year-Olds," *New England Journal of Medicine* 328 (1993): 153–58.

48. J. S. Meyer, B. W. Judd, T. Tawakina, et al., "Improved Cognition After Control of Risk Factors for Multi-Infarct Dementia," *Journal of the American Medical Association* 256 (1986): 2203–9.

49. N. Pancharuniti, C. A. Lewish, H. E. Sauberlich, et al., "Plasma Homocysteine, Folate, and Vitamin B_{12} Concentrations and Risk Factors for Early Onset Coronary Artery Disease," *American Journal of Clinical Nutrition* 59 (1994): 940–48.

50. P. A. Bastenie, L. Van Haelst, M. Bonnyns, et al., "Preclinical Hypothyroidism: A Risk Factor for Coronary Heart Disease," *Lancet* 1, no. 7692 (1971): 203–4.

51. L. A. Rybaczyk, M. J. Bashaw, D. R. Pathak, S. M. Moody, R. M. Gilders, and D. L. Holzschu, "An Overlooked Connection: Serotonergic Mediation of Estrogen-Related Physiology and Pathology," *BMC Women's Health* 5, no. 1 (2005): 12.

52. M. L. Ancelin and K. Ritchie, "Lifelong Endocrine Fluctuations and Related Cognitive Disorders," *Current Pharmaceutical Design* 11, no. 32 (2005): 4229–52.

53. V. W. Henderson, "Estrogen-Containing Hormone Therapy and Alzheimer's Disease Risk: Understanding Discrepant Inferences from Observational and Experimental Research," *Neuroscience* 138, no. 3 (2006): 1031–39.

54. B. B. Sherwin, "Estrogen and/or Androgen Replacement Therapy and Cognitive Functioning in Surgically Menopausal Women," *Psychoneuroendocrinology* 13 (1988): 345–57.

55. G. Bertschy, D. De Ziegler, and F. Bianchi-Demicheli, "Mood Disorders in Perimenopausal Women: Hormone Replacement or Antidepressant Therapy?" [French], *Revue Médicale Suisse* 1, no. 33 (2005): 2155–56, 2159–61.

56. M. L. Morgan, I. A. Cook, A. J. Rapkin, A. F. Leuchter, "Estrogen Augmentation of Antidepressants in Perimenopausal Depression: A Pilot Study," *Journal of Clinical Psychiatry* 66, no. 6 (2005): 774–80.

57. B. B. Sherwin, "Affective Changes with Estrogen and Androgen Replacement Therapy in Surgically Menopausal Women," *Journal of Affective Disorders* 14 (1988): 177–87.

CHAPTER 19. Living with Thyroid Eye Disease

1. C. A. Gorman, R. S. Bahn, and J. A. Garrity, "Ophthalmopathy," in *Werner and Ingbar's The Thyroid*, 6th ed., edited by L. E. Braverman and R. D. Utiger, 657–76 (Philadelphia: Lippincott, 1991).

2. B. J. Major, B. E. Busuttil, and A. G. Frauman, "Graves' Ophthalmopathy: Pathogenesis and Clinical Implications," *Australian and New Zealand Journal of Medicine* 28 (1998): 39–45.

3. D. L. Kendler, J. Lippa, and J. Rootman, "The Initial Clinical Characteristics of Graves' Orbitopathy Vary with Age and Sex," *Archives of Ophthalmology* 111 (1993): 197–201.

4. J. Tallstedt, G. Lundell, O. Tørring, et al., "Occurrence of Ophthalmopathy After Treatments of Graves' Hyperthyroidism," *New England Journal of Medicine* 326 (1992): 1733–38.

5. B. Bush, *Barbara Bush: A Memoir* (New York: St. Martin's Press, 1994).

6. M. Farid, A. C. Roch-Levecq, L. Levi, B. L. Brody, D. B. Granet, and D. O. Kikkawa, "Psychological Disturbance in Graves' Ophthalmopathy," *Archives of Ophthalmology* 123, no. 4 (2005): 491–96.

7. P. Perros, A. L. Cromble, and P. Kendall-Taylor, "Natural History of Thyroid-Associated Ophthalmopathy," *Clinical Endocrinology* 42 (1995): 45–50.

8. R. S. Bahn, "Assessment and Management of the Patient with Graves' Ophthalmo-pathy," *Endocrine Practice* 1, no. 3 (1995): 172–78.

9. I. B. Hales and F. F. Rundle, "Ocular Changes in Graves' Disease: A Long-Term Follow-up Study," *Quarterly Journal of Medicine* 29 (1960): 113–26.

10. G. B. Bartley, V. Fatourechi, E. F. Kadrmas, et al., "The Treatment of Graves' Oph-thalmopathy in an Incidence Cohort," *American Journal of Ophthalmology* 121 (1996): 200–6.

11. M. J. Shih, S. L. Liao, and H. Y. Lu, "A Single Transcutaneous Injection with Botox for Dysthyroid Lid Retraction," *Eye* 18, no. 5 (2004): 466–69.

12. I. A. Petersen, J. P. Kriss, I. R. McDougall, et al., "Prognostic Factors in the Radio-therapy of Graves' Ophthalmopathy," *International Journal of Radiation Oncology/ Biology/Physics* 19 (1990): 259–64.

13. C. M. Ng, H. K. Yuen, K. L. Choi, et al., "Combined Orbital Irradiation and Sys-temic Steroids Compared with Systemic Steroids Alone in the Management of Moderate-to-Severe Graves' Ophthalmopathy: A Preliminary Study," *Hong Kong Medical Journal* 11, no. 5 (2005): 322–30.

14. L. Baldeschi, I. M. Wakelkamp, R. Lindeboom, M. F. Prummel, and W. M. Wier-singa, "Early Versus Late Orbital Decompression in Graves' Orbitopathy: A Retro-spective Study in 125 Patients," *Ophthalmology* 113, no. 5 (2006): 874–78.

15. A. Eckstein, B. Quadbeck, G. Mueller, A. W. Rettenmeier, R. Hoermann, K. Mann, P. Steuhl, and J. Esser, "Impact of Smoking on the Response to Treatment of Thyroid Associated Ophthalmopathy," *British Journal of Ophthalmology* 87, no. 6 (2003): 773–76.

16. M. F. Prummel, W. M. Wiersinga, M. Mourits, et al., "Effect of Abnormal Thyroid Function on the Severity of Graves' Ophthalmopathy," *Archives of Internal Medicine* 150 (1990): 1098–1101.

17. E. A. Bouzas, P. Karadimas, G. Mastorakos, and D. A. Koutras, "Antioxidant Agents in the Treatment of Graves' Ophthalmopathy," *American Journal of Ophthalmology* 129, no. 5 (2000): 618–22.

18. L. Bartalena, C. Marocci, F. Bogazzi, et al., "Relation Between Therapy for Hyperthy-roidism and the Course of Graves' Ophthalmopathy," *New England Journal of Medi-cine* 338, no. 2 (1998): 73–78.

19. L. Bartalena, C. Marocci, F. Bogazzi, et al., "Use of Corticosteroids to Prevent Pro-gression of Graves' Ophthalmopathy After Radioiodine Therapy for Hyperthyroid-ism," *New England Journal of Medicine* 321 (1989): 1349–52.

20. N. Sonino, M. E. Girelli, M. Boscaro, et al., "Life Events in the Pathogenesis of Graves' Disease," *Acta Endocrinologica* 128 (1993): 293–96.

21. B. Shine, P. Fells, O. M. Edwards, et al., "Association Between Graves' Ophthalmo-pathy and Smoking," *Lancet* 335 (1990): 1261–63.

CHAPTER 20. My T4/T3 Approach

1. W. M. Wiersinga, "Thyroid Hormone Replacement Therapy," *Hormone Research* 56, suppl. 1 (2001): 74–81.

2. R. W. Rees-Jones and P. R. Larsen, "Triiodothyronine and Thyroxine Content of Des-iccated Thyroid Tablets," *Metabolism* 26 (1977): 1213–18.

3. S. N. Bjerke, T. Bjoro, and S. Heyerdahl, "Psychiatric and Cognitive Aspects of Hy-pothyroidism" [Norwegian], *Tidsskrift for den Norske Laegenforening* 121, no. 20 (2001): 2373–76.

4. M. Alevizaki, E. Mantzou, A. T. Cimponeriu, C. C. Alevizaki, and D. A. Koutras, "TSH May Not Be a Good Marker for Adequate Thyroid Hormone Replacement Therapy," [German], *Wiener Klinische Wochenschrift* 117, no. 18 (2005): 636–40.

5. H. F. Escobar-Morreale, F. E. Escobar del Rey, M. J. Obregon, and G. Morreale de Escobar, "Only the Combined Treatment with Thyroxine and Triiodothyronine Ensures Euthyroidism in All Tissues of the Thyroidectomized Rat," *Endocrinology* 137 (1996): 2490–502.

6. G. Hennemann, R. Docter, T. J. Visser, P. T. Postema, and E. P. Krenning, "Thyroxine Plus Low-Dose, Slow-Release Triiodothyronine Replacement in Hypothyroidism: Proof of Principle," *Thyroid* 14, no. 4 (2004): 271–75.

7. R. Bunevicius, G. Kazanavicius, R. Zalinkevicius, and A. J. Prange Jr., "Effects of Thyroxine as Compared with Thyroxine Plus Triiodothyronine in Patients with Hypothyroidism," *New England Journal of Medicine* 340 (1999): 424–29.

8. S. Grozinsky-Glasberg, A. Fraser, E. Nahshoni, A. Weizman, and L. Leibovici, "Thyroxine-Triiodothyronine Combination Therapy Versus Thyroxine Monotherapy for Clinical Hypothyroidism—Meta-Analysis of Randomized Controlled Trials," *Journal of Clinical Endocrinology and Metabolism* 91, no. 7 (2006): 2592–99.

CHAPTER 21. The ThyroLife Diet for Successful Long-Term Weight Loss and Healthy Metabolism

1. R. Arem, *The Protein Boost Diet* (New York: Atria, 2012).

2. R. de Cassia Goncalves Alfenas, J. Bressan, and A. Cardoso de Paiva, "Effects of Protein Quality on Appetite and Energy Metabolism in Normal Weight Subjects," *Arquivos Brasileiros de Endocrinologia and Metabologia* 54, no. 1 (2010): 45–51.

3. Y. Zhang, K. Guo, R. E. LeBlanc, et al., "Increasing Dietary Leucine Intake Reduced Diet-Induced Obesity and Improves Glucose and Cholestrol Metabolism in Mice via Multimechanisms," *Diabetes* 56, no. 6 (2007): 1647–54.

4. E. P. Plaisance et al., "Dietary Methionine Restriction Increases Fat Oxidation in Obese Adults with Metabolic Syndrome," *Journal of Clinical Endocrinology and Metabolism* 96, no. 5 (2011): 836–40.

5. D. K. Layman, "The Role of Leucine in Weight Loss Diets and Glucose Homeostasis," *American Society for Nutritional Sciences* 133, no. 1 (2003): 261S–67S.

6. C. S. Johnston, "Strategies for Healthy Weight Loss: From Vitamin C to the Glycemic Response," *Journal of the American College of Nutrition* 24, no. 3 (2005): 158–65.

7. S. E. La Fleur, A. Kalsbeek, J. Wortel, et al., "A Daily Rhythm in Glucose Tolerance: A Role for the Suprachiasmatic Nucleus," *Diabetes* 50, no. 6 (2001): 1237–43.

8. W. Huang, K. M. Ramsey, B. Marcheva, and J. Bass, "Circadian Rhythms, Sleep, and Metabolism," *Journal of Clinical Investigation* 121, no. 6 (2011): 2133–41.

9. B. Dziedzic, J. Szemraj, J. Bartkowiak, and A. Walczewska, "Various Dietary Fats Differentially Change the Gene Expression of Neuropeptides Involved in Body Weight Regulation in Rats," *Journal of Neuroendocrinology* 19, no. 5 (2007): 364–73.

10. G. Taubes, *Good Calories, Bad Calories* (New York: Knopf, 2007); G. S. Birketvedt, M. Shimshi, E. Thom, and J. Florholmen, "Experiences with Three Different Fiber Supplements in Weight Reduction," *Medical Science Monitor* 11, no. 1 (2005): PI5–8.

11. J. W. Anderson, P. Baird, R. H. Davis Jr., et al., "Health Benefits of Dietary Fiber," *Nutrition Reviews* 67, no. 4 (2009): 188–205.

12. M. Wilders-Truschnig, H. Mangge, C. Lieners, et al., "IgG Antibodies Against Food

Antigens Are Correlated with Inflammation and Intima Media Thickness in Obese Juveniles," *Experimental and Clinical Endocrinology and Diabetes* 116, no. 4 (2008): 241–45.

13. M. P. Montgomery, F. Kamel, T. M. Saldana, et al., "Incident Diabetes and Pesticide Exposure Among Licensed Pesticide Applicators: Agricultural Health Study, 1993–2003," *American Journal of Epidemiology* 167, no. 10 (2008): 1235–46.

14. G. B. Post, P. D. Cohn, and K. R. Cooper, "Perfluorooctanoic Acid (PFOA), an Emerging Drinking Water Contaminant: A Critical Review of Recent Literature," *Environmental Research* 116 (2012): 93–117.

15. R. Estruch, M. A. Martinez-Gonzales, D. Corella, et al., "Effects of a Mediterranean-Style Diet on Cardiovascular Risk Factors," *Annals of Internal Medicine* 145, no. 1 (2006): 1–12.

16. M. Martinez-Tome, A. M. Jimenez, S. Ruggieri, N. Frega, R. Strabbioli, and M. A. Murcia, "Antioxidant Properties of Mediterranean Spices Compared with Common Food Additives," *Journal of Food Protection* 64, no. 9 (2001): 1412–19.

17. F. A. Scheer, M. F. Hilton, C. S. Mantzoros, and S. A. Shea, "Adverse Metabolic and Cardiovascular Consequences of Circadian Misalignment," *Proceedings of the National Academy of Sciences* 106, no. 11 (2009): 4453–58.

18. J. Louis-Sylvestre, A. Lluch, F. Neant, and J. E. Blundell, "Highlighting the Positive Impact of Increasing Feeding Frequency on Metabolism and Weight Management," *Forum of Nutrition* 56 (2003): 126–28.

19. W. Huang, K. M. Ramsey, B. Marcheva, and J. Bass, "Circadian Rhythms, Sleep, and Metabolism," *Journal of Clinical Investigation* 121, no. 6 (2011): 2133–41.

20. A. K. Kant and B. I. Graubard, "Eating Out in America, 1987–2000: Trends and Nutritional Correlates," *Preventive Medicine* 38, no. 2 (2004): 243–49.

21. M. Hermanussen, A. P. Garcia, M. Sunder, M. Voigt, V. Salazar, and J. A. Tresguerres, "Obesity, Voracity, and Short Stature: The Impact of Glutamate on the Regulation of Appetite," *European Journal of Clinical Nutrition* 60, no. 1 (2006): 25–31.

22. H. Benson, J. F. Beary, and M. P. Carol, "The Relaxation Response," *Psychiatry: Journal for the Study of Interpersonal Processes* 37, no. 1 (1974): 37–46.

23. L. Rapoport, M. Clark, and J. Wardle, "Evaluation of a Modified Cognitive-Behavioural Programme for Weight Management," *International Journal of Obesity and Related Metabolic Disorders* 24, no. 12 (2000): 1726–37.

24. D. Shahar, D. Schwarzfuchs, D. Fraser, et al., "Dairy Calcium Intake, Serum Vitamin D, and Successful Weight Loss," *American Journal of Clinical Nutrition* 92, no. 5 (2010).

25. P. Flachs, O. Horakova, P. Brauner, et al., "Polyunsaturated Fatty Acids of Marine Origin Upregulate Mitochondrial Biogenesis and Induce Beta-Oxidation in White Fat," *Diabetologia* 48, no. 11 (2005): 2365–75.

26. D. Parra, A. Ramel, N. Bandarra, et al., "A Diet Rich in Long Chain Omega-3 Fatty Acids Modulates Satiety in Overweight and Obese Volunteers During Weight Loss," *Appetite* 51, no. 3 (2008): 676–80.

27. B. Halliwell, "Oxygen Radicals: A Common Sense Look at Their Nature and Medical Importance," *Medical Biology* 62, no. 2 (1984): 71–77.

28. G. DiMartino, M. G. Matera, B. De Martino, et al., "Relationship Between Zinc and Obesity," *Journal of Medicine* 24 (1993): 177–83.

29. M. J. Berry and P. R. Larsen, "Role of Selenium in Thyroid Hormone Actions," *Endocrine Reviews* 13, no. 2 (1992): 207–19.

30. S. V. Vladeva, D. D. Terzieva, and D. T. Arabadjiiska, "Effects of Chromium on the

Insulin Resistance of Patients with Type II Diabetes Mellitus," *Folia Medica* 47, Nos. 3–4 (2005): 59–62.

31. C. S. Johnston, "Strategies for Healthy Weight Loss: From Vitamin C to the Glycemic Response," *Journal of the American College of Nutrition* 24, no. 3 (2005): 158–65.

32. H. R. Mogul, S. J. Peterson, B. I. Weinstein, S. Zhang, and A. L. Southren, "Metformin and Carbohydrate-Modified Diet: A Novel Obesity Treatment Protocol: Preliminary Findings from a Case Series of Nondiabetic Women with Midlife Weight Gain and Hyperinsulinemia," *Heart Disease* 3, no. 5 (2001): 285–92.

33. T. L. Lenz and W. R. Hamilton, "Supplemental Products Used for Weight Loss," *Journal of the American Pharmaceutical Association* 44, no. 1 (2004): 59–67.

34. I. Hininger-Favier, R. Benaraba, S. Coves, et al., "Green Tea Extract Decreases Oxidative Stress and Improves Insulin Sensitivity in an Animal Model of Insulin Resistance, the Fructose-Fed Rat," *Journal of American College of Nutrition* 28, no. 4 (2009): 355–61.

35. M. S. Westerterp-Plantenga, M. P. Lejeune, and E. M. Kovacs, "Body Weight Loss and Weight Maintenance in Relation to Habitual Caffeine Intake and Green Tea Supplementation," *Obesity Research* 13, no. 7 (2005): 1195–204.

36. V. P. Menon and A. R. Sudheer, "Antioxidant and Anti-inflammatory Properties of Curcumin," *Advances in Experimental Medicine and Biology* 595 (2007): 105–25.

37. W. Suwannaphet, A. Meeprom, S. Yibchok-Anun, and S. Adisakwattana, "Preventive Effect of Grape Seed Extract Against High-Fructose-Diet-Induced Insulin Resistance and Oxidative Stress in Rats," *Food and Chemical Toxicology* 48, no. 7 (2010): 1853–57.

38. E. Roti, R. Minelli, and E. Gardini, "The Use and Misuse of Thyroid Hormone," *Endocrine Reviews* 14, no. 4 (1993): 401–23.

39. G. D. Braunstein, R. Koblin, M. Sugawara, et al., "Unintentional Thyrotoxicosis Factitia Due to a Diet Pill," *Western Journal of Medicine* 145 (1986): 388–91.

40. F. Ohno and K. Miyoshi, "Clinical Observations on Thyreoidismus Medicamentosus Due to Weight-Reducing Pills in Japan," *Endocrinologica Japonica* 18 (1971): 321–23.

41. H. Wyatt, "Strategies to Fight Weight Regain," presented at the 93rd Annual Meeting of the Endocrine Society, Boston, June 4, 2011.

CHAPTER 22. My Thyroid Mind-Body Program

1. M. J. Nyirenda, D. N. Clark, A. R. Finlayson, J. Read, A. Elders, M. Bain, K. A. Fox, and A. D. Toft, "Thyroid Disease and Increased Cardiovascular Risk," *Thyroid* 15, no. 7 (2005): 718–24.

2. W. J. W. Morrow, J. Homsy, and J. A. Levy, "The Influence of Nutrition on Experimental Autoimmune Disease," in *Nutrient Modulation of the Immune Response*, edited by S. Cunningham-Rundles, 153–67 (New York: Dekker, 1993).

3. M. Messina and G. Redmond, "Effects of Soy Protein and Soybean Isoflavones on Thyroid Function in Healthy Adults and Hypothyroid Patients: A Review of the Relevant Literature," *Thyroid* 16, no. 3 (2006): 249–58.

4. B. B. Sherwin, "Affective Changes with Estrogen and Androgen Replacement Therapy in Surgically Menopausal Women," *Journal of Affective Disorders* 14 (1988): 177–87.

5. A. L. Williams, D. Katz, A. Ali, C. Girard, J. Goodman, and I. Bell, "Do Essential Fatty Acids Have a Role in the Treatment of Depression?" *Journal of Affective Disorders* 93, nos. 1–3 (2006): 117–23.

6. V. E. Kelley, A. Ferretti, S. Izui, et al., "A Fish Oil Diet Rich in Eicosapentaenoic Acid Reduces Cyclooxygenase Metabolites and Suppresses Lupus in MRL/1pr Mice," *Journal of Immunology* 134 (1985): 1914–19.

7. B. D'Avanzo, E. Ron, C. La Vecchia, et al., "Selected Micronutrient Intake and Thyroid Carcinoma Risk," *Cancer* 79 (1997): 2186–92.

8. O. Olivieri, D. Girelli, M. Azzini, et al., "Low Selenium Status in the Elderly Influences Thyroid Hormones," *Clinical Science* 89 (1995): 637–42.

9. J. S. Hampl, C. A. Taylor, and C. S. Johnston, "Vitamin C Deficiency and Depletion in the United States: The Third National Health and Nutrition Examination Survey, 1988 to 1994," *American Journal of Public Health* 94, no. 5 (2004): 870–75.

10. K. Asayama and K. Kato, "Oxidative Muscular Injury and Its Relevance to Hyperthyroidism," *Free Radical Biology and Medicine* 8 (1990): 293–303.

11. V. Bacic Vrca, F. Skreb, I. Cepelak, Z. Romic, and L. Mayer, "Supplementation with Antioxidants in the Treatment of Graves' Disease; The Effect on Glutathione Peroxidase Activity and Concentration of Selenium," *Clinica Chimica Acta* 341, nos. 1–2 (2004): 55–63.

12. M. Kornitzer, F. Valente, D. De Bacquer, J. Neve, and G. De Backer, "Serum Selenium and Cancer Mortality: A Nested Case-Control Study Within an Age- and Sex-Stratified Sample of the Belgian Adult Population," *European Journal of Clinical Nutrition* 58, no. 1 (2004): 98–104.

13. P. D. Whanger, "Selenium and the Brain: A Review," *Nutritional Neuroscience* 4, no. 2 (2001): 81–97.

14. M. J. Berry and P. R. Larsen, "The Role of Selenium in Thyroid Hormone Action," *Endocrine Reviews* 13 (1992): 207–19.

15. R. Gärtner, B. C. Gasnier, J. W. Dietrich, B. Krebs, and M. W. Angstwurm, "Selenium Supplementation in Patients with Autoimmune Thyroiditis Decreases Thyroid Peroxidase Antibodies Concentrations," *Journal of Clinical Endocrinology and Metabolism* 87, no. 4 (2002): 1687–91.

16. J. F. Bach, "The Multi-Faceted Zinc Dependency of the Immune System," *Immunology Today* 2 (1981): 225–27.

17. C. W. Levenson, "Zinc: The New Antidepressant?" *Nutrition Reviews* 64, no. 1 (2006): 39–42.

18. W. B. Alshuaib and M. V. Mathew, "Vitamins C and E Modulate Neuronal Potassium Currents," *Journal of Membrane Biology* 210, no. 3 (2006): 193–98.

19. A. Coppen and C. Bolander-Gouaille, "Treatment of Depression: Time to Consider Folic Acid and Vitamin B$_{12}$," *Journal of Psychopharmacology* 19, no. 1 (2005): 59–65.

20. K. Lechner, M. Fodinger, W. Grisold, A. Puspok, and C. Sillaber, "Vitamin B$_{12}$ Deficiency. New Data on an Old Theme" [German], *Wiener Klinische Wochenschrift* 117, no. 17 (2005): 579–91.

21. A. L. Williams, A. Cotter, A. Sabina, C. Girard, J. Goodman, and D. L. Katz, "The Role for Vitamin B-6 as Treatment for Depression: A Systematic Review," *Family Practice* 22, no. 5 (2005): 532–37.

22. R. Salerno-Kennedy and K. D. Cashman, "Relationship Between Dementia and Nutrition-Related Factors and Disorders: An Overview," *International Journal for Vitamin and Nutrition Research* 75, no. 2 (2005): 83–95.

23. J. E. Maras, O. I. Bermudez, N. Qiao, P. J. Bakun, E. L. Boody-Alter, and K. L. Tucker, "Intake of Alpha-Tocopherol Is Limited Among US Adults," *Journal of the American Dietetic Association* 104, no. 4 (2004): 567–75.

24. A. Cherubini, A. Martin, C. Andres-Lacueva, et al., "Vitamin E Levels, Cognitive

Impairment and Dementia in Older Persons: The InCHIANTI Study," *Neurobiology and Aging* 26, no. 7 (2005): 987–94.

25. C. Hatzigeorgiou, A. J. Taylor, I. M. Feuerstein, L. Bautista, and P. G. O'Malley, "Antioxidant Vitamin Intake and Subclinical Coronary Atherosclerosis," *Preventive Cardiology* 9, no. 2 (2006): 75–81.

26. K. Hensley, E. J. Benaksas, R. Bolli, et al., "New Perspectives on Vitamin E: Gamma-Tocopherol and Carboxyethylhydroxychroman Metabolites in Biology and Medicine," *Free Radical Biology and Medicine* 36, no. 1 (2004): 1–15.

27. T. Mano, K. Iwase, R. Hayashi, et al., "Vitamin E and Coenzyme Q Concentrations in the Thyroid Tissues of Patients with Various Thyroid Disorders," *American Journal of the Medical Sciences* 315, no. 4 (1998): 230–32.

28. F. Ogura, H. Morii, M. Ohno, T. Ueno, S. Kitabatake, N. Hamada, and K. Ito, "Serum Coenzyme Q10 Levels in Thyroid Disorders," *Hormone and Metabolism Research* 12, no. 10 (1980): 537–40.

29. W. K. Al-Delaimy, E. B. Rimm, W. C. Willett, M. J. Stampfer, and F. B. Hu, "Magnesium Intake and Risk of Coronary Heart Disease Among Men," *Journal of the American College of Nutrition* 23, no. 1 (2004): 63–70.

30. M. B. Zemel, "Regulation of Adiposity and Obesity Risk by Dietary Calcium: Mechanisms and Implication," *Journal of the American College of Nutrition* 21, no. 2 (2002): 146S–51S.

31. E. C. Claud and A. W. Walker, "Bacterial Colonization, Probiotics, and Necrotizing Enterocolitis," *Journal of Clinical Gastroenterology* 42 (Suppl. 2) (2008): S46–52.

32. J. A. Bravo, P. Forsythe, M. V. Chew, et al., "Ingestion of Lactobacillus Strain Regulates Emotional Behavior and Central GABA Receptor Expression in a Mouse via the Vagus Nerve," *Proceedings of the National Academy of Sciences* 108, no. 38 (2011): 16050–55.

33. P. P. Smyth and L. H. Duntas, "Iodine Uptake and Loss—Can Frequent Strenuous Exercise Induce Iodine Deficiency?" *Hormone and Metabolism Research* 37, no. 9 (2005): 555–58.

34. N. R. Rose, A. M. Saboori, L. Rasooly, et al., "The Role of Iodine in Autoimmune Thyroiditis," *Clinical Reviews in Immunology* 17 (1997): 511–17.

35. H. R. Harach and E. D. Williams, "Thyroid Cancer and Thyroiditis in the Goitrous Region of Salta, Argentina, Before and After Iodine Prophylaxis," *Clinical Endocrinology* 43 (1995): 701–6.

36. M. F. Holick, E. S. Siris, N. Binkely, et al., "Prevalence of Vitamin D Inadequacy Among Postmenopausal North American Women Receiving Osteoporosis Therapy," *Journal of Clinical Endocrinology and Metabolism* 90, no. 6 (2005): 3215–24.

37. M. F. Holick, "Vitamin D: Important for Prevention of Osteoporosis, Cardiovascular Heart Disease, Type 1 Diabetes, Autoimmune Diseases, and Some Cancers," *Southern Medical Journal* 98, no. 10 (2005): 1024–27.

38. F. M. Gloth III, W. Alam, and B. Hollis, "Vitamin D Versus Broad Spectrum Phototherapy in the Treatment of Seasonal Affective Disorder," *Journal of Nutrition, Health, and Aging* 3, no. 1 (1999): 5–7.

39. G. Tamer, S. Arik, I. Tamer, and D. Coksert, "Relative Vitamin D Insufficiency in Hashimoto's Thyroiditis," *Thyroid* 21, no. 8 (2011): 891–96.

40. T. Yasuda, Y. Okamoto, N. Hamada, K. Miyashita, M. Takahara, F. Sakamoto, T. Miyatsuka, et al., "Serum Vitamin D Levels Are Decreased and Associated with Thyroid Volume in Female Patients with Newly Onset Graves' Disease," *Endocrine* 42, no. 3 (2012): 739–41.

41. C. Ernst, A. K. Olson, J. P. Pinel, R. W. Lam, and B. R. Christie, "Antidepressant Effect of Exercise: Evidence for an Adult-Neurogenesis Hypothesis?" *Journal of Psychiatry and Neuroscience* 31, no. 2 (2006): 84–92.
42. R. Arem, *The Protein Boost Diet* (New York: Atria, 2012).
43. I. A. Holm, J. E. Manson, K. B. Michels, E. K. Alexander, W. C. Willett, and R. D. Utiger, "Smoking and Other Lifestyle Factors and the Risk of Graves' Hyperthyroidism," *Archives of Internal Medicine* 165, no. 14 (2005): 1606–11.
44. N. Knudsen, I. Bulow, P. Laurberg, H. Perrild, L. Ovesen, and T. Jorgensen, "High Occurrence of Thyroid Multinodularity and Low Occurrence of Subclinical Hypothyroidism Among Tobacco Smokers in a Large Population Study," *Journal of Endocrinology* 175, no. 3 (2002): 571–76.
45. S. Yoshida and M. E. Gershwin, "Autoimmunity and Selected Environmental Factors of Disease Induction," *Seminars in Arthritis and Rheumatism* 22, no. 6 (1993): 399–419.
46. C. C. Chow and C. S. Cockram, "Thyroid Disorders Induced by Lithium and Amiodarone: An Overview," *Adverse Drug Reactions and Acute Poisoning Reviews* 9, no. 4 (1990): 207–22.
47. F. Monzani, N. Caraccio, A. Dardano, and E. Ferrannini, "Thyroid Autoimmunity and Dysfunction Associated with Type I Interferon Therapy," *Clinical and Experimental Medicine* 3, no. 4 (2004): 199–210.
48. K. C. McCowen, J. R. Garber, and R. Spark, "Elevated Serum Thyrotropin in Thyroxine-Treated Patients with Hypothyroidism Given Sertraline" (letter), *New England Journal of Medicine* 337, no. 14 (1997): 1010–11.

RESOURCES

DOMESTIC ORGANIZATIONS

HORMONE HEALTH NETWORK (PUBLIC EDUCATION ABOUT HORMONE-RELATED CONDITIONS)
www.hormone.org
8401 Connecticut Avenue, Suite 900
Chevy Chase, MD 20815-5817
Telephone: 1-800-HORMONE

THE THYROID FOUNDATION OF AMERICA
www.allthyroid.org
One Longfellow Place, Suite 1518
Boston, MA 02114
Telephone: 1-800-832-8321

GRAVES' DISEASE & THYROID FOUNDATION
www.gdatf.org
PO Box 2793
Rancho Santa Fe, CA 92067
Telephone: 1-877-643-3123
Email: info@gdatf.org

AMERICAN THYROID ASSOCIATION, PATIENT RESOURCES
www.thyroid.org
6066 Leesburg Pike, Suite 550
Falls Church, VA 22041
Telephone: 1-800-THYROID

LIGHT OF LIFE FOUNDATION (FOR THYROID CANCER PATIENTS)
www.checkyourneck.com
PO Box 163
Manalapan, NJ 07726
Telephone: 609-409-0900
Email: info@checkyourneck.com

THYCA: THYROID CANCER SURVIVORS' ASSOCIATION, INC.
www.thyca.org
PO Box 1545
New York, NY 10159-1545
Telephone: 1-877-588-7904
Email: thyca@thyca.org

THE KELLY G. RIPKEN PROGRAM
http://thyroid-ripken.med.jhu.edu
Johns Hopkins Medicine
1830 E. Monument Street, Suite 333
Baltimore, MD 21287
Telephone: 1-888-595-2131

INTERNATIONAL ORGANIZATIONS

THYROID FOUNDATION OF CANADA
www.thyroid.ca
PO Box 298
Bath, ON K0H 1G0, Canada
Telephone: 1-800-267-8822 in Canada

THYROID FEDERATION INTERNATIONAL (RESOURCE FOR PEOPLE INTERESTED IN STARTING A LOCAL PATIENT ORGANIZATION)
www.thyroid-fed.org
PO Box 471
Bath, ON K0H 1G0, Canada
Telephone: 613-544-8364
Email: tfi@thyroid-fed.org

BRITISH THYROID FOUNDATION
www.btf-thyroid.org
One Sceptre House, Suite 12
Hornbeam Square North, Hornbeam Park
Harrogate, HG2 8BP, UK
Telephone: +44 (0) 1423 810093
Email: info@btf-thyroid.org

THYROID EYE DISEASE (TED) HEAD OFFICE
www.tedct.co.uk
P.O. Box 1928
Bristol, BS37 0AX, UK
Telephone: +44 (0) 7469921782
E-mail: info@tedct.org.uk

ASSOCIATION FRANÇAISE DES MALADES DE LA THYROÏDE
www.asso-malades-thyroide.org
BP 1-82 700 Bourret, France
Telephone: +33 (0) 5 63 27 50 80
Email: asso.thyroide@gmail.com

SCHILDDRÜSEN-LIGA DEUTSCHLAND E.V.
www.schilddruesenliga.de
Johamiter GmbH, Waldkrankenhaus
Waldstrasse 73
53177 Bonn, Germany
Telephone: 0228 386 9060
Email: info@schilddruesenliga.de

THYREOIDEA LANDSFORENINGEN
www.thyreoidea.dk
Strandkrogen 4A
3630 Jaegerspris, Denmark

SCHILDKLIER ORGANISATIE NEDERLAND
www.schildklier.nl
Postbus 60
3940 AB Doorn, The Netherlands
Telephone: +31 085-489 12 36
Email: info@schildklier.nl

STOFFSKIFTEFORBUNDET
www.stoffskifte.org
Fr. Nansen plass 9, N-0160
Oslo, Norway
Telephone: 011+ 47 22 94 1010
Email: post@stoffskifte.org

SKÖLDKÖRTELFÖRENINGEN
www.skoldkortelforeningen.se
Box 5183
121 18 Johanneshov, Sweden
Email: info@skoldkortelforeningen.se

THYROID FOUNDATION OF ST. PETERSBURG
42 Chaykovsky Street
St. Petersburg 191123, Russia
Email: gasparyan@peterlink.ru

AUSTRALIAN THYROID FOUNDATION
www.thyroidfoundation.org.au
Suite 2, 8 Melville Street
Parramatta NSW, 2150, Australia
Telephone: +61 2 9890 6962
Email: info@thyroidfoundation.org.au

INSTITUTO DA TIREOIDE
www.indatir.org.br
Telephone: (5511) 3032-3090
R conselheiro Brotero 353, sala 36
São Paulo—SP—CEP 01154-000, Brazil
Email: duvidas@indatir.org.br

EDUCATIONAL WEBSITES

MYTHYROID.COM
An evidence-based, patient-centered website by Dr. Daniel J. Drucker, University of
Toronto, Mount Sinai Hospital, and Toronto General Hospital, devoted to diseases of the
thyroid
www.mythyroid.com

ENDOCRINEWEB.COM
Discusses thyroid, parathyroid, and endocrine disorders
www.endocrineweb.com

THYROID DISEASE MANAGER
Online educational source for clinicians
www.thyroidmanager.org

THYROID-INFO.COM
Unbiased news, books, support from patient advocate Mary Shomon
www.thyroid-info.com

DIRECTORIES FOR THYROID SPECIALISTS

AMERICAN THYROID ASSOCIATION
www.thyroid.org
6066 Leesburg Pike, Suite 550
Falls Church, VA 22041
Telephone: 1-800-THYROID

AMERICAN ASSOCIATION OF CLINICAL ENDOCRINOLOGISTS
www.aace.com
245 Riverside Avenue, Suite 200
Jacksonville, FL 32202
Telephone: 904-353-7878

THE ENDOCRINE SOCIETY
www.endocrine.org
8401 Connecticut Avenue, Suite 900
Chevy Chase, MD 20815
Telephone: 301-941-0200

FIBROMYALGIA ORGANIZATIONS

NATIONAL FIBROMYALGIA ASSOCIATION
www.fmaware.org
3857 Birch Street, Suite 312
Newport Beach, CA 92660
Phone: 714-921-0150
Email: nfa@fmaware.org

AMERICAN FIBROMYALGIA SYNDROME ASSOCIATION, INC.
www.afsafund.org
PO Box 32698
Tucson, AZ 85751
Telephone: 520-733-1570
Email: kthorson@afsafund.org

CHRONIC FATIGUE SYNDROME ORGANIZATIONS

SOLVE ME/CFS INITIATIVE
www.solvecfs.org
5455 Wilshire Boulevard, Suite 1903
Los Angeles, CA 90036
Telephone: 704-364-0016

NATIONAL CFIDS FOUNDATION
www.ncf-net.org
103 Aletha Road
Needham, MA 02492
Telephone: 781-449-3535
Email: info@ncf-net.org

AUTOIMMUNE DISORDER ORGANIZATIONS

AMERICAN AUTOIMMUNE RELATED DISEASES ASSOCIATION
www.aarda.org
22100 Gratiot Avenue
Eastpointe, MI 48021
Telephone: 586-776-3900

ARTHRITIS FOUNDATION
www.arthritis.org
1355 Peachtree Street NE, Suite 600
Atlanta, GA 30309
Telephone: 1-844-571-HELP

LUPUS FOUNDATION OF AMERICA, INC.
www.lupus.org
National Office
2121 K Street NW, Suite 200
Washington, DC 20037
Telephone: 202-349-1155
Email: info@lupus.org

SJÖGREN'S SYNDROME FOUNDATION
www.sjogrens.org
6707 Democracy Boulevard, Suite 325
Bethesda, MD 20817
Telephone: 1-800-475-6473

SCLERODERMA FOUNDATION
www.scleroderma.org
300 Rosewood Drive, Suite 105
Danvers, MA 01923
Telephone: 1-800-722-HOPE

NATIONAL ADRENAL DISEASES FOUNDATION
www.nadf.us
505 Northern Boulevard
Great Neck, NY 11021
Telephone: 516-487-4992

MENTAL HEALTH ORGANIZATIONS

NATIONAL INSTITUTE OF MENTAL HEALTH (NIMH)
www.nimh.nih.gov
Office of Communications
6001 Executive Boulevard, Room 8184, MSC 9663
Bethesda, MD 20892-9663
Telephone: 1-866-615-6464
Email: nimhinfo@mail.nih.gov

NATIONAL ALLIANCE ON MENTAL ILLNESS
www.nami.org
3803 N. Fairfax Drive, Suite 100
Arlington, VA 22203
Telephone: 1-800-950-NAMI

MENTAL HEALTH AMERICA (FORMERLY THE NATIONAL MENTAL HEALTH ASSOCIATION)
www.nmha.org
500 Montgomery Street, Suite 820
Alexandria, VA 22314
Telephone: 703-684-7722

DEPRESSION AND BIPOLAR SUPPORT ALLIANCE
www.dbsalliance.org
55 E. Jackson Boulevard, Suite 490
Chicago, IL 60604
Telephone: 1-800-826-3632

INTERNATIONAL FOUNDATION FOR RESEARCH AND EDUCATION ON DEPRESSION (IFRED)
www.ifred.org
PO Box 17598
Baltimore, MD 21297
Email: info@ifred.org

AMERICAN PSYCHOLOGICAL ASSOCIATION
www.apa.org
750 First Street NE
Washington, DC 20002-4242
Telephone: 1-800-374-2721

AMERICAN PSYCHIATRIC ASSOCIATION
www.healthyminds.org
1000 Wilson Boulevard, Suite 1825
Arlington, VA 22209
Telephone: 703-907-7300
Email: apa@psych.org

ANXIETY AND DEPRESSION ASSOCIATION OF AMERICA
www.adaa.org
8701 Georgia Avenue, Suite 412
Silver Spring, MD 20910
Telephone: 240-485-1001

THE ANXIETY NETWORK
www.anxietynetwork.com

INTERNATIONAL OCD FOUNDATION
www.iocdf.org
PO Box 961029
Boston, MA 02196
Telephone: 617-973-5801
Email: info@iocdf.org

FREEDOM FROM FEAR (ANXIETY AND DEPRESSION RESOURCE ORGANIZATION)
www.freedomfromfear.org
308 Seaview Avenue
Staten Island, NY 10305
Telephone: 718-351-1717
Email: help@freedomfromfear.org

POSTPARTUM DEPRESSION ORGANIZATIONS

POSTPARTUM SUPPORT INTERNATIONAL
www.postpartum.net
6706 SW 54th Avenue
Portland, OR 97219
Telephone: 1-800-944-4773

MASSACHUSETTS GENERAL HOSPITAL CENTER FOR WOMEN'S MENTAL HEALTH
Perinatal and Reproductive Psychiatry Program
Simches Research Building
185 Cambridge Street, Suite 2200
Boston, MA 02114
www.womensmentalhealth.org

INFERTILITY ORGANIZATIONS

PATH2PARENTHOOD
www.path2parenthood.org
305 Madison Avenue, Suite 901
New York, NY 10017
Telephone: 1-888-917-3777
Email: info@path2parenthood.org

RESOLVE: THE NATIONAL INFERTILITY ASSOCIATION
www.resolve.org
7918 Jones Branch Drive, Suite 300
McLean, VA 22102
Telephone: 703-556-7172
Email: info@resolve.org

NUCLEAR MEDICINE ORGANIZATIONS

SOCIETY OF NUCLEAR MEDICINE AND MOLECULAR IMAGING
www.snmmi.org
1850 Samuel Morse Drive
Reston, VA 20190-5316
Telephone: 703-708-9000

SUPPORT FOR SPOUSES ORGANIZATIONS

WELL SPOUSE ASSOCIATION
www.wellspouse.org
63 West Main Street, Suite H
Freehold, NJ 07728
Telephone: 1-800-838-0879

CAREGIVER ACTION NETWORK
www.caregiveraction.org
1130 Connecticut Avenue NW, Suite 300
Washington, DC 20036-3904
Telephone: 202-454-3970
Email: info@caregiveraction.org

FAMILY CAREGIVER ALLIANCE
www.caregiver.org
235 Montgomery Street, Suite 950
San Francisco, CA 94104
Telephone: 1-800-445-8106
Email: info@caregiver.org

**AMERICAN ASSOCIATION OF SEXUALITY EDUCATORS,
COUNSELORS AND THERAPISTS**
www.aasect.org
1444 I Street NW, Suite 700
Washington, DC 20005
Telephone: 202-449-1099
Email: info@aasect.org

INDEX

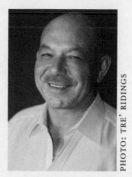

RIDHA AREM, M.D., is a world-renowned endocrinologist and director of the Texas Thyroid Institute, located at the Texas Medical Center in Houston. For years he served as chief of endocrinology and metabolism at Ben Taub Hospital. He also served as clinical professor of medicine at Baylor College of Medicine and medical director of the Endocrine Laboratory at Methodist Hospital.

Dr. Arem has greatly contributed to thyroid-related research and is the author of many peer-reviewed articles published in prestigious medical journals. He was the founder and editor in chief of *Clinical Thyroidology,* an official publication of the American Thyroid Association, and is the author of *The Protein Boost Diet* (Atria, 2013), a popular book that provides the fundamentals of the ThyroLife Diet detailed in this book.

Over the years, Dr. Arem has lectured healthcare professionals in numerous national and international educational programs on thyroid and hormonal issues.

TexasThyroidInstitute.com

ThyroidWellness.com

AremWellness.com

ABOUT THE TYPE

This book was set in Garamond, a typeface originally designed by the Parisian type cutter Claude Garamond (c. 1500–61). This version of Garamond was modeled on a 1592 specimen sheet from the Egenolff-Berner foundry, which was produced from types assumed to have been brought to Frankfurt by the punch cutter Jacques Sabon (c. 1520–80).

Claude Garamond's distinguished romans and italics first appeared in *Opera Ciceronis* in 1543–44. The Garamond types are clear, open, and elegant.